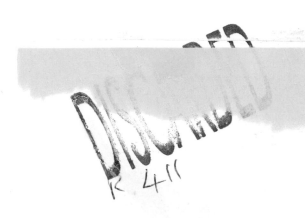

The Selection and Performance of Radiologic Equipment

The Selection and Performance of Radiologic Equipment

Edited by

William R. Hendee, Ph.D.

Professor and Chairman
Department of Radiology
University of Colorado
  Health Sciences Center
Denver, Colorado

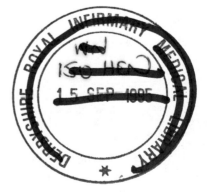

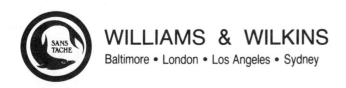

WILLIAMS & WILKINS
Baltimore • London • Los Angeles • Sydney

Editor: George Stamathis
Associate Editor: Carol Eckhart
Copy Editor: Andrea Clemente
Design: Bert Smith
Illustration Planning: Reginald Stanley
Production: Raymond E. Reter

Copyright ©, 1985
Williams & Wilkins
428 E. Preston Street
Baltimore, Md 21202, U.S.A.

Printed in the United States of America

Library of Congress Cataloging in Publication Data

Main entry under title:

Selection and performance of radiologic equipment.

Includes index.
1. Radiology, Medical—Instruments—Testing. 2. Radiology, Medical—
Instruments—Standards. I. Hendee, William R. [DNLM: 1. Radiology—
instrumentation.
WN 150 S464]
RC78.5.S45 1985   616.07′57′028   84-20957
ISBN 0-683-03958-X

Composed and printed at the
Waverly Press, Inc.

85 86 87 88 89
10 9 8 7 6 5 4 3 2 1

Preface

On October 1, 1983, 30% of the acute care hospital beds in the United States were encompassed by the Prospective Payment System (PPS) for Hospital Services.* Over the ensuing year, institutions containing most of the remaining acute care beds fell under the System. Without doubt, provisions of the PPS, and the changes these provisions are expected to stimulate in the private sector of health care reimbursement, are restricting the delivery of health care in the United States in a radical fashion. The long-term consequences of this restructuring process promise to be more significant than any other singular event in the history of medicine in this country.

Under the Prospective Payment System, hospitals are paid for patient services by assignment of Diagnostic Related Groups (DRGs), rather than on the basis of actual costs incurred during patient care. The DRG approach classifies patient diagnoses into 23 major categories based on organ systems. These categories are subdivided into a total of 467 distinct headings, each of which is termed a DRG. Patients in the same DRG are expected to elicit similar clinical responses so that approximately equal resources of the hospital will be utilized in the care of each patient. Reimbursement for this care is determined by a prescribed formula that excludes any direct consideration of the actual costs of caring for any particular patient.

With the PPS approach to health care reimbursement, Departments of Radiology are transformed instantaneously from profit-generating activities within the hospital into cost centers that are financial liabilities if they are not nurtured carefully and managed effectively. Critical to effective management is the recognition that radiology is a high technology enterprise accompanied by high capitalization and operating costs. Because it is a referral, rather than a primary care, service, radiology does not control the flow of most patients into its facilities. No more vulnerable position can be envisioned for a clinical specialty as the nation enters the era of prospective payment.

Effective departmental management is the key to survival of radiology departments in the new era of prospective payment. Among the many management issues of concern is the acquisition of radiologic equipment. In most hospitals, the costs of acquiring, operating, and maintaining radiologic equipment constitute a significant portion of the hospital budget. With the new system of reimbursement limitations, reductions in this portion of the budget are inevitable.

To develop more cost-effective radiology services without compromising their quality requires a carefully planned and orderly process for the selection, evaluation, and maintenance of radiologic equipment. Work in this area over the past decade at the University of Colorado has yielded a program that is both cost and medically effective. By and large, it is the University of Colorado program that is described in this text. From the many comments and letters received as a result of papers delivered and published about various aspects of the Colorado program, we know that it is adaptable to other institutions in different settings. By publication of this text, we are hopeful that additional institutions will benefit from the approaches to equipment acquisition, operation, and maintenance that have been so helpful to us.

The Colorado approach to radiologic equipment has been modified continuously over the years in response to innumerable suggestions from many colleagues, friends, and users of the approach. Although it is impossible to identify these persons individ-

---

* Title VI of Publication 98-21: Social Security Amendments of 1983.

ually, it is important to at least thank them collectively. We also wish to thank three individuals in our department: Mrs. Carol Cottle and Mrs. Barb Freeman for typing what must have appeared at times to be an unlimited number of manuscripts, and Mrs. Linda Taylor for all her efforts in keeping the book organized, the figures, tables and references straight, and the authors productive.

Contributors

Richard L. Banjavic, Ph.D.
Denver, Colorado

Robert K. Cacak, Ph.D.
Hospital Physicist
St. Paul Hospital
Dallas, Texas

Carolyn E. Finster, B.S.
Department of Radiology Administration
University of Colorado Health Sciences
    Center
Denver, Colorado

William R. Hendee, Ph.D.
Professor and Chairman
Department of Radiology
University of Colorado Health Sciences
    Center
Denver, Colorado

Geoffrey S. Ibbott, M.S.
Medical Physicist
Department of Radiology
University of Colorado Health Sciences
    Center
Denver, Colorado

David A. Owen, B.S.E.E.
Department of Radiology
University of Iowa Hospital
Iowa City, Iowa

Raymond P. Rossi, M.S.
Senior Instructor
Department of Radiology
University of Colorado Health Sciences
    Center
Denver, Colorado

Ann L. Scherzinger, Ph.D.
Assistant Professor
Department of Radiology
University of Colorado Health Sciences
    Center
Denver, Colorado

Victor M. Spitzer, Ph.D.
Assistant Professor
Department of Radiology
University of Colorado Health Sciences
    Center
Denver, Colorado

Steven R. Wilkins, Ph.D.
Department of Radiology
St. Anthony's Hospital
Denver, Colorado

Contents

CHAPTER ONE

Introduction to Equipment Selection

WILLIAM R. HENDEE, Ph.D.

Organized medicine rapidly is approaching a period of unparalleled opportunity, challenge, and risk. In 1970, total health care expenditures in the United States constituted 7.6% of the gross national product (GNP). By 1980, the percentage had risen to 9.4%, an increase of almost 2% in a GNP that grew substantially over the same period. In one decade, the cost of personal health care rose from $65.3 billion in 1970 to $217.9 billion in 1980, an increase of 333%. Even when corrected to 1980 dollars, the rate of growth in health care expenditures is substantial. In the same period, federal support of health care in the United States climbed from $14.5 billion in 1970 to $62.5 billion in 1980, an increase of 431%.

Many factors have contributed to the dramatic increase in the cost of health care. The general inflation of the United States economy has contributed to the increased cost; however, the costs of medical supplies and equipment have increased at a rate greater than that of general inflation and show no sign of stabilizing in the near future. Many technological advances have evolved over the past 10 yr, and they add to the cost of health care, as well as to its value for the sick and injured. In the arena of technological advances, radiology has been among the leading medical disciplines over the past 10 yr and is likely to maintain this forefront position over the decade of the 1980s as well. The country has experienced a declining but still finite population growth, as well as a gradual aging of the population, and both of these factors contribute to the cost of health care. Principally through government benefits, health care has become more accessible to us all, and especially to those in the lower income brackets. Although improved accessbility to health care is a notable achievement, its impact on health care costs should not be ignored. Finally, a major influence on health care costs has been the substantial salary increases awarded to health care personnel, especially to those in the lower personnel categories of hospitals and medical clinics across the country. In spite of major technological advances, medicine is still a labor-intensive industry, and labor costs consume a significant and increasing portion of the health care dollar.

The rapid increase in health care costs has not escaped the attention of the United States public. In 1981 a survey was conducted by the American Medical Association that identified cost as the principal concern of the consumers of health care. As perceived by the public, medical costs are more of a problem than any other health care issue including accessibility, quality, and depersonalization.

In response to this public concern, efforts to control health care costs by regulation were initiated at federal and state levels in the 1970s. Among these efforts were the establishment of regional Health Systems Agencies (HSAs) to regulate the acquisition of major items of medical equipment and the expenditure of substantial funds for capital construction, and the creation of a Federal Office of Technology Assessment to advise the Health Care Finance Administration on Medicare reimbursement of charges for medical procedures of extraordinary cost or questionable efficacy. These attempts to curtail health care costs have been only marginally effective at best, and recent administrative changes at the federal level have resulted in a reduced emphasis on governmental regulation of the health care industry. On the other hand, proof of efficacy before reimbursement of charges for medical procedures can be anticipated for the future, especially for those procedures associated with ancillary services, such as laboratory and radiology.

These types of issues, rooted solidly in the fundamental economics of health care delivery, present momentous challenges for organized medicine in the decade of the

1980s. The two major challenges identified for this decade by the American Medical Association are:

1. To develop a cost-effective approach to health care delivery; and
2. To resist inappropriate economics that compromise the quality of health care.

Nowhere are these challenges more apparent and more significant than in the discipline of radiology.

Approximately a decade ago, radiology entered a period of unparalleled development that has been heralded by many as a technological revolution. In part, this development represents little more than the discovery of the medical imaging field by the microelectronics and computer industries. Even so, significant advances in the technology of medical imaging have occurred over the past 10 yr. The impact on radiology has been substantial, and there are no signs, other than economic, that the impact will not grow significantly over the next decade. Among the radiological innovations that were virtually unheard of at the beginning of the 1970s are digital radiography, transmission computed tomography, emission computed tomography, including positron tomography, real-time ultrasound, and magnetic resonance. On the horizon are methods such as quantification of data from ultrasound and computed tomography, and possibly such techniques as transillumination (diaphonography) and the use of radiolabeled antibodies for both cancer detection and treatment. There is little question but that the final three decades of the 20th century promise to constitute one of the most exciting periods in the evolution of radiology. Unfortunately, this evolution could not have arrived at a more unfortunate time in terms of the health care economy.

Because of the collision courses of advancing technology, increasing costs, and limited financial resources, radiology faces some difficult issues over the next few years. One of these issues is the efficacy of radiologic procedures. No longer can radiology afford the luxury of justifying a procedure because it provides additional information about the patient without asking if the information influences the care of the patient, the possibility of survival, and an improved quality of life. Radiologic procedures also

should be evaluated in terms of their cost effectiveness as well as their ratios of benefit vs risk and hazard. Some radiologic procedures must be identified as competing with others; the adage that all radiologic procedures are complementary must be recognized as an outmoded concept. An important need, largely unaddressed at this time, is the delineation of preferred pathways for triaging patients through the multiplicity of examinations available today in a modern radiology program. In addition, techniques should be developed to provide a radiologic consensus concerning particular patients so that the referring physician receives a collective diagnostic opinion from radiology rather than a multitude of disparate views from separate imaging centers within the department. As an adequate number, and in some specialty areas a surplus, of physicians develops over the next few years, struggles over radiologic "turf" will intensify. These struggles will be accentuated by increased competition for health care dollars among all the medical specialties.

In addition to these issues, radiology is faced with some major problems associated with the high cost of present equipment and the even higher cost of some of the newer modalities for diagnosis and treatment. Included among these problems are the responsibilities of maintaining radiologic facilities in a reasonable way, replacing radiologic equipment at the most suitable time, adding new modalities whenever their efficacy and cost effectiveness is proven, and upgrading existing equipment to improve patient care. Satisfying these responsibilities is increasingly difficult as constraints on financial resources continue to escalate. Increasingly, decisions regarding the maintenance, replacement, and upgrading of radiology facilities reflect compromises based on limited resources. To be most effective, these decisions require a carefully planned approach to equipment purchase in radiology that is designed to provide adequate patient care in the most cost-effective manner possible. In most institutions, for example, it no longer is acceptable to approach the purchase of radiologic equipment with the assumption that the finest (and usually most expensive) system available commercially will be purchased since that system has the greatest likelihood of providing satisfactory clinical performance. Instead, eco-

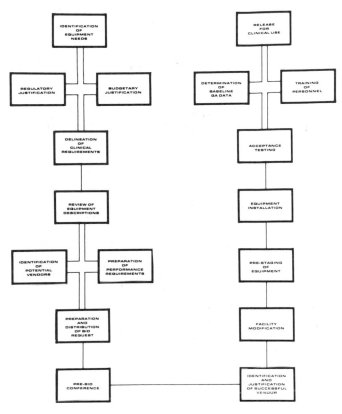

Figure 1.1. Microcosting analysis of cost and hospital charge for a PA and lateral chest examination. Approach to equipment purchases, installation, and maintenance presented in the text.

nomic constraints often require that the purchaser choose the system that is adequate to satisfy the clinical needs at the most reasonable price available. In adopting the latter approach, the purchaser should specify the technical characteristics of system performance in some detail to the supplier and should verify upon installation that the system satisfies the performance criteria agreed upon by purchaser and supplier at the time of purchase.

The objective of equipping and maintaining a radiology service in the most intelligent and cost-effective manner possible is not an easy goal to attain. Its pursuit probably is accomplished best with a carefully planned sequence of operations that addresses all aspects of the planning and purchase process, including performance identification, specification, verification, and maintenance. One such approach that has been developed as a collaborative enterprise of purchaser and supplier and that has proven effective in the clinical setting is described in this text. Depending on local circumstances and re-

sources, the approach presented here can be supplemented, modified, or used in whole or in part to develop a cost-effective approach to equipment purchase and maintenance in radiology. Of course, the approach is adaptable as well to equipment needs outside of radiology.

The approach to equipment purchase, installation, and maintenance presented in this text is separated into several sequential activities. These activities are described in Figure 1.1, where each of the headings constitutes a separate chapter or section in the text. In each of the chapters, a brief introduction to the activity is followed by a detailed presentation of the approach extracted from the different modalities of radiology (roentgenography, nuclear medicine, ultrasound, computed tomography, and radiation therapy). Modifications to the approaches based on local circumstances are encouraged, and those that are found to be particularly useful would be of considerable interest to the authors of the text. We look forward to learning of these modifications.

CHAPTER TWO

Identification of Clinical Needs

WILLIAM R. HENDEE, Ph.D., RAYMOND P. ROSSI, M.S.,
VICTOR M. SPITZER, Ph.D., RICHARD L. BANJAVIC, Ph.D.,
ROBERT K. CACAK, Ph.D., and GEOFFREY S. IBBOTT, M.S.

INTRODUCTION

The decision to purchase a particular diagnostic imaging system can be based on a number of factors. Some of these factors may be related directly to improved quality and cost effectiveness of imaging services; others may be somewhat more ethereal, but nonetheless important to the overall strategy of the institution and the improvement of its position within the medical community. Examples of the former factors include the addition of equipment to provide needed services to an expanding patient population, the replacement of equipment with a history of frequent breakdowns and undependable performance, and the acquisition of equipment to offer new services of proven clinical efficacy and cost effectiveness. Somewhat less obvious, but still justifiable reasons for equipment purchase include enhancement of the prestige and referral pattern of the institution within the community, reduction of the legal liability of the institution because of the unavailability of certain medical imaging services, and maintenance of a facility that is sufficiently up-to-date to attract and retain the highest quality personnel at both the professional and staff levels.

To help balance the many factors influencing an equipment purchase decision, the multiyear plan for equipment purchase is very helpful. Such a plan extended over a 7-yr period is illustrated in Figure 2.1. This plan should be used as a guide, rather than as an inflexible mode of operation. For example, if all equipment purchases cannot be accommodated in a particular year because of limited resources, then the plans for succeeding years should be changed to incorporate those items deleted from the purchase list. Also, a new modality may develop more rapidly or slowly than originally anticipated, and its year of acquisition may shift from time to time, depending on the best estimate of when the modality will mature to clinical application.

For each imaging unit in the radiology service, a record should be maintained of the cause, frequency, and duration of unit failure, as well as the cost of restoring the unit to operation (Fig. 2.2). These records are helpful in establishing and modifying the schedule for equipment replacement and for

1983–1984
DX—2) Patient information system
    4) Urographic tables 2/tomographic
CT—1) CT scanner
RT—3) Treatment planning system
Department—Departmental Remodeling—CT Scanner
1984–1985
DX—General R&F room 2212
    ER radiology replacement
    Operating room cysto system
CT—Patient scheduling system
RT—4 MV accelerator
NM—LFOV camera and computer replacement
US—Real-time scanner
Department—Continuation of Radiology Remodeling Requested in 1983–1984
1985–1986
DX—General R&F room 2209
    General R&F room 2219
    Neuroangiography
    Special skull unit—room 2210
RT—18 MV accelerator
NM—Multiplane tomographic scanner
    Mobile camera and computer replacement
US—Echocardiography system with 2D strip ultrasound
1986–1987
DX—General R&F room 2210
1987–1988
NM—Tomographic camera replacement

Figure 2.1. Example of a multiyear plan for the replacement of capital equipment. Abbreviations used are: Dx, diagnosis; RT, radiotherapy; NM, nuclear medicine; US, ultrasound.

Date	Description of equipment malfunction	Corrective action taken	Repair cost	Equipment downtime (hr)
9/5/78	Film changer hold down clamps broken.	Installed new floor plate for changer hold down.	$850	24
9/7/78	Medrad syringe falling off table mount.	Adjust syringe attachment mechanism.	N/C	½
9/21/78	70-mm photospot camera inconsistent. Possible focal spot problem.	70-mm system checks OK. Large focal spot of AP found to be out of specification.	$180	4
10/11/78	Injector fails to maintain pressures at low flow rate.	Flow module found to be defective and replaced.	$291	1
10/12/78	Carry out complete preventive maintenance (PM) on lateral and AP changers	Changer PM performed and adjusted for current studies.	$461	8
10/27/78	Injector head movement not smooth.	Problem determined to be in power amp module—new one required.	$204	2
11/10/78	Scout films during runoff jamming. Densities varying. Stepper malfunctioning.	Repaired AP Elema. Take-up tray. Adjusted stepper techniques. Determine consistency of exposure.	$184	4
11/13/78	Pressure transducer diaphragm damaged.	Evaluate unit and sent to manufacturer for repair. Repair not possible.	$50	None
8/13/78	Medrad injector not delivering correct inject volume.	Volume module replaced.	$145	2½
12/4/78	Medrad will not draw up contrast.	Replaced fuse in power amp module.	$83	2
12/7/78	Injector not working properly.	Possibly defective flow module. Scheduled for evaluation.	N/C	2

Figure 2.2. Representative maintenance record for an x-ray facility. N/C, no charge.

justifying the acquisition of replacement equipment to individuals with regulatory or budgetary control over the purchase (see Chapter 3). From these records, estimates can be made of patient revenue lost and of the overloading of parallel facilities caused by the failure of specific imaging units. They are also helpful in documenting the quality of maintenance and repair on individual units in the service. Further discussion of maintenance records is provided in Chapter 9.

In the justification of replacement needs, an analysis can be valuable of the deficiencies of present equipment, including a review of current procedures and whether they yield results of desired quality (1). For a radiographic unit, for example, are exposure times too long to control patient motion, suggesting that a higher power rating is needed for the x-ray generator? Would smaller focal spots provide improved im-

ages, or would the accompanying increase in exposure time produce unacceptable patient motion? Could the power rating of the generator be combined with the selection of focal spots and screen-film combinations to yield a reasonable compromise among all three quantities at an acceptable cost? Are grid ratios too high, creating problems with mechanical alignment, increased exposures and tube loading, or are they too low, yielding insufficient reduction of scatter radiation? Is automatic exposure control necessary or desirable? How often is it used on the present equipment?

All too frequently, a lack of understanding of technical specifications by the equipment purchaser and an unfamiliarity with specific clinical requirements on the part of the equipment supplier combine to produce overexpenditures for medical imaging equipment and unfulfilled expectations of equipment performance (2). Answers to questions such as those in the preceding paragraph can provide valuable insight into the requirements for replacement (and new) equipment. Analysis of the rate of repeat examinations also is useful in identifying problems which could be resolved by the proper choice of equipment. To illustrate the issues discussed above and to provide some guidance to considerations important in the identification of equipment requirements, Tables 2.1 through 2.5 provide a listing of key points on a component basis for typical roentgenographic imaging equip-

Table 2.1
Considerations in Identifying Equipment Requirements: X-Ray Generators and X-Ray Tubes

X-ray generators
  Phase and wave form
  Power rating (kW = kVp × mA)
  Switching method and capability
  Timing modes
    Manual (range and increment)
    Automatic exposure control (AEC)
    Grid-controlled
  Technique selection
    Three point (kVp, mA, t)
    Two point (kVp, mAs)
    One point (kVp, AEC, falling load)
  High-speed rotor controllers
  Tube current
    Manual (range, increment, focal spot selection)
    Falling load (continuous, stepped)
    Accuracy, linearity, independence of kilovolt peak (kVp)
    Voltage regulation
    Auto primary
    Phase drop out
    kVp (range increment)
    Accuracy independence of milliamperage

X-ray tubes
  Focal spot size/growth
  Power rating
    Single radiographic
    Rapid sequence radiographic
    Cinefluoroscopic
  Anode heat storage capacity
  Anode cooling
    Housing heat storage capacity
    Housing cooling rate and method
  Anode angle/field coverage
  Leakage radiation
  Anode rotation speeds
  Stator configurations

Table 2.2
Considerations in Identifying Equipment Requirements: Tables, Tube Supports, and Grids

Tables/patient handling devices
  Degree of tilt
  Travel—head/foot; side/side
  Flat top
  Curve top
  Accessories
    Foot boards
    Braces
    Cassette holders
  Tomo adaption capability
  Reciprocating grid mechanisms
  Type of locks
  Power assist
Tube supports
  Overhead/floor standing
  Mechanical rigidity
  Safety mechanisms
  Tube angulation
  Travel within room
  Bridge passing capability
  Auto tracking with image receptor (servo drive)
  Maximum and minimum heights
  Indicators
Grids
  Type
  Ratio
  Interspace material

Table 2.3
Considerations in Identifying Equipment Requirements: Beam Restriction Systems

Radiographic
  Positive beam limitation
  Size
  Operator control
  Numerical indicators
  Operational indicators
  Off-focal radiation reduction design

Fluoroscopic
  Auto tracking
  Corresponding to imaging mode being used
  Size and shape

ment. Similar listings for other imaging modalities are available in the following sections of this chapter.

Additional considerations in equipment purchase include any space, financial, and time constraints imposed on the acquisition process. Adequate space often is a problem when contemplating replacement equip-

Table 2.4
Considerations in Identifying Equipment Requirements: Fluoroscopic Imaging Systems

Image intensifier	Input phosphor material type
	Single or multiple field
	Size
Automatic brightness control	Type
	kVp
	mA
	kVp ↑, mA ↑
	mA ↑, kVp trail
	Sensing
	Area
	Detection
Spot film system	Front load
	Back load
	Format selection/display
	Masks/compression cones
	Size
Photospot systems	Format size
	Roll or cut
	Patient identification
	Film supply indicators
	Extra take-up magazine
	Frame rate
Cine systems	Format size
Videotape recorders	
Videodisc recorders	

Table 2.5
Considerations in Identifying Equipment Requirements: Automatic Exposure Control Systems/Vertical Wall Boards/Accessories

Automatic exposure control systems
   Minimum controllable exposure time
   Detector type
   Location—pre/post cassette
   Single field
   Multiple field
   Field combination
   Density control
   Adaptability to multiple film/screen combination

Vertical cassette holders
   Multisizing/single size
   Height adjustment
   Grid
   AEC

Accessories
   Cassettes/screens
   Lead aprons
   Others

Table 2.6
Recommended Labeling Parameters for Pulser-Transducer Asembly-Receiver Systems

1. Absolute maximum ultrasonic power.
2. Absolute maximum spatial peak-temporal average intensity (SPTA).
3. Absolute maximum spatial peak-pulse average intensity (SPPA).
4. Pulse repetition frequency (PRF).
5. Absolute maximum spatial average-temporal average intensity (SATA) in the same plane and with the same control settings used to measure the absolute maximum spatial peak-temporal average intensity.
6. Center frequency and fractional bandwidth of all transducer assemblies.
7. Focal length, focal area, and depth of focus for focused transducer assembly.

ment that must be housed within an existing room. Obviously, funding limits may impose a ceiling on the cost of equipment that can be purchased. In an inflationary economy, increases in price during the interim between the allocation of funds and the final decision on the desired equipment often present a problem to the purchaser. For this reason, it is often wise to identify the clinical needs to be addressed by the equipment before requesting funds for its purchase. In this manner a realistic estimate of costs can be obtained and adjusted for anticipated cost increases. Time constraints such as delivery and installation times, facility renovation time, and equipment down time also are important factors to be considered during the identification of clinical needs.

One of the first tasks facing the potential purchaser of medical imaging equipment is the identification of equipment require-

ments in terms of the intended clinical applications (3, 4). Fulfillment of this task assures the user that a particular item of equipment will meet the demands of the clinical environment. Theoretically, the approach to this task should be straightforward; the purchaser simply would match the technical specifications for a specific equipment item to the clinical tasks to be performed with the equipment. If the equipment is intended for x-ray examination of

Table 2.7
Comparison of Clinical Needs to Ultrasound System Capabilities

Clinical needs	System requirement
Parallel serial slices through organ of choice	Articulated arm scanner
Frame rate fast enough to discern heart valve motion	Real-time scanner which includes frame rate of about 30/sec or greater
Portability for echocardiographic studies outside of diagnostic clinic area	Portable real-time scanner with attached linear or sector array
Small facility with only one room suitable for placement of ultrasound system	Articulated arm static scanner with attached real-time linear or array or sector scan abilities
High ob/gyn patient load in small clinic	Small, sequential linear array for gross observational and, perhaps, some simple measurements if calibrated calipers present
Management of expression of patient concern over biological effects due to diagnostic ultrasound	All static and real-time scanners equipped with console control of pulser or power levels
Desire to do tissue analysis (qualitative or quantitative) using reflected signals	Enough transducer assemblies present over broad enough frequency range which can provide their depth of field over a sufficient region of interest
More detail in scans of in utero fetal structures	High (e.g., 5 to 7.5 MHz) frequency transducer assemblies of a suitable diameter whose beam can penetrate far enough to place the focal plane at depths of 5 to 7 cm.

the gastrointestinal (GI) tract, for example, then clinically acceptable images for this region of anatomy should be demonstrable with a prototype assembly of the equipment. Unfortunately, complete information is not available concerning the degree of spatial resolution, contrast resolution, noise suppression, etc., essential for clinical diagnosis with any specific imaging modality and application. Hence, a different approach to this problem must be utilized.

Absolutely essential to the identification of equipment requirements for a given clinical application are extensive discussions involving all the individuals who will use the equipment or who are interested in or knowledgeable about it. Among these individuals are physicians, technologists, administrators, representatives of equipment vendors, physicists, service engineers, and outside consultants. Each of these individuals can contribute to the identification of equipment requirements. Physicians will know the range of clinical examinations to be accommodated by the equipment and will be able to identify certain operational and per-

formance features that will facilitate the equipment's use. Technologists are directly involved in using the equipment, and their advice is essential to decisions about desired operational characteristics, convenience features, and room layout. Administrators should be consulted for financial, regulatory, and space constraints on the equipment acquisition. Representatives of equipment vendors can provide advice about the types of equipment available for the intended applications and about advances that might impact on the selection of particular equipment. Radiological physicists and engineers can interpret the technical specifications of the vendors, prepare specifications for equipment performance to be incorporated into the bid document, and evaluate the serviceability and probable reliability of the equipment. It may also be helpful to involve consultants in the equipment selection process, especially when these persons can provide an independent perspective on the equipment needs of a department.

To enhance communication among the individuals involved in the equipment selection process, it is usually desirable to arrange scheduled meetings. During these meetings the issues that will influence the acquisition of equipment can be reviewed and documented. In formulating the clinical requirements for a medical imaging system, several issues need to be carefully addressed. Initially, the type of radiology practice should be considered. In a large teaching hospital, for example, many individuals with different levels of experience may be involved in the use of the equipment. In this setting, simplicity of operation of the equipment may be a desirable feature. Operational simplicity may be less important in a small community hospital or private office where only a small number of individuals use the equipment. Another consideration is the types of patients (i.e., the "patient mix") to be examined with the equipment. For example, equipment designed for adult studies might not be well suited for pediatric work; if chest roentgenograms constitute a significant fraction of the work load, a dedicated chest unit might be a wise investment.

The volume of studies expected for the equipment is an important consideration that can influence the selection of both operational features and overall design of the equipment. Some equipment that may be suitable for low-volume applications may prove operationally inconvenient and mechanically unreliable in applications with a high patient turnover. The range of examinations to be performed with the equipment also may impact on its desired characteristics. The performance requirements for a general purpose radiographic room intended for a wide range of examinations would be greatly different from those for a room dedicated to a single examination such as chest roentgenography. Consideration should also be given to the suitability of the equipment for backup service for other facilities in the department or, in some circumstances, its portability for studies in other locations.

After the issues described above have been thoughtfully considered, individuals involved in the selection process should have an excellent idea of the clinical needs to be addressed by the desired equipment. A description of these needs should be incorporated in the bid document to be distributed to potential vendors. This description should include a brief statement of the desired equipment and should identify the types of procedures to be performed, anticipated patient mix, examination volume, any special equipment constraints, and the image receptors and processing techniques to be employed. In the statement of clinical needs any minimum or "must have" equipment features also should be included, together with any special constraints such as financial, delivery, service, space or utilities limitations that may be present. Examples of statements of clinical needs for various imaging modalities constitute the remainder of this chapter.

ROENTGENOGRAPHY
General Equipment Requirements

The equipment shall be a general purpose radiographic/fluoroscopic unit with provisions to perform the normal range of radiographic and fluoroscopic examinations, including: gallbladders, upper and lower gastrointestinal studies, endoscopic retrograde cholangiopancreatograms, colon studies, barium enemas, cervical and lumbar myelograms, arthrograms, hysterosalpingograms, and routine radiographic studies, such as spines, abdomens, etc. The equipment shall provide backup capability for chest examinations. The anticipated work load is 35 patients/day. The bidded equipment shall be of sufficient construction and of a heavy duty nature to handle this projected work load in a reliable manner. The film-screen combination currently employed has a relative speed of 200.

Specific Equipment Requirements

Outlined below are specific performance requirements for the radiographic/fluoroscopic unit. The requirements have been stated in a form to facilitate response by all potential vendors. In responding to these requirements, the potential vendor shall supply the most complete specifications (e.g., product data sheets) available.

X-RAY GENERATOR

The x-ray generator shall be of the three-phase, 6- or 12-pulse type. The power rating shall be 100 kW minimum, with a capacity of 800 mA at 125 kilovolts peak (kVp) being acceptable and a maximum secondary voltage of 150 kVp. Independent control is required of both the radiographic and fluoroscopic x-ray tubes, including technique factor display. For film recording of fluoroscopic images (spot film/photospot), selection of either the small or large focal spot is required. Primary solid-state contacting, automatic line voltage regulation, automatic kVp and space charge compensation, and generator overload and x-ray tube overload protective circuitry are required. Asynchronous/forced termination timing and manual timing to a minimum of at least 5 msec are required. Automatic exposure control of the trifield type, capable of providing adequately controlled exposures down to 5 msec or less, is required. Anatomical programming is not desired.

Tube current/focal spot loading of the constant load or continuously falling load type is acceptable. Rapid acceleration rotor control with capability for high-speed rotation is required. Time delay from rotation activation to high-speed rotation shall not exceed 1.5 sec. The generator is to provide all required control functions for both radiographic and fluoroscopic imaging modes and will include all standard cabling and accessories.

X-RAY TUBES

X-ray tubes of the rotating anode type are required for both the radiographic and fluoroscopic imaging modes. Nominal focal spot sizes for both tubes shall be in the 0.6- to 0.7-mm range for the small focal spot and in the 1.2- to 1.5-mm range for the large focal spot. The power rating of the large focal spot shall match the available generator power, as closely as possible, in the 60- to 120-kVp range. A minimum anode heat storage capacity of 300,000 heat units (HU) and a minimum housing heat storage capacity of 1,500,000 HU are required. Anode heat load indication and tube warm-up protective circuitry are required. Full coverage of 17-inch film dimensions at a 40-inch distance from source to image receptor is required. Exposure counters for the radiographic and fluoroscopic tubes are desired, as is a total elapsed fluoroscopic tube on-time indicator. Complete tube rating charts for the x-ray tubes are to be included.

PATIENT HANDLING/SUPPORT TABLE

A patient handling and support table with 90°/90° tilt capability and a four-way power

driven flat top is required. A radiographic Bucky, including a high-speed reciprocating grid mechanism with 10:1 aluminum interspace grid, trifield automatic exposure control pickup assembly, and cassette-size sensing tray, is required. The table shall be capable of being driven and tilted simultaneously. Table controls are to be located on both the table side and the spot film device. Table shall incorporate a design for the spot film device (described below) that allows free float of the total fluoroscopic imaging assembly. Automatic centering of table and horizontal stop (defeatable) for angulation are required. Variable extension of the table top as a function of table angulation with automatic pull back are required. Table accessories shall include foot board, shoulder braces, myelographic boots, hand grips, head holder, urological leg supports, compression band, and cross-table cassette holder.

RADIOGRAPHIC TUBE SUPPORT/ RADIOGRAPHIC BEAM RESTRICTION SYSTEM

The radiographic tube support shall be a ceiling-mounted, bridge suspension type. The tube support shall be mechanically rigid and equipped with a safety mechanism to prevent the tube from falling in case of lock failure. Tube support shall permit motion of the tube along the entire length of the table and positioning of the tube within the room for use with a wall-mounted cassette holder. Positive locking mechanism shall be provided for centering the x-ray tube with respect to the under table image receptor and the wall-mounted cassette holder. Tube and column rotation shall be 90°/90°. When the x-ray tube is positioned for a cross-table film, the suspension shall permit the focal spot of the x-ray tube to be placed at least 12 inches below the tabletop. Positive locks are required for a nominal source-image receptor distance (SID) of 40 inches with the table either horizontal or vertical, and for nominal SIDs of 40 and 72 inches with respect to the wall-mounted cassette holder. A light localizing, rectangular, positive beam limitation (PBL) system is required. The PBL system shall provide a continuous range of SIDs in conjunction with the under table image receptor with the table horizontal, a single SID (40 inches) in conjunction with the under table image receptor with the table vertical, and two SIDs (40 and 72 inches) in conjunction with the wall-mounted cassette holder. Manual override of the PBL system is required. Numerical indication of SID and numerical indication of field size as a function of SID and cassette centering are required.

WALL-MOUNTED VERTICAL CASSETTE HOLDER

A wall-mounted, multisizing, vertical cassette holder is required. The cassette holder shall be equipped with a trifield automatic exposure control system pickup and a 10:1, 103 line/inch, aluminum interspace, stationary grid. The automatic exposure control pickup shall be postgrid, but precassette.

FLUOROSCOPIC IMAGING SYSTEM

The fluoroscopic imaging system shall include the following components:

Spot Film Device

A mechanically rigid spot film device is required that is capable of supporting a multimode image intensifier, TV camera, small format film camera, and associated optics without overhead suspension (i.e., free float). The spot film device shall be properly integrated to the patient support/handling table. The spot film device shall be of the power-assist type and shall provide control of all table motions, spot film mode selections, fluoroscopic exposure initiation, and spot film or photospot exposure initiation. The spot film device shall be of the front and/or rear loading type. Preprogram capability is desired to provide 1:1, 2:1 longitudinal, 2:1 transverse, and 4:1 and 6:1 formats with program sequence override. A 9:1 capability also is desired. Automatic collimation to the selected spot film mode with automatic masking is preferred. The spot film device should include a movable compression cone and grid. A myelographic stop for the spot film device is required. The spot film device should provide maximum clearance from the radiographic table when in the parked position. A switch to dim the room lights shall be provided on the spot film device.

Image Intensifier

A cesium iodide, dual or trifield image intensifier is required that incorporates light distribution optics for both the TV camera and the small format film recording camera. Controls for selecting imaging modes shall be located at the position of the fluoroscopist.

Automatic Brightness Control System

An automatic brightness control system for use in conjunction with the image intensifier is required. Control of fluoroscopic technique factors (if applicable) must be available at the fluoroscopist's position. A clear indication of fluoroscopic technique factors shall be visible at the fluoroscopist's position. Fluoroscopic exposure initiation is to be accomplished by a switch at the spot film device and/or a foot switch. Brightness hold mode is required.

TV Chain

The closed circuit television chain shall be of the 525-line type and shall employ a vidicon (antimony trisulfide or lead monoxide) TV camera. A wall- (preferred) or cart-mounted 14-inch or 17-inch 525-line TV monitor is required. The size of the monitor shall depend on its final location within the room.

Small Format Film Recording Camera

A 100 to 105 mm, roll or cut film camera is required for photospot imaging. Capability for 1 frame/sec to 6 frames/sec is required. Positive patient identification for recorded photospot films shall be incorporated in the camera. A film supply indicator is required. The camera system shall be equipped with two takeup magazines and, for cut film units, shall provide a minimum of 50 frames of unexposed film. Frame rate selection is to be located at the fluoroscopist's position. Photospot exposure initiation should be controlled by a switch located on the spot film device and/or by a second position of the fluoroscopic foot switch.

Videotape Recorder

A ¾-inch cassette video recorder for recording of fluoroscopic studies is required. The recorder shall be interlocked to the fluoroscopic exposure control switch so that tape transport and recording occurs only during fluoroscopy. Playback shall be accomplished through the TV monitor used for fluoroscopy. In the playback mode, stop frame and single frame advance are required.

NUCLEAR MEDICINE

Nuclear medicine enjoys the availability of a wide variety of scintillation camera designs and options and some highly specialized detector systems for high patient volume and unusual studies. Characterization of the available patient population and referring physician interest is essential in the identification of the equipment most suitable for an efficient department. A moderate amount of ancillary equipment must also be considered (e.g., xenon traps, isotope calibrators, survey meters, probes, well counters, and fume hoods). Clinical needs in nuclear medicine should be reviewed to establish the types of ancillary equipment needed. In this chapter the scintillation camera configuration is emphasized.

Imaging Equipment

The number of scintillation cameras a department needs to meet the requirements of general patient population mixes and normal referral patterns is on the order of 1/100 beds. As another rough estimate, 10 to 15 examinations/day can be performed on a single camera. For multiple camera departments, different camera configurations usually should be available to provide imaging capabilities over a wide range of clinical studies. The need for mobile service should be evaluated and weighed against the higher cost and limited capabilities of mobile cameras.

For stationary cameras, the patient load may dictate the camera size or field of view. Cancer centers, institutions with large numbers of patients with pulmonary disease, and those with high numbers of liver and renal patients dictate a large field of view camera (15- to 21-inch diameter), whereas heavy cardiac and pediatric caseloads can benefit from the improved performance of smaller cameras (10- to 12-inch diameter). Large numbers of gallium-67 and indium-111 studies may be served best by a thick crystal ($\frac{1}{2}$ inch). Cameras designed for low energy isotopes, on the other hand, provide improved spatial resolution because of a thin-

ner crystal ($\frac{1}{4}$ inch). Minor improvements in resolution obtained by increasing the number of photomultiplier tubes are balanced mainly against available finances. The choice of collimators also may be influenced by the patient population. Two or three medium- and high-energy collimators may be warranted if ^{67}Ga, ^{111}In, and ^{131}I studies are performed in reasonable numbers. Some departments may compromise sensitivity and resolution by using only one collimator for both medium- (^{67}Ga and ^{111}In) and high-energy (^{131}I) isotopes. If a small field of view camera is the only imaging instrument in the department, then diverging collimators may be in order. For low-energy work (^{99m}Tc, ^{201}T, ^{123}I, and ^{133}Xe), low and high resolution (high and low sensitivity, respectively) collimators are normally used. The highest resolution imaging capability available (usually used for imaging small organs) is provided by a pinhole collimator; this collimator is frequently used for thyroid, pediatric, and bone and joint imaging. For departments with severe space restrictions, collimator storage can be a problem for large field of view cameras. Storage arrangements range from side-by-side collimator storage, requiring floor space in excess of the area represented by all the collimators, to storage modules that stack the collimators on top of each other. A recent innovation in some large cameras is the core replacement collimator where only the inner core (field of view) and a very thin supporting frame are exchanged. This exchange is usually done by hand.

Some other camera options to consider are: (a) a multichannel energy analyzer (MCA), which is of great benefit for teaching and is highly desirable for routine use with isotopes containing multiple photopeaks; (b) magnification mode to increase resolution for a field of view smaller than that of the entire camera; (c) displacement of the region of image magnification from the center of the camera to facilitate cardiac stress work and pediatric imaging near the edge of the detector housing; (d) count density termination to produce reproducibly good photographic images of organs rather than of entire fields of view; and (e) multiple energy windows which are particularly useful for ^{67}Ga imaging.

Additional analysis of the department

work load may reveal that whole body scanning capability would increase patient throughput (Fig. 2.3). Several techniques are available for whole body scanning. They include camera movement, table movement, and, for small rooms, coordinated and simultaneous movement of camera and table. A jumbo field of view camera is another consideration for departments with a large number of whole body scans. These cameras have a 21-inch field of view and can produce a whole body scan with a single pass over the patient in place of the two to three passes required by smaller field of view cameras.

Tomographic capability is a final consideration in the acquisition of a scintillation camera. This decision is based on diagnostic accuracy rather than patient load. Two major tomographic modalities are available; both impose additional performance requirements (linearity and uniformity) on the detector.

The first tomographic method is limited angle tomography with a multiview colli-

mator attached to a standard scintillation camera (Fig. 2.4). These systems require no additions to the scintillation camera other than the multiview collimator. One major advantage of the multiview approach is its ability to image dynamic processes, since all views are acquired simultaneously. The competing technique for tomography is a rotating detector that provides 360° tomography. Motors and electronics for rotation are added to the camera, and a counterbalanced detector suspension normally is employed. Rotating systems range from very simple construction, not very different from a conventional camera, to massive gantries, much like those used for transmission computed tomography. The latter approach may utilize either one or two detector heads (Fig. 2.5).

Archival storage of nuclear medicine images traditionally has been on photographic film. Cathode ray tube (CRT) and photographic camera systems are available in wide ranges of price and performance. Polaroid

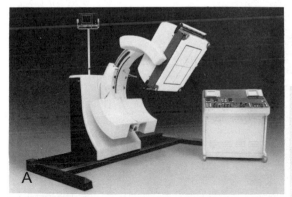
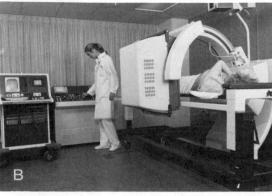
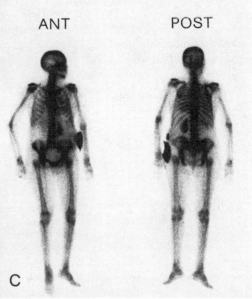

Figure 2.3. Whole body imaging is accomplished by moving the camera long the base rails (*A*) or with a moving table (*B*). The entire skeletal image in one picture is the result (*C*). (*A*, Courtesy of Technicare Corp.; *B*, Courtesy of Toshiba Corp.; *C*, Courtesy of Picker Corp.)

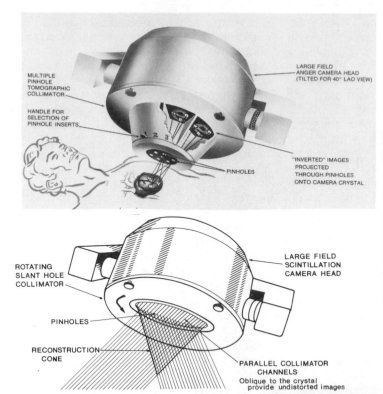

Figure 2.4. Two versions of limited angle tomography (requiring only a collimator and software) include the seven-pinhole technique which collects all tomographic views simultaneously (*upper*) and the rotating slant hole collimator technique (*lower*) which obtains depth information while the collimator rotates on the camera face during scintigraphic data acquisition.

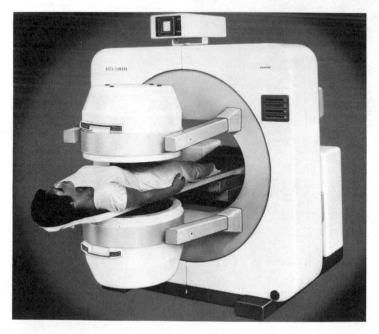

Figure 2.5. At the opposite end of the price spectrum from the units shown in Figure 2.4 is the double headed 360° tomographic system. Two detector heads rotate through 180° and therefore collect data in half the time of a single head system rotating through 360°. (Courtesy of Siemens.)

film has been replaced almost entirely by 5- × 7- or 8- × 10-inch transparent film to yield greater contrast. Camera systems with fine dot CRTs (≤0.007 inch) provide a wide range of image formats on film to accommodate both low count density fast flow studies and high count density static images. Stand alone image formatters are available, as well as more compact (mirrored) models built into the scintillation camera console.

Some of the newer photographic systems offer both direct analog input from the scintillation camera and digital input from a computer or from the end stage of one of the newer digital scintillation cameras.

The nuclear medicine computer is evolving from an image enhancement tool to an integral part of the scintillation camera. The computer is currently required for tomographic and most cardiac imaging applications; however, direct utilization of digital images on the computer monitor as a replacement for film for diagnostic imaging is still in its infancy. As other imaging modalities in radiology begin to accommodate image interpretation directly from computer monitors, then the compatibility of software and hardware among modalities will become important.

Other diagnostic instrumentation may include single probe detectors for thyroid uptake measurements, well counters and liquid scintillation counters for in vitro procedures, and possibly scanning probes for bone densitometry (Fig. 2.6). Multidetector systems (16 to 32 detectors) are available for highly specialized regional cerebral blood flow measurements (Fig. 2.7), and specialized nonimaging cardiac probes (two concentric detectors for ventricular and background blood pool measurements) (Fig. 2.8) can be obtained for highly specialized patient populations.

The most costly ancillary equipment may be the gas delivery and trapping systems used most often for lung ventilation imaging. The type of system to be utilized may be dictated by the number of anticipated lung studies per year and by radiation safety considerations for the technologists. Apparatus ranges from disposable gas bags for very low numbers of studies to charcoal filter systems that may be refrigerated for higher trapping efficiency (Fig. 2.9). The shielding required around the trap depends on whether ^{133}Xe or ^{127}Xe is used; consequently, the diagnostic preference for these isotopes must be established.

In a full service nuclear medicine department, other instrumentation may include an isotope calibrator for documentation of the injected radiation dose, survey meters

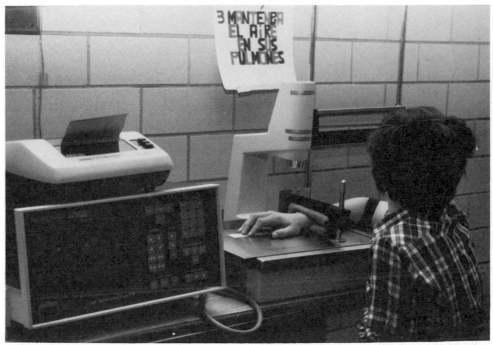

Figure 2.6. Bone density maps are produced by scanning the gamma ray source along the forearm and measuring the transmitted radiation with the single detector moving in coordination with the source. Larger systems are also available for scanning the spine. (Courtesy of National Jewish Hospital and Asthma Center.)

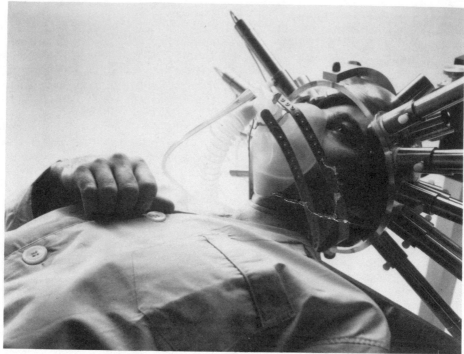

Figure 2.7. Regional cerebral blood flow (RCBF) can be determined from the time-varying radio-activity measured by the multiple probes positioned about the brain. The patient inhales radioactive xenon gas, which enters the bloodstream and perfuses the brain. A 32-probe system is shown, but similar systems with 8 and 16 probes are available. (Courtesy of Harshaw Chemical Company.)

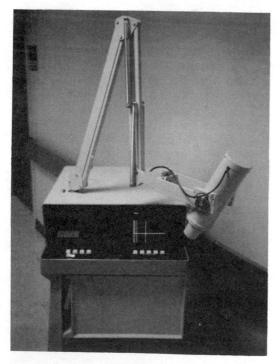

Figure 2.8. A small, inexpensive dual detector system (Nuclear Stethoscope) placed over the left ventricle is designed to indicate cardiac function. The inner crystal registers radioactivity in the left ventricle, and the surrounding (donut-shaped) crystal indicates background activity. (Courtesy of BIOS, Inc.)

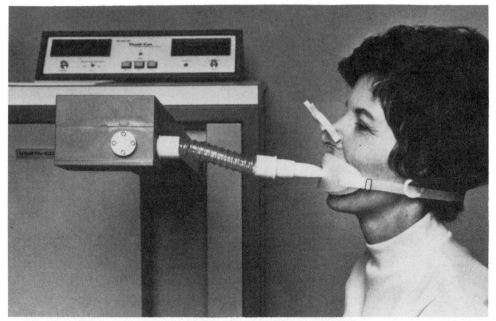

Figure 2.9. Pulmonary function and blood perfusion (see Fig. 2.7) studies may involve the use of radioactive gases. The system pictured is for storage and administration of the gas by inhalation and the subsequent trapping of the radioactive gas exhaled. Water and oxygen content can be controlled in most systems. (Courtesy of RADX.)

for monitoring contaminated and storage areas, and area monitors in hot labs for indication of nearby high activity (Fig. 2.10). Cardiac stress equipment consisting of supine bicycle and treadmill devices are needed for stress-gated and thallium redistribution studies, respectively. A high quality R-wave trigger is also needed for gated cardiac studies, and a complete EKG monitor would be appropriate for stress-gated work. Other gating devices to "freeze out" respiratory motion are also available.

ULTRASOUND

Technological advances have had as much effect in diagnostic ultrasound instrumentation as in any other modality of roentgenographic imaging. The instrumentation has progressed from the wash tubs and renovated B-29 gun turrets containing large quartz scanning crystals used as little as 30 yr ago (5) to the electronically sophisticated, commerically produced miniature ceramic crystals and polymers employed today in clinical facilities around the world. Furthermore, the quality of diagnostic sonograms has improved significantly as the technology

has become increasingly sophisticated. Today the sonologist has at his or her disposal equipment varying from static articulated arm B-mode systems that can image serial planes through any region of the body to small, self-contained linear array units no larger than the proverbial "breadbox" (6). The key feature is that the quality of the images is relatively independent of the system chosen. The variety of ultrasound instrumentation available necessitates a clear identification of the clinical needs to be addressed by the instrumentation. Several examples of clinical needs as selection criteria for ultrasound equipment are given in this section.

Static vs. Real-Time Scanners

In the ultrasound clinic, the estimated volume of various examinations (i.e., neonatal brain scanning, carotid imaging or flow analysis, echocardiographic procedures in both children and/or adults, general upper abdominal procedures including studies of the liver, gallbladder, spleen, kidneys or pancreas, general lower abdominal and pelvic procedures which include examinations

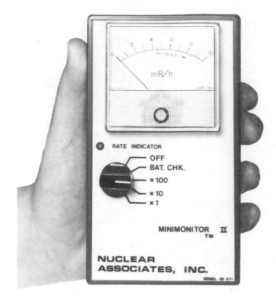

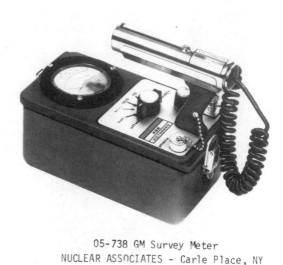

05-738 GM Survey Meter
NUCLEAR ASSOCIATES - Carle Place, NY

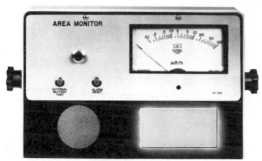

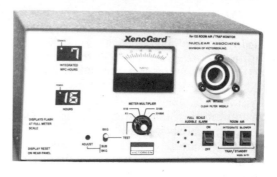

Figure 2.10. Hand-held survey meters (*above*) for periodic measurement of possible radioactive spills are required for nuclear medicine departments. Area monitors (*below*) for continuous monitoring of background radiation are desirable for radiopharmaceutical preparation areas and radioactive gas-dispensing rooms. (Courtesy of Nuclear Associates.)

of the bladder and genitalia, and studies of the breast, thyroid, or suspected superficial masses) influences the purchase of a static or real-time scanner, the latter either a stationary or portable real-time mechanical sector system or a sequential or phased linear array. Also, the need for dedicated instead of multipurpose units is influenced by the work load. Today, most equipment is modular, so that electronic problems can be isolated to a certain board, and a substitute board can be inserted to avoid prolonged downtime. If an original board is replaced, however, a quick check on the calibration and registration of the system is advisable to ensure that nothing else in the pulser-transducer-receiver-scan converter-image chain has been affected.

Depending on the projected work load, the user may wish to consider optional features, such as the presence of relocatable electronic calipers on the display or access to variations in preprocessing and postprocessing of the echo signals into and out of the scan converter. Also, the presence of a separate freeze frame control on real-time units can give an image of the heart in midbeat so that the intraventricular valves can be studied and the presence of abnormal growths or fluid collection within the pericardial sac can be identified.

A last concern in ultrasound imaging is the manner in which hard copy images are made from a video display. In most centers, the older technique of Polaroid photography of the video image has been replaced by multiformat camera imaging from a flat-faced CRT onto an 8- × 10-inch x-ray film. The signal sent to the camera is independent of the image on the video display, so that the camera should be adjusted to produce the most diagnostically informative echo possible. The number of images per film is selectable from 1 to 9. If a real-time sector system is present, an additional visual recording device such as a videotape or videodisc recorder aids in preserving the constantly changing image.

The purchaser should consider space limitations in the acquisition of new equipment. For example, the room space available can be a major factor in determining whether a general purpose static B-mode system with added real-time scanning capability could be purchased in place of a dedicated portable system. Also, the ability to control room lighting and adequate regulation of the environment (i.e., humidity and air conditioning to regulate temperature fluctuations to within a few degrees of 22°C) are necessary features to acquire the most diagnostically relevant imaging results. In addition, the division of larger rooms into smaller scanning areas often is attainable by use of curtains or room dividers.

Other necessities for ultrasound examining rooms are adequate shelving and cabinet facilities to store items (such as linens, towels, "linen savers," examining gowns, coupling gels, and mineral oil) that must be used during an ultrasound study. Also, a sink is helpful when the sonographer is cleaning up after an examination.

Articulated Arm Static B-Scanner

The articulated arm static B-scanner is most efficient in acquiring image information over a large field of view, in serial planes if necessary, when organ or patient motion (e.g., heart motion or breathing) do not present a problem. Typical applications include: survey scans of the thyroid (7), liver (8), gallbladder (9), spleen (10), kidneys (11), pancreas (12), prostate (13), pelvic region (14), great vessels in the retroperitoneum (15), ob/gyn studies both with and without a fetus present (16), postmastectomy chest wall measurements for radiation therapy, and tumor delineation before therapy (17). By proper use of a single crystal static B-

scan transducer assembly (e.g., by using an internal, external, or water-path standoff), scans can be obtained of superficial structures such as the breast (18), testes (19), superficial body surfaces (20), and suspected superficial tumors. In any examination, the proper transducer assembly (i.e., frequency, active element diameter, and focal characteristics) must be chosen if sonograms of satisfactory diagnostic quality are to be obtained. Since a static B-mode scanner should reliably handle a work load of 20 or more patients per day, a thorough program of quality assurance must be maintained (21). Such a program permits continuous optimum system performance and hence fewer repeated studies. Even though no deleterious biological effects of ultrasound have been verified at diagnostic levels, provision of certain acoustic output and transducer assembly parameters have been recommended (22). These parameters are given in Table 2.6 and extend to all types of diagnostic ultrasound equipment (i.e., mechanical sector scanners, electronically phased linear array sector scanners, electronically sequenced linear arrays, and dedicated TM-mode (Time-Motion mode) systems.

Real-Time Scanners

There are some ultrasound examinations where organ motion is an important consideration (e.g., echocardiographic studies (23), fetal life monitoring (24), and quantitative blood flow measurements (25)). For these applications, real-time scanners are necessary. The nature of the study and the information desired usually dictate the specific piece of equipment used. A simple sequential linear array providing about 20 frames (images)/sec on the video monitor is ideal for lower power scanning of in utero fetal structures. These units provide images in oblique planes and can be placed in therapy treatment rooms for periodic verification of the position of the radiation field with respect to the tumor and any radiation-sensitive organs (26).

If the long, rectangular aperture (e.g., 64 elements at 3.5 MHz, approximately 1 cm × 12 cm) of a conventional linear array is inadequate for a study where smaller acoustic entrance dimensions are required, then a shorter (32 element) linear array, phased while sequencing to provide a "pie slice" field of view, can be employed. This approach is especially useful in echocardiography examinations where a small aperture, wide field of view, and medium depth of penetration are preferred (27). The number of cardiovascular studies a department expects to perform may suggest the acquistion of a dedicated real-time phased array. The need to move the unit from floor to floor or from room to room imposes an extra requirement of portability on such a unit.

There may be occasions where no type of linear array real-time scanner meets an institution's needs (e.g., when it is necessary to do abdominal real-time scanning such as longitudinal planes through the liver and right kidney where the lower ribs inhibit complete contact between the transducer assembly and the skin). Here, a mechanically driven sector scanner is the system of choice, because it provides the required flexibility. When equipped with properly calibrated calipers, this system can also be used to predict fetal gestational age by anatomic measurements such as the BPD (fetal biparietal diameter) (28).

Once the clinical needs have been identified, a choice must be made between stand alone, portable real-time units and real-time add-ons to fixed static scanners. In exercising this choice, care must be taken to verify that the add-on systems yield imaging performance parameters (i.e., sensitivity, linearity, precision in measurements, reproducibility, and spatial resolution) equivalent to those of a compatible stand alone real-time system (see Chapter 7).

CONCLUSION

The following questions should always be addressed to verify that intended equipment purchases match identified clinical needs.

1. Is system sensitivity large enough to permit adequate penetration of the interrogating pulsed beam without reducing its center frequency and thus sacrificing spatial resolution?
2. Is the work load of echocardiographic studies heavy enough to merit the purchase of more dedicated real-time systems suitable for cardiac studies?
3. Are the manufacturer's transducer as-

semblies adequate when compared with newer, more efficient quarterwave and multimatching layer designs?
4. Is there a need for increased portability in present units to satisfy the needs, for example, for more ultrasound scanning procedures desired for premature labor cases on the hospital's labor deck?
5. Are there any external means to vary the amplitude or time duration of the excitation pulse to the transducer to provide the sonographer with some control over the unit's acoustic output and thus exposure to the patient?

By answering queries such as these, the potential buyer can develop a table where "Clinical Needs" are listed on the left-hand side and a "System Requirement" is listed on the right-hand side. Completion of this table is the first step in determining if additional diagnostic ultrasound equipment is needed in the department and, if so, what type. An example of such a comparison chart is given in Table 2.7.

COMPUTED TOMOGRAPHY SCANNERS

A computed tomography (CT) scanner is one of the more expensive and technically complex items of radiologic equipment commonly purchased by hospitals and radiology clinics. It was introduced into the market in the early 1970s and has been quickly integrated into the medical imaging arena because of its unique imaging abilities. The success of the CT scanner is exemplified by the creation of two journals dedicated primarily to the clinical and technical aspects of the field. (Di Chiro G (ed): *Journal of Computer Assisted Tomography.* New York, Raven Press; Ledley RS (ed): *Computerized Radiology* (formerly *Computerized Tomography.* New York, Pergamon Press.)

The advantages that CT scanners enjoy are numerous and include the following:

1. Ability to image subtle differences in soft tissue. This capability is particularly true inside the skull, although the utility of CT to discriminate soft tissues in the body also has been amply demonstrated.

2. Ability to display images in a "slice" format. This eliminates the confusion of superimposed images of over- and underlying tissues found in conventional radiographs.
3. Wide dynamic range. In a single image, information regarding dense and lucent tissues is present. By adjustment of the gray level monitor, all tissue densities can be displayed.

Selection of a CT scanner, as with any purchase of major imaging equipment, should be undertaken with considerable forethought, planning, and analysis of the needs and constraints of the institution. It is especially important to consider the needs of personnel using the equipment at an early stage in the decision-making process (29–31), as it becomes difficult, if not impossible, to change the unit to accommodate last minute desires once the purchase decision has been finalized and the mechanics of purchasing have commenced.

This section does not presume to answer the question: "Which CT scanner shall I buy?" Instead, it offers suggestions of which questions to ask and from whom to seek answers so that an intelligent and logical choice may be made. Frequently, several desirable features are either not available or affordable, and compromises with regard to scanner selection and site preparation are inevitable. The section is divided into three parts that may be summarized in the form of questions:

1. Who gives input regarding the choice of a CT scanner?
2. What are the constraints of the institution?
3. What features of CT scanners are relevant to the selection?

Who Gives Input Regarding the Choice of a CT Scanner?

PHYSICIAN

The physician is the primary interpreter of clinical CT images. Consequently, he is able to specify the imaging needs in terms of the anatomical features that need to be discriminated and the level of image quality required. For example, is a whole body CT scanner required or is a dedicated head unit sufficient? Are high spatial resolution characteristics necessary to perform detailed studies of the inner ear and spine?

The physician's knowledge of past referral patterns and anticipated work loads can be invaluable. Is the population of patients rather routine or does the patient mix dictate versatility (and probably added expense) of a more flexible instrument? In a busy department or clinic, patient throughput is another factor to be considered.

In private practice, the physician may function as a business manager as well as an interpreter of images. In these cases economic considerations, some of which are described below, are important and may compromise decisions based purely on technical factors.

PHYSICIST

For the selection of complex equipment such as a CT scanner, a physicist is essential to provide in-depth technical support and advice. The physicist may be an in-house physicist or a consultant. An individual with a thorough knowledge of CT scanners is particularly well suited to measuring performance parameters and to making comparative evaluations between various models prior to purchase. He/she can be invaluable in translating a qualitative description of the institution's needs into a quantitative specification of imaging performance. The physicist can also be helpful in designing the CT suite and prescribing radiation shielding where required.

TECHNOLOGIST

Frequently the technologist has the major burden of patient contact during a CT exam and is most familiar with the operation of the CT scanner. This individual can suggest patient handling features that are beneficial to technologists and to patients. A careful selection of the console layout, patient bed operation, and other safety and convenience features may ultimately result in smoother patient flow, reduced fatigue, and better morale.

ADMINISTRATOR AND BUSINESS MANAGER

These individuals can assist with the fiscal aspects of selecting and purchasing a CT scanner and can provide valuable information concerning contractual and fiscal negotiations. Monetary and space constraints are often specified by an administrator or business manager, and the quality and versatility of a CT scanner often depend on constraints identified by them. Patient volume and revenue ultimately dictate the limits of scanner cost. Questions of whether to lease or buy can be fielded by these individuals or others knowledgeable about current banking conditions and potential tax advantages. They can also provide assistance in the preparation of an application for a Certificate of Need, when necessary, and can supply fiscal and referral data for such a document.

ARCHITECTS

An architect can assist in the design and location of the CT unit. Remodeling suggestions can be provided within the constraints of space and money. Requirements for electrical power, air conditioning, water and floor loading should be integrated into the design based upon the manufacturer's recommendations.

VENDORS

The marketing representatives of manufacturers can provide information on the scanners available, the features each of them has, and the costs of the features. Frequently they can provide technical performance specifications, as well.

PROFESSIONAL COLLEAGUES

Other imaging physicians, physicians from referring services, physicists, and technologists may be consulted on the features and characteristics they have found useful in CT scanners. If familiar with a particular scanner, they can often provide insight into the routine operation of the scanner and provide information that is not readily apparent from sales demonstrations. Pointed inquiries of colleagues about their "likes and dislikes" of a particular scanner may yield valuable information. Users can also answer questions regarding a manufacturer's service capabilities and the dedication of the manufacturer to keep the CT scanner updated with new software and hardware features.

What Are the Constraints of the Institution?

Requirements and constraints within the hospital or clinic may be broadly categorized into three groups: space, money, and time. These items are summarized in detail below.

SPACE REQUIREMENTS

The floor space required for a CT scanner includes space for support facilities, as well as space for the scanner and control room. The location of these support facilities relative to the CT suite is important to the smooth and efficient flow of patients.

One possible design for a complete CT scan suite is shown in Figure 2.11.

Scanner Room

This room contains the scanner gantry, patient bed, and any auxiliary equipment specified by the manufacturer. Typically, the scanner room, the control room, and the equipment room occupy about 650 sq ft. Sufficient space should be provided to accommodate patient gurneys and physiological monitoring equipment, when required. Doorways should permit passage of gurneys and wheelchairs. Radiation shielding may be required in some of the walls and doors, especially for heavy volume sites. For low and medium volume CT suites, radiation shielding beyond plasterboard is frequently not necessary on many, perhaps even all, of the walls. The gantry is heavy, and additional support of the floor may be necessary if the scanner is not located at ground level.

Control Room

The control room is the area from which the CT examination is controlled. It should be located to provide an unobstructed view of the patient, usually through a window. The room size should be large enough to permit free movement of several people. One scanner configuration that is often employed uses a separate diagnostic console located in a remote area of the room. This console permits the physician to view images without interference with scanner operation.

Equipment Room

This area houses the computers, electronics, and x-ray generators and requires atten-

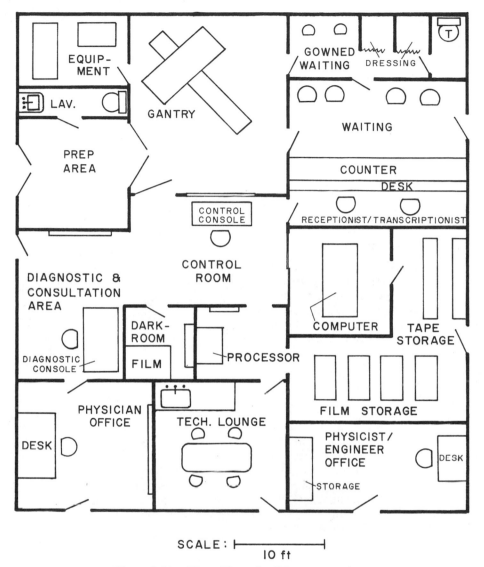

Figure 2.11.   Floor Plan of a CT scanner suite.

tion only infrequently. The equipment area should be easily accessible to the control room, but acoustically insulated from it. In general, substantial amounts of heat are generated in this room, and additional air conditioning and a raised "computer floor" are frequent requirements. Some manufacturers are designing scanner configurations that require no additional equipment area or an area of reduced size. For these scanners, a small electronics cabinet is often required in the control or scanner room, and additional air conditioning in these areas may be antic-

ipated. For any configuration of the equipment area, the manufacturer should supply engineering details of air conditioning requirements, flooring, etc.

Patient Preparation Area

A small patient preparation area adjacent to the scan room provides an area where the next patient can be prepared for a CT examination during the latter stages of the preceding patient's examination. This area is particularly beneficial for CT scanners that offer additional gurneys that can be detached from the gantry. An added benefit, in terms of throughput, may be realized by having a patient immediately available when the preceding patient's examination has been completed. A patient preparation area also provides nonambulatory patients with privacy while awaiting examination.

Waiting Room

An ambulatory patient reception and waiting area is suggested for the comfort and convenience of these patients. This area is especially important in a clinical environment where most of the patients are ambulatory.

Reading and Consultation Room

It is desirable to designate an area outside of the control room as a reading area. This enables the radiologist to interpret the images, dictate reports, and consult with other physicians without disturbing or being disturbed by normal functioning of the control area. Space should be provided for a viewing console, light boxes, and for temporary storage of patient files.

File Room

As in conventional radiographic areas, a location for the storage of patient files is required near the CT area. Since CT scanner hard copy images are usually of uniform size, it may be more efficient to store them separately from the storage area for conventional examinations. Proximity to the CT scan area and reading room provides efficient access. In some installations, floppy disks may be stored in the same file as film. Many of the same precautions must be observed for floppy disks as with magnetic tape storage.

Magnetic Tape Storage Area

For those installations that store images on magnetic tape as well as film, an area must be provided for proper storage of magnetic tape. The storage area for magnetic tapes should be cool, dry, and free from reasonably strong magnetic fields. This last requirement precludes locations near electric motors, transformers, and magnetic resonance scanners.

Dark Room and Processor

This area should be located reasonably close to the control room to provide quick access to the processing of films generated by the multiformat camera.

Offices

An office for the physician and physicist should be provided in the vicinity of the CT suite, permitting clinical and technical problems to be addressed conveniently and promptly.

Technologists' Lounge

This area serves many purposes. It may contain lockers for uniforms, coats, and other personal items. A table and comfortable chairs are suggested for lunch and coffee breaks. An area of this type located conveniently to the CT suite encourages personnel to confine their eating and drinking to this area and reduces the problems of food, liquids, and cigarette smoke in the control room, where they are hazards to the computer system.

Storage Areas

A security area may be provided for the storage of clinical supplies, test equipment, and spare parts for the CT scanner. Providing the service engineer with a location for his tools and parts may encourage him to keep extra scanner parts at the institution, thereby eliminating shipping times for frequent repair items and reducing overall downtime.

FINANCIAL REQUIREMENTS

In planning for the acquisition of a CT scanner and its operation, one must allow for capital costs and some other costs that may be less than obvious.

CT Scanner and Optional Equipment

Obviously, the capital cost of purchasing the scanner must be considered, as well as the selected options. Shipping and transportation costs are sometimes overlooked; occasionally they will be assumed by the manufacturer, at least in part, through negotiation.

Physics Test Equipment

These items include instruments and phantoms for acceptance testing, quality assurance, and periodic calibrations. A dosimetry system is required for determining patient dose. An instrument for measuring scattered and leakage radiation is also suggested.

Remodeling and Renovation

Renovation costs are frequently incurred prior to installation of a CT scanner. These costs may include installation of larger air conditioning and ventilation systems, electrical power lines, water and sewer lines, and oxygen and gas outlets. Constructing new walls or moving old walls may be required. Some of the walls, doors, and windows may require radiation shielding. Carpeting, draperies, and acoustical ceilings help to reduce noise from an operating scanner. Cupboard space for storing supplies and a work counter and desk space for scanner personnel should be included. Also, decorator items (e.g., wall hangings) and furniture for the waiting areas, lounges, control room, and offices should be included. Finally, the cost of file and tape racks should not be overlooked.

Salaries and Overhead

A significant cost in the operation of a CT scanner is the salaries of technologists, physicists, receptionists, secretaries, orderlies, and dictation transcribers. For some installations, especially those with more than one scanner, an in-house service engineer may be economically feasible.

Operating Expenses

There are many other items loosely categorized as "supplies" that are essential to the operation of a CT suite. These include radioopaque contrast media, hypodermic syringes and needles, drugs, emergency equipment, tape, gauze, bandages, and other hospital supplies. Bedding, patient gowns, and laundry must be included. Stationery supplies for bookkeeping, patient scheduling, billing, and reports must be considered. In addition, the costs generally included in the "overhead" category are: utilities, telephone, housekeeping, and general maintenance of the suite.

Service

The service costs for a CT scanner may be significant. Depending on the resources of the installation, it may be desirable to employ an in-house engineer who is capable of repairing and calibrating the CT scanner. The cost of all parts must be considered when the in-house method is chosen. A small on-site inventory of spare failure-prone parts may be a prudent investment.

It may be more efficient, if not less expensive, to contract for service with the manufacturer or with an independent service group. A service contract usually includes the cost of essentially all parts except x-ray tubes. The time of day that service is normally available may be negotiated with the service organization. Service at night or on weekends is sometimes contractable at substantially higher costs. A typical annual cost for 40 hr/week service, excluding x-ray tubes, is 6 to 8% of the purchase price of the scanner. Considering that the cost of each tube may be several thousands of dollars, x-ray tubes alone can add significantly to the overall service budget.

TIME REQUIREMENTS

A smooth installation of a CT scanner with a minimum of last-minute unexpected surprises requires proper orchestration of prepurchasing tasks, purchasing, room preparation, and installation. The provision of adequate time for these tasks minimizes frustration with architects, site planners, the manufacturer, and institutional personnel who operate and test the scanner.

Certificate of Need

Depending on the requirements of local health planning agencies, purchase of a CT scanner may require submission of an application for a Certificate of Need (CON). Preparation of this document may require a few weeks of proper documentation of the institution's needs. Proper planning must consider preparation time for the CON application, deadlines for submission, review by the planning agency, and public hearings concerning the CON application.

Selection

Selection of a CT scanner should be based upon a number of clinical and technical criteria described in the next section. This process involves investigating the types and models of scanners currently on the market and choosing the type that most closely matches the needs of the institution.

Manufacturer Lead Time

It is rare that a manufacturer can provide instant off-the-shelf delivery of a CT scanner. More frequently, the manufacturer requires a time period before he can deliver a scanner, typically a number of months. In extreme cases, particularly for models that are in a developmental or prototype stage, the delivery time conceivably could be as long as a year or more from the time of purchase. Whatever the time required, this period should be used for site preparation and renovation. For those installations that are replacing an old scanner and wish to maintain continuous CT scanning service during remodeling, a short term lease of a mobile CT system may be a reasonable solution.

Installation

A period of time is required after delivery to assemble, test, and calibrate a CT scanner. Usually the installation can be completed in 2 to 8 weeks, depending on the manufacturer and the complexity of the model. Near the end of this period, acceptance testing is recommended. The physicist will require a few 8-hr days to complete the tests and to make recommendations to the manufacturer regarding areas of suboptimal performance.

Training Period

Before a full patient schedule is attempted on a new installation, a training and "de-bugging" period is suggested. During this period, the temptation to schedule a full load of patients should be resisted. One or two patients per day over the first few days will permit the technologists to become familiar with scanner operation and will allow time to establish an examination routine without the pressure of a backlog of scheduled patients. Undoubtedly, certain adjustments in procedure and additions to the supplies stock will be necessary. Many electronic and mechanical components fail during their first few hours of use; a light patient schedule permits repairs to be made without rescheduling large numbers of patients. As familiarity and reliability are established, more patients per day can be added until a full load is achieved.

What Features of CT Scanners Are Relevant to the Selection?

A number of considerations determine the type of CT scanner required by a specific institution. The general characteristics of a scanner are broadly categorized according to institution in Table 2.8. Most institutions fall in more than one category, and considerable overlap may exist in the general characteristics sought in a CT scanner. Frequently, all desirable features are not available on a particular scanner, and compromises are required.

Specific characteristics of CT scanners are divided into three categories: hardware features, software features, and other clinical features (Table 2.9). Frequently, items in the following tables do not fit entirely into one or the other of these categories, and overlap is common.

Table 2.8
General Characteristics of a CT Scanner

Type of institution	Characteristics
Research/teaching	1. Accessibility to software for manipulating and processing images 2. Versatility 3. High resolution and good image quality 4. Research features
High volume clinic	1. Ease of use 2. High throughput features 3. Reliability 4. Ease of service 5. Multiple consoles
Low volume clinic	1. Lower cost 2. Reliability, particularly if in a remote area

RADIATION THERAPY

In most radiation therapy departments, the major pieces of equipment can be divided into three categories: treatment units, simulators, and treatment planning computers. Equipment in these categories is generally complex, expensive, and provided by a number of manufacturers. Selection of a suitable item is a formidable task, but careful consideration of the requirements of the clinical service can help ensure that a reasonable choice is made.

Treatment Units

The decision to offer radiation therapy services creates the initial requirement for a treatment unit. This decision is based upon patient care, financial factors, and population statistics and is dealt with elsewhere in this book. Once one or more treatment units are in place, the need may arise to replace these units or add to additional units. This need usually stems from the inability of existing equipment to provide the capabilities thought necessary by the department. For example, the growing undependability or outright failure of a treatment unit may necessitate its replacement. If repair of the unit is impractical or not cost-effective, justification for its replacement should be straightforward.

In some situations, however, installation of a new treatment unit may be necessary, even if an existing unit (or units) is functioning properly. Whether the existing unit is replaced may depend on space limitations or other factors.

The need for a new treatment unit often is a reflection of deficiencies in existing units which prevent the incorporation of new techniques into the clinical service. For example, the availability of electron beams has become an essential feature of a comprehensive radiation therapy service. Increases in patient load may demand acquisition of an additional treatment unit. Recommendations of maximum capacity for treatment units may be found in the CROS "Blue Book" (33) and HSA publications (34). Changes in the composition of patient load may necessitate replacement or addition of treatment units. For example, increased referrals of patients with carcinoma of the prostate supports the installation of an accelerator providing a high-energy photon beam. Trends in treatment technique may have a similar effect. For example, the desirability of total skin electron beam therapy for treatment of mycosis fungoides may prompt the decision to install an accelerator that provides low-energy electrons.

The decision to install new equipment may be tempered by several additional factors, such as the cost of the equipment and service, limitations in space and personnel, and plans of other facilities in the region to add or upgrade radiation therapy. Additionally, those responsible for the decision must consider the capability of an existing facility to accommodate the new equipment. Services such as electrical power, water, air conditioning, and radiation shielding may have to be supplemented. Should the necessary expansion of these services be impractical, construction of a new facility might be considered.

Similar considerations must be deliberated when selecting the maximum energy of a new treatment unit. While there is a tendency nationwide toward the selection of higher beam energies, improvements in therapeutic effectiveness often are difficult to demonstrate at the higher energies. The maximum energy should be selected with the objective of actual patient benefit in terms of parameters such as percent depth dose, skin sparing, beam sharpness, etc. These factors should be compared to disadvantages such as increased cost, increased space requirements, increased personnel requirements (for example, in-house service technicians), greater shielding requirements, and additional problems such as neutron production occurring with the use of high-energy x rays.

Decisions also must be made regarding specific aspects of performance of the new treatment unit. While most therapy units sold today are mounted isocentrically with the axis of rotation 100 cm from the radiation source, used and reconditioned equipment is available that provides other specifications. Occasionally, facility limitations or patient load requirements may make a stand-mounted unit, or an 80-cm isocentric unit, a practical alternative to a new 100-cm unit.

The need to treat patients in unusual positions may influence the purchase decision. Treatment at long distances for total body irradiation preempts the use of a fixed beam stop and requires suitable shielding. Simi-

Table 2.9
Hardware Features of CT Scanners

Features	Qualities to consider
1. Head or body scanner	Whole body scanners can examine any part of the anatomy, although they are considerably more expensive than dedicated head scanners. Manufacturers of both types usually consider their whole body model to be "top of the line," and therefore body scanners are more likely to have desirable features: faster, better images, more versatile software, etc. Examinations of head and bodies have been shown to occur in the U.S. at the ratio of 3:1 (32)
2. Scan speed	Generally, faster speeds are needed in bodies to reduce motion (respiration) artifacts. Scan speeds generally range from 1 to 240 sec, depending on model. Extremely long scan speeds can reduce patient throughout.
3. Spatial resolution	Higher resolution is required for fine detail studies (e.g., inner ear, spine). Currently, ability to see detail as small as 0.5 mm is possible with some scanners.
4. Contrast resolution	Ability to discriminate subtle differences in tissue (e.g., white vs gray matter in brain, lesions in certain organs). This particular characteristic is difficult to quantify.
5. Tilting gantry	Permits images of patients at angles other than perpendicular to patient axis. Some manufacturers offer a tilting table in lieu of a tilting gantry. The latter system permits the elevation of the patient's feet, convenient for some myelographic procedures. A table that pivots about a vertical axis through the scan plane is also offered by some manufacturers.
6. Variable kVp and/or filtration	Permits dual energy scans that are useful in tissue characterization studies. Also, some types of x-ray filters distribute the dose more uniformly over the patient.
7. Variable mA	Permits increase or decrease in patient dose with a corresponding reduction or increase in image noise.
8. Tube type	A rotating anode is generally capable of a higher flux density of rays which permits a higher dose in a shorter scan and subsequently a less noisy image. Rotating anode tubes generally have heat-loading limitations that may limit the number of consecutive scans. Patient throughput and some dynamic studies may be limited. Stationary anode tubes, on the other hand, can usually be scanned continuously without a heat-loading problem at the cost of somewhat increased noise in the image.
9. Variable scan width	Wider scan widths generally produce less noisy images, and fewer scans are required to cover the anatomical region to be examined. Narrow slice widths improve the visibility of small anatomical details and reduce partial volume effects.
10. Anatomical localization system	Useful for defining anatomy to be scanned and establishing protocol (number of scans, scan width, gantry/bed angle).
11. Detachable patient bed (gurney)	This feature plus an extra bed increases throughput by permitting a second patient to be positioned on the table while the first patient is being scanned.
12. Data storage service(s)	Current data and reconstructed images are usually stored on a computer disk, either a "hard" disk or a "floppy" disk. A hard disk is not easily removed from the system, and the images and data stored on it must be transferred or discarded when it is filled. If the data are to be saved, they must be transferred from the hard disk to a floppy disk or a magnetic tape for archival storage. Magnetic tape is not as convenient as floppy disks for archival storage, but the cost per image stored is less. This mode of data storage requires space in addition to the usual patient file storage.

Table 2.9—Continued

Features	Qualities to consider
13. Multiformat camera	This device produces an image on film from an image on a TV screen. Film formats may be selected from common sizes (e.g., 8 × 10 inch or 11 × 14 inch), and the number of images on each film may be fixed or varied, depending on the model of the camera. Larger film sizes usually permit a series of images to fit on fewer films. However, smaller film may be easier to handle and store. Polaroid cameras are optional on some systems.
14. Radiation field indicators	These are usually one or more fields of light indicating the position of the radiation field. Sometimes the light field is coincident with the x-ray beam in the gantry; in some models, however, the light field is external to the gantry at a well-defined distance from the x-ray beam. In the latter case, the patient is positioned with the light field, then moved to the location of the x-ray beam.
15. Dynamic scanning capabilities	This feature provides rapid successive scans through a particular region of anatomy. After reconstruction, the sequence of generated images permits viewing of anatomical changes as a function of time. For example, the flow of a contrast medium through a specified organ may be monitored over a period of several scans. Some systems utilize data collected during only a fraction of the scan to reconstruct an image. The image is not as good as that reconstructed from data for a complete scan; however, by using fractions of scan data, several images, each distinct in time, may be reconstructed from a single scan. Some manufacturers offer the option of physiologic gating to reconstruct an image from data obtained during a selected portion of the cardiac cycle. A rapid sequence of images reconstructed from successive phases of the heart cycle can give the appearance of a beating heart.
16. Control and viewing consoles	Some manufacturers configure their CT scanners so that the diagnostic console and the control console are side by side in a single cabinet. Other models present an additional cabinet for the diagnostic console so that it may be in a separate location from the control console. Depending on space constraints, one configuration may be more desirable than another. For example, if the radiologist wishes to examine images while patient scanning is in progress, the former configuration may be convenient because of the proximity of the technologist directing the scans. The type of configuration should be chosen with some foresight regarding the operation of the CT suite.
17. Reconstruction time	Although reconstruction time may appear to be a software feature, the time for reconstruction actually depends on the size and speed of the computers and the amount of data sampled in the scan. The latter usually depends on the scan speed and the number of detectors in the scanner. Typical reconstruction times range from nearly instantaneous to about 1 min. The patient volume may dictate, to some extent, the reconstruction speed required, although reconstruction speed is probably not the primary factor for determining patient throughput.

larly, the desire to treat patients in the seated position may eliminate a beam stop. An unwillingness to invest time in extensive operator training or to provide in-house service capability may make a simpler unit of proven performance more attractive.

A final consideration in the identification of the clinical requirements for a new treatment unit hinges on the proposed use of the unit. A department that will be relying on the new unit to carry a heavy work load may be well advised to select one of the more simple, dependable units. Such a choice should help reduce downtime and the accompanying frustration and revenue loss. In particular, single unit departments probably should avoid complex units that are susceptible to high downtime. In contrast, a department with an active research program may select a more complex unit with capabilities for innovative treatment techniques. Generally, these are departments better equipped to tolerate the increased frequency of tuning and greater downtime of the more complex treatment units.

SIMULATOR

Most persons involved in radiation therapy believe that a simulator is an essential item in a department that provides curative megavoltage radiation therapy. In past years, only a small number of simulators has been available, making selection of an appropriate unit relatively easy. Today, however, there are a number of simulators to choose from. These units provide a wide variety of capabilities and prices.

The purchase of a simulator most often is prompted by the desire to monitor a course of therapy to assure that the treatment plan is being followed. Used in this fashion, a simulator improves upon the documentation provided by treatment verification (port) films. For this purpose, a simulator need not be extremely complex. However, some simulators are installed with the intent of actually developing treatment plans as well as documenting the adherence to a plan developed by other techniques. Simulators for developing treatment plans are more complex because they should permit manipulation of the simulator with a minimum of inconvenience.

A trend toward more complex treatments, perhaps accompanied by the installation of a complex treatment unit, may accelerate the decision to install a simulator. Installation of a simulator also may be stimulated by a patient load that has grown sufficiently large to limit the time available for setting up new patients on the treatment unit(s). A complex or unusual treatment may require an hour or more for the initial treatment setup. Performing this setup on a simulator rather than a treatment unit increases the treatment capacity of the unit. The corresponding increase in revenue may partially offset the cost of the simulator.

Finally, the possible legal handicap imposed by the lack of a simulator cannot be overlooked. For at least certain treatment regimes, it has been demonstrated that possible complications may be reduced if simulation is performed prior to treatment (35). If these improvements are verified in other institutions, the use of a simulator may become accepted as a standard of practice in radiation therapy.

The specific equipment requirements of a simulator are determined by its intended use. A simulator which is acquired only for treatment verification and documentation purposes can be rather simple. Such simulators require neither fluoroscopy nor a wide range of target-to-axis distances (TAD). At least one simulator is manufactured expressly for treatment verification and documentation.

Departments considering the installation of a limited simulator should review their patient load and their requirements for treatment planning. Should the patient mix change or the complexity of treatment arrangements increase, a simulator which is intended only for documentation may not be adequate.

On the other hand, simulators intended for treatment planning must necessarily be more complex. These simulators are often used to develop optimum treatment plans in a dynamic fashion, and fluoroscopy provides a means to speed up this process. The presence of an image intensifier sometimes limits the vertical motion of the treatment couch, and a wider range of TADs is required to accommodate a full range of treatment distances. The use of treatment units with different isocenter distances also requires a suitable range of TADs. To properly simulate the treatment of patients at extended treatment distances, an even wider range of TADs may be required.

Another major difference among simulators is the degree of operator convenience. Simulators vary widely in this respect, from ones which provide mechanical scales and extremely limited motor-driven controls, to microprocessor-driven simulators that move components automatically to avoid collisions and that provide digital displays of all parameters in various locations. The appropriate degree of complexity in a simulator is a trade-off between desirable features and the cost and required amount of service. As one would expect, the more complex a system becomes, the more service usually is required, and the greater the requirement for preventive maintenance. A department should consider its willingness to provide the required service commitment before purchasing a complex simulator. At the same time, it should be recognized that a piece of equipment which is inconvenient and tedious to use most likely will not be used often, if at all.

The primary advantage of a simulator in radiation therapy planning is the visualization of structures that are generally difficult to locate on port films or verification films taken with the accelerator. In evaluating the need for a simulator, a department should consider the frequency of situations in which the patient anatomy cannot be visualized sufficiently to ensure that treatment fields are placed correctly. The incidence of even a small number of such occurrences probably justifies the use of a simulator, especially if the cases involve risk to the spinal cord.

The space and facility requirements for a simulator are comparable to those for a treatment unit. A large room is needed, since the dimensions of a simulator often exceed those of a treatment unit. The control room should be spacious enough to provide comfortable working conditions. It should be situated to provide easy access directly into the simulator room and also allow movement between physicians' offices and the treatment units without passing through the simulator room. The control room should be equipped with view-boxes located away from the primary control area. The control room should provide a viewing window that is large enough to permit visual monitoring of the patient, but small enough to furnish the patient with a sense of privacy. The fluoroscopy monitor should be located where it can be viewed by several people.

TREATMENT PLANNING COMPUTER

In radiation therapy, a treatment planning computer is felt to be a requirement, rather than a luxury (36). With the possible exception of departments providing palliative treatments only, a computer is required for a sizable fraction of the work load.

A department should be able to justify purchase of a treatment planning computer on the basis that it represents a minimum level of quality care. Present standards for accuracy in dose delivery essentially demand the use of a computer to take into account individual variations among patients. While the technology of treatment planning computers is ever changing and is generally considered, even today, to be somewhat less than optimum, most treatment planning systems do a reasonably good job of computing dose distributions for patients.

A department wishing to upgrade or add to its present treatment planning capability might point to an increase in patient load as evidence that the request is justified. It is important to recognize, however, that an increase in computational speed does not necessarily result in a significant decrease in the overall time required to generate a treatment plan, since the computational time usually is only a small fraction of the entire process. Large departments sometimes find that an additional computer may be required. A cost-effective alternative which is often employed is the purchase of a second data-entry terminal and the operation of the computer in a time-sharing mode. This approach allows two (or more) treatment planning technologists to work simultaneously, often with little observable increase in the time required to generate a treatment plan.

The features required for a treatment planning computer may vary somewhat from one department to another. For example, a number of mechanisms for patient data entry are required. Most systems marketed today are equipped with magnetic tape drives, so that CT scans may be entered directly. This capability is essential for situations that consider patient geometry and tissue density in planes other than that containing the central axis of the radiation beam. These techniques are becoming available and represent the beginning of three-dimensional treatment planning. Data from CT may not always be available for each patient, so a device is required to enter patient contours obtained by other means. Virtually all treatment planning systems are equipped with digitizing devices for this purpose. Similar devices are used to enter the shape of irregular fields to perform Clarkson integrations and to enter the locations of implanted radioactive sources. Users should be cautious when selecting a digitizer to ensure that reasonable accuracy is provided. Of course, the user must also ensure that the images from which contours and heterogeneity information are taken are also spatially undistorted.

The overall computing requirements of a department should be considered when reviewing treatment planning systems that are commercially available. It is possible that a single computer purchased primarily for treatment planning may also have other capabilities, such as support of a tumor registry or a patient scheduling program. It is also possible that computer equipment presently available in the service can be interfaced with a new system to expand the capabilities of both. These and other considerations can influence the purchase decision and should be reviewed carefully.

The capability of a treatment planning system is dictated largely by its software complement. Analysis of available systems should consider not only the programs available for treatment planning (although these obviously are the highest priority) but also any other desired functions such as tumor registry, patient scheduling and billing, word processing, and general-purpose high-level (e.g., FORTRAN) programming. Once these requirements have been decided upon, the configuration of the hardware will be largely (although not completely) determined. For example, the desire to enter CT image data directly into the computer may require the addition of a magnetic tape drive. Such a requirement may eliminate from contention smaller computer systems without tape drive capability. If word processing software is required, a high-quality printer probably should be specified. Many treatment planning systems do not automatically include a suitable printer.

Once a general idea of the hardware configurations and software capabilities has been reached, consideration can be given to the requirements of personnel and space. Clearly, a more complex system will be more demanding of the operator. A department must often choose between a system that is easy to learn and straightforward to operate but that is quite inflexible, and a system that has many possibilities for extending its capabilities but requires an experienced computer operator and frequent maintenance.

The department must keep in mind that all computer systems require space, not just for the computer and its peripherals, but for storage of ancillary devices (such as an isodose plotter) and spare parts. In addition, space is required for related activities such as film viewing and the preparation of patient contour information. Larger, more complex computer systems clearly require more space. In some cases special preparations must be made, such as antistatic carpeting, raised flooring, additional electrical power, and increased air conditioning.

References

1. Rossi RP, Hendee, WR: Exchange of information between the purchaser and supplier of radiological imaging equipment. *Proceedings of the Society for Photooptical Instrumentation Engineers.* Bellingham, WA, SPIE, 1976, vol 96, pp 385–388.
2. Thompson TJ: *Primer of Clinical Radiology.* Boston, Little, Brown, 1973.
3. Thompson TJ: *A Practical Approach to Modern X-ray Equipment.* Boston, Little, Brown, 1978.
4. Stone T: Equipment acquisition procedures. *Proceedings of the Society for Photooptical Instrumentation Engineers.* Bellingham, WA, SPIE, 1977, vol 127, pp 167–171.
5. Holmes JR: Diagnostic ultrasound during the early years of A.I.U.M. *J Clin Ultrasound* 8:299, 1980.
6. Weinstein BJ: Abdominal, Ob/Gyn. In Ziskin MC (ed): *Sonic Exchange,* ed 6, Bethesda, MD, American Institute of Ultra in Medicine, 1982.
7. Swaenepoel L, Demeester-Mirkine N, Sacre R, et al: Ultrasound examination of the thyroid. *ROFO* 137:12, 1982.
8. Taylor KJW, Carpenter DA, Hill CR, et al: Gray scale ultrasound imaging: the anatomy and pathology of the liver. *Radiology* 119:415, 1976.
9. Fleischer AC, Muhletaler CA, Jones TB: Sonodetection of gallbladder perforation. *South Med J* 75:606, 1982.
10. Weinberger G, Mitra SK, Yoeli G: Ultrasound diagnosis of splenic vein thrombosis. *J Clin Ultrasound* 10:345, 1982.
11. Brandt TD, Neiman HL, Dragowski MJ, et al: Ultrasound assesment of normal renal development. *J Ultrasound Med* 1:49, 1982.
12. Arger PH, Mulhern CB, Bonavita JA et al: An analysis of Pancreatic sonography in suspected pancreatic disease. *J Clin Ultrasound* 7:91, 1979.
13. Greenberg M, Neiman HL, Brandt TD, et al: Ultrasound of the prostate. Analysis of tissue texture and abnormalities. *Radiology* 141:757, 1981.
14. Fleischer AC, Walsh JW, Jones JW III, et al: Sonographic evaluation of pelvic masses: Method of examination and role of sonography relative to other imaging modalities. *Radiol Clin North Am* 20:397, 1982.
15. Harter LP, Gross BG, Callen PW, et al: Ultrasonic evaluation of abdominal aortic thrombus. *J Ultrasound Med* 1:315, 1982.
16. Matadial L, Sang RH: Ultrasound in obstetrics and

gynaecology. *East Indian Med J* 30:178, 1981.

17. Plesner J, Badcock PC, Leeman S: The accuracy of ultrasound scanning for radiotherapy field planning. Paper presented at Tumour Ultrasound 1977, London, 1977.

18. Brascho DJ: Ultrasound of the female breast: current state of the art. *Ala J Med Sci* 19:83, 1982.

19. Miskin M, Martin B, Brain J: Ultrasonographic examination of scrotal masses. *J Urol* 117:243, 1977.

20. Marich KW, Ramsey SD, Wilson DA, et al: An improved medical ultrasonic imaging system for scanning peripheral anatomy. *Ultrasound Imaging* 3:309, 1981.

21. Banjavic RA: Design and maintenance of a quality assurance program for diagnostic ultrasound equipment. *Semin Ultrasound* 4:10, 1983.

22. American Institute of Ultrasound in Medicine (AIUM): *AIUM/NEMA (National Electrical Manufacturers Association) Safety Standard for Diagnostic Ultrasound Equipment.* Washington, DC or Bethesda, MD, AIUM/NEMA Standards Publication No. UL1-1981, 1981.

23. Wells, PNT: *Biomedical Ultrasonics.* New York, Academic Press 1977, pp 300.

24. Campbell K, MacNeill I, Patric J: Time series analysis of ultrasonic observations of gross fetal body movements during the last 10 weeks of pregnancy. *Ultrasound Imaging* 3:330, 1981.

25. Moritake K, Handa H, Izumi H, et al: Experimental study on quantitative flow measurement by a doppler flowmeter with a sound-spectrograph. *Neurol Res* 3:363, 1981.

26. Banjavic RA: Ultrasound in the radiotherapy department; past, present and furture. In Fullerton GD, Zagzebski JA (eds): *Medical Physics of CT and Ultrasound.* New York, American Institute of Physics, 1980, pp 469.

27. Shattuck DP, von Ramm OT: Compound scanning with a phased array. *Ultrasound Imaging* 4:93, 1982.

28. Smazal SF, Weisman LE, Hopper KD, et al: Comparative analysis of ultrasonographic methods of gestational age assessment. *J Ultrasound Med* 2:147, 1983.

29. Nickoloff EL: What to look for when buying CT equipment. *Appl Radiol* 11:3, 69–74, 1982.

30. Kelsey CA, Berardo PA, Smith AR, et al: CT scanner selection and specification for radiation therapy. *Med Phys* 7:555–558, 1980.

31. Margulis AR, Boyd DP, Axel L: The desirable properties of computed tomography scanners. *Radiology* 134:261, 1980.

32. Hughes GMK: National survey of computed tomography unit capacity. *Radiology* 135:669–703, 1980.

33. Committee for Radiation Oncology Studies: *Criteria for Radiation Oncology in Multidisciplinary Cancer Management.* National Cancer Institute, National Institutes of Health, Feb 1981.

34. Health Planning and Resources Development Act of 1974 (PL 93-641), Jan 4, 1975.

35. Dritschilo A, Sherman D, Bahman E, et al: The cost effectiveness of a radiation therapy simulator: a model for the determination of need. *Int J Radiat Oncol Biol Phys*, 5:243–247, 1979.

36. Steward JR, Hicks JA, Boone MLM: Computed tomography in radiation therapy. *Int J Radiat Oncol Biol Phys* 4:313–324, 1978.

CHAPTER THREE

Justifying the Purchase of Radiologic Equipment

CAROLYN E. FINSTER, B.S., and WILLIAM R. HENDEE, Ph.D.

Introduction

Purchases of radiologic equipment are among the more expensive propositions facing a hospital. Hence, the radiology department should be prepared to provide considerable justification for its requests.

There are many issues to be addressed in a purchase justification. The mission and goals of the institution establish the first level of justification. Topics such as a description of the institution, its organization, purpose and goals, admissions policy, modes of reimbursement, number of beds, and types of services and patients should be considered in answering the question "What is my institution and what does it wish to become?"

Other questions encountered in preparing a justification of radiologic equipment include: What is the budget and funding process? What types of radiological services are present, and what types are desired? How do the services fit into the existing and projected community health care systems? Answers to questions such as these are helpful in justifying the expenditure of large amounts of money for equipment.

Economic justification is one of the more important issues related to equipment purchase. Another concern of equal, if not greater importance is the quality of care to patients. Patient care should be the ultimate focus of all services in a hospital, including those in a radiology service.

After addressing the issues described above, the question should also be raised of possible alternatives to acquiring a particular piece of equipment.

The Institution

A complete description of the institution should be furnished as background information in justifying the purchase of radiologic equipment. The description should include an explanation of the organizational structure of the institution and the authority under which it operates (i.e., state legislature, board of directors, as part of a chain of hospitals, etc.). Other important features are the admissions policy and the mixture of patient types. For example, if the hospital is a trauma center, certain types of radiologic equipment may be needed for the emergency room. Other data needed for the justification include the average number of patient days, occupancy rate, and bed capacity (newborn, pediatric, surgical, etc.).

Further concerns to be included in a description of the institution are any anticipated changes from past patterns of care that might affect the work load, case mix, or types of procedures performed in the radiology department. For example, a new service such as neurosurgery may open 20 new beds over the next 12 months. This increase in capacity could have a profound effect on radiology, especially neuroradiology and computed tomography.

Also important are the institution's funding processes and budgetary constraints. Most hospitals compile a budget from data on past and projected patient revenues and from anticipated revenue sources such as community bonds, investments, gifts, and, for governmental institutions, tax subsidies. Many hospitals fund the acquisition of capital equipment from funds set aside as a "depreciation account." The sources of revenue available to fund the acquisition of capital equipment and the anticipated schedule of their availability are essential to the development of a multiyear plan for the replacement of present equipment and the acquisition of new equipment.

Also important to an equipment justification is a profile of the radiology service. This profile should present historical data describing the types and numbers of studies performed, together with projections of future alterations in data trends associated with changes within the hospital or the radiology service. Of particular importance are anticipated changes in performance of the radiology service associated with new technology and with variations in reimbursement policies imposed by third party carriers and governmental agencies. The growing emphasis on cost effectiveness is becoming increasingly important in profiling a radiology department.

Need for Specific Equipment

If the desired equipment is to replace existing equipment, a brief history of the existing equipment and an explanation for its replacement are needed. If the desired equipment is an addition to present facilities, then a justification in terms of improved patient care, increased revenue, etc., is desirable. Some of the questions to be addressed in preparing these documents are:

1. What is the equipment presently in use in the department?
2. What is the maximum work load capacity of the equipment?
3. What is the failure rate of the equipment?
4. What downtime is experienced as a result of equipment failure?
5. What are the repair costs and losses in patient revenue associated with equipment failure?
6. Are there patient risks that accompany equipment failure?
7. Is equipment performance so unsatisfactory that patient care is compromised?
8. How often are patients transferred to another room or institution because the equipment is inoperable or is operating unsatisfactorily.
9. What is the cost of these transfers financially, as well as in terms of patient risk and inconvenience?

In the preparation of an equipment justification, it often is helpful to contract for the services of an outside recognized professional consultant in radiologic equipment, provided that such an individual is not available within the institution. A consultant can provide an independent appraisal of the present status of equipment in the department and the need for new or replacement equipment. Often this appraisal is helpful in supporting the documentation prepared internally within the department. Frequently it is helpful to department directors and hospital administrators to have corroborating evidence to support their recommendations. Lists of consultants with special expertise in radiologic equipment are available from organizations such as the American Association of Physicists in Medicine* and the American College of Radiology.†

Additional demands on radiologic equipment may surface in certain types of hospitals. These demands include educational, research, and community needs. Representatives of teaching hospitals might argue that they require state-of-the-art equipment because they admit many patients with more complex medical problems than those experienced by average patients in a community hospital. Furthermore, it can be argued that medical students and housestaff in the teaching hospital require the most up-to-date and sophisticated equipment on which to train. At a number of hospitals, especially those affiliated with medical schools, extensive programs in clinical research are conducted. These programs may benefit the hospital in several ways, including an improved understanding of the fundamental characteristics of human health and disease, the development of improved diagnostic and treatment methods, the design of improved equipment, and an enhanced reputation as an institution offering state-of-the-art medicine.

Finally, the question of community needs should be addressed. Is the institution the only location in the region where certain highly specialized radiologic procedures are available? Does the institution serve principally as a primary or as a tertiary health care center for the region? Is there a level of expertise in the institution that is not dupli-

* American Association of Physicists in Medicine, c/o American Institute of Physics, 335 East 45th St., New York, NY 10017.
† American College of Radiology, 6900 Wisconsin Avenue, Chevy Chase, MD 20015.

cated elsewhere in the vicinity? These are the types of questions that should be considered in addressing the needs of the community.

Economic Justification

The sources of revenue and the mix of patients that provides the revenue should be considered carefully. The following data should be included in any economic justification:

Number of patients
Average length of stay
Separation of patients into various age groups
Occupancy rate

Other factors that might be important in analyzing the present and future patient mix include:

Community growth and aging patterns.
Highway and housing construction, the siting of new industries, etc.
The fraction of patients who are covered by health insurance, the number of Medicare and Medicaid patients, the number of indigent patients, etc.

An example of a hospital's reimbursement pattern is shown in Table 3.1.

In part, the patient mix of an institution is dependent upon the utilization and referral patterns of physicians in the community and the medical specialties offered by the institution. An urban hospital surrounded by physicians' offices will draw a certain concentration of patients. A small hospital in a rural or small town setting draws its patient population over a larger, but less populated, geographical locale. One of the prominent influences on the patient population of an institution is the physicians who have staff privileges in the institution.

Whenever a new or replacement item of equipment is contemplated, the radiology service should assess the impact of the equipment on radiology revenue and expenses. Equipment that provides a new type of study will generate additional revenue; however, income from procedures that are replaced by the new study must be subtracted from the additional revenue. For any item of equipment, possible expenses include those listed in Table 3.2.

An analysis of expenses and revenue associated with a new item of radiologic equipment is depicted in Table 3.3.

A simple method to compute the break-even charge for a new technology is to take the annual budget of direct and indirect costs, increase this budget by an appropriate amount to compensate for the average fractional reimbursement rate for the institution, and divide the adjusted budget by the projected annual work load. The result is the break-even point for computing hospital charges. The procedure is outlined in Table 3.4.

Presented in Table 3.5 is an example of billings for an assumed charge of $560 per MR examination, using the patient mix that was described in Table 3.1.

Table 3.1
Analysis of Revenue by Sponsor

Sponsor type	Inpatient (%)	Outpatient (%)
Medicare	19.6	21.7
Medicaid	8.6	9.1
Pending Medicaid	10.0	3.9
Other states' Medicaid	1.3	0.2
Blue Cross	6.2	5.6
Other commercial insurance	21.1	
Other government agencies	2.2	1.3
Nongovernment agencies	1.6	3.2
Grants and contracts	2.9	1.1
Self-pay	25.4	52.9
Other	1.1	1.0
	100.0	100.0

Table 3.2
Expenses of Operating a Radiology Service

1. Lease payments
2. Regular payroll—staff
3. Miscellaneous payroll—overtime and on-call
4. Service/maintenance contracts
5. Expendable supplies
6. Medical supplies
7. Office supplies
8. Utilities (water, electricity, etc.)
9. Film and processor supplies
10. Renovation of hospital space
11. Miscellaneous expenses

Table 3.3
Analysis of Expenses and Revenue Associated with a New Item of Radiologic Equipment

Equipment:	Harshaw Chemical Analyzer for cerebral blood flow studies[a]	$ 130,000.00
New staff:	One registered nuclear medicine technologist	$ 18,000.00
Service contract:	Estimated as 10% of purchase price (following 1-yr warranty	$ 13,000.00
Medical supplies:	Xenon $37.50/study	$ 13,500.00
Office supplies:	N/A	0
Utilities:	Part of indirect costs	0
Supplies:	$5.00/study	$ 1,800.00
		$ 176,300.00
New procedures anticipated:	360 × $240	$ 86,400.00

[a] Paid for in approximately 2 yr.

Table 3.4
Computation of Break-Even Charge for a Particular Imaging Technology

Assumptions	
Examinations per year:	2,500
Total expenses (direct and indirect):	$ 1,400,000

$$\frac{\text{Expenses}}{\text{Volume}} = \text{Charge to patient}$$

$$\frac{\$\ 1,400,000}{2,500} = \$560/\text{per cxam}$$

Table 3.5
Anticipated Various Sources for MR Examinations[a]

	% of outpatients	No. of examinations[b]	Charges billed[c]
Medicare	21.7	543	$304,080
Medicaid	13.0	325	$182,000
Other states' Medicaid	0.2	5	$2,800
Blue Cross	5.6	140	$78,400
Government agencies	4.5	113	$63,280
Self-pay	52.9	1,323	$740,880
Other	2.1	51	$28,560
	100	2,500	$1,400,000

[a] Assuming all patients are outpatients for this example.
[b] Total volume = 2,500.
[c] Charge/study = $560.

What the percentage breakdown of sources of reimbursement means in terms of actual reimbursement depends on each institution's rate of reimbursement from each payor. Shown in Table 3.6 is a hypothetical example of the reimbursement from different payors.

Lease vs Purchase?

The Economic Recovery Act of 1981 provided some changes in the Federal tax laws that encourage institutions to use leasing arrangements for the acquisition of expensive items of equipment. Under the Recovery Act, certain tax benefits of leasing are more easily transferred to the lessee. In addition, the Act removed all restrictions on the transfer of the 10% investment tax credit to the lessee. Sometimes there are advantages other than financial for leasing rather than purchasing radiology equipment. In an era of rapidly changing technology, leasing provides the opportunity for an institution to upgrade its equipment at moderate cost during the leasing period or at its conclusion. By leasing, a department can decrease its likelihood of being saddled with outdated equipment.

There are many who feel that leasing rather than purchasing equipment is a hedge against inflation because payments for leased equipment can be made with pretax dollars. Furthermore, in an inflationary period payment is made in dollars of constantly depreciating value when the lease is extended over a lengthy period. In deciding whether to finance new equipment with a loan or through a lease, there are several questions that should be addressed. For example, some banks offer floating point loans; a loan of this type may require much higher payments, should the Federal Reserve Board tighten its money supply during the term of the loan. On the other hand, leasing companies usually require an above average rate of interest. With a leasing arrangement, the down payment otherwise required for a bank loan can be invested. With many leasing companies, used equipment can be traded in, and upgrades to the equipment usually can be negotiated without difficulty. When a loan is negotiated with a bank, the lendor usually is not interested in the equipment; hence, a bank usually will not offer the advantages of trade-in and upgrading (1).

On the other side of the coin is the question of price and expected useful life of the equipment. If the expected life of the equipment is longer than the lease period, the outright purchase of the equipment may be more cost-effective than leasing (2).

Alternatives to Sole Acquisition

An option to the purchase or lease of equipment by one institution is the sharing of equipment among institutions. In some metropolitan areas, hospitals are joining together in the acquisition of expensive radiology equipment; often they have mutual agreements to share certain facilities and to refer patients to the hospital with the greater capability to care for specific problems. In

Table 3.6
Reimbursement from Different Types of Payors

Payor type	Reimbursement rate		Net revenue
Medicare charges × Medicare reimbursement rate	$304,080 × 1.25	=	$380,100
Medicaid charges × Medicaid reimbursement rate	$182,000 × 1.00	=	$182,000
Blue Cross (BC) charges × BC liability × BC contractual agreement	$78,400 × 0.80 × 0.95	=	$59,584
Government agency charges × Government reimbursement rate	$63,280 × 0.80	=	$50,624
Self-pay charges × reimbursement rate	$740,880 × 0.40	=	$296,352
Other charges	$28,560 × 0.75	=	$21,420
	Net revenue total	=	$990,080

some cases it is more cost-efficient, as well as more effective in terms of patient care, for hospitals to share services rather than to offer competitive services in all areas.

With the spiraling costs of health care and the imposition of regulations designed to control health care costs, the cost effectiveness of new equipment acquisitions will become an increasingly important issue. No longer will it be possible to establish hospital charges on the basis of the cost of procedures, including the use of radiologic equipment. In the future the level of reimbursement, rather than patient charges, will be the critical issue. Careful analysis by radiology personnel and hospital administrators will be required to address this issue effectively.

Quality Of Care

Quality of care is one of the more challenging issues to address in the purchase of new radiologic equipment. In some cases, new equipment can have an impressive impact on patient care. For example, few would argue that computed tomographic imaging has had a major influence on the delivery of quality health care in this country. Among the patient care considerations for new equipment are:

Reduced invasiveness of procedures
Decreased patient inconvenience
Reduced morbidity
More rapid diagnosis
More definitive diagnosis
Decreased radiation dose

Other considerations regarding the quality of patient care include the way in which the radiology department is integrated with the rest of the hospital. Are the capabilities of the radiology staff similar to those of other medical services? For example, it might be inappropriate to purchase an MR Imaging Unit at this time in an institution where neurology and neurosurgery are not strong referring services.

Another important aspect of quality patient care is continuing education. Hospital personnel should be permitted to maintain and improve their knowledge and skills on a continuing basis, especially in a discipline such as radiology, where the technology is changing rapidly. Quality care is strongly dependent upon the ability and motivation of employees of the institution; recognition of the employees' importance and support of their continuing education are essential features in a quality assurance program.

Acknowledgment. Thanks are extended to Ms. Debra Ann Ginsburg, Assistant Director, University Hospital, Denver, for initial inspiration and encouragement to undertake this chapter.

References

1. Grossman, R: Leasing versus buying equipment. *Appl Radiol* Nov/Dec:69–72, 1983.
2. Seale DL, Keats TE: Planning of radiological department. In Karmano M, Stieve FE, (eds): *Leasing—Another Way to Finance X-Ray Equipment*, International Symposium, Finland, August, 1972. Stuttgart, FRG, Stuttgart, 1974.

CHAPTER FOUR

Preparation of Performance Specifications

WILLIAM R. HENDEE, Ph.D., RAYMOND P. ROSSI, M.S.,
VICTOR M. SPITZER, Ph.D., RICHARD A. BANJAVIC, Ph.D.,
ROBERT K. CACAK, Ph.D., GEOFFREY S. IBBOTT, M.S.

INTRODUCTION

Once the clinical needs for the radiologic imaging equipment have been identified and compared to descriptions of the equipment available from various vendors, the development of performance specifications for the equipment can be initiated. Usually these specifications are prepared in two forms, entitled General Equipment Requirements and Specific Equipment Requirements. Examples of both types of requirements for various modalities of radiologic equipment are provided below.

In the development of equipment specifications, certain levels of performance are established that represent a synthesis of manufacturer's technical specifications, industry standards, governmental regulations, and the experience of the institution and of the individual preparing the specifications (1–4). These performance levels should be achievable by most, if not all, manufacturers of equipment in the assembly of off-the-shelf components; i.e., the equipment specifications and performance levels should not be so restrictive that some manufacturers are excluded from submitting a bid and others are forced to select components that exceed the usual characteristics of their product line. In addition, each vendor should understand that exception may be taken to any specific equipment requirement proposed by the institution, provided that the vendor substitutes and justifies an alternate specification.

A performance specifications document is helpful in at least two ways in assuring that purchased equipment performs satisfactorily. First when identical information is requested from all vendors, comparison of many performance variables is facilitated. Second, since the vendor has supplied the

technical performance information, the document is contractual, and the institution may insist that the purchased equipment performs at least as well as stated by the vendor. As part of this process, vendors should be informed that acceptance tests will be used to demonstrate that the actual performance of the equipment after delivery meets or exceeds the stated specifications. Acceptance tests are described in a later chapter.

The vendor should understand that formal acceptance will be based on the full operation of all systems and satisfactory clinical application, as well as technical data. Satisfactory clinical application implies that a few patients will be examined (or treated) on a trial basis prior to final acceptance, and that these patient studies do not constitute acceptance of the unit.

Before discussing the aspects of equipment performance that are related directly to imaging capabilities, three issues that are important but not well suited to specific performance specifications should be considered. These issues are electrical and mechanical specifications for the equipment and specifications related to state and federal regulations. These specifications are determined primarily by the design of the equipment and should be specified by the vendor.

Electrical

Since all radiological systems require a source of electrical power for operation, the specific requirements for this source should be supplied by the vendor and must be compatible with the capabilities of the institution. The number, voltage, phase, isolation and kilovolt rating of required power sources must be understood, because inadequate power sources frequently are the explanation for inadequate performance of equipment. A particularly important specification is the required precision of the supplied power. For satisfactory performance, radiologic equipment often requires line voltage regulation to better than 95%. For most imaging systems, this requirement necessitates separate electrical lines from those supplying power to elevators, lighting, or other components that cause current surges and consequent voltage drops in power lines. For some systems (e.g., ultrasound equipment), the presence of electrical noise on power lines may affect the overall signal to noise ratio of the measurements used for image construction.

Mechanical

In the identification of the type of equipment most suitable for a particular application, a review of the mechanical specifications for the equipment is appropriate. These specifications should include environmental constraints, such as the space available for the equipment, the temperature and humidity requirements for proper operation, and the shielding necessary to prevent excessive radiation exposures in nearby facilities or to ensure proper operation of the equipment (e.g., radio frequency (rf) shielding for a magnetic resonance imaging (MRI) unit.

As an example of mechanical specifications, an examination table for radiographic studies is considered. Mechanical specifications might include such items as degree of angulation (cranial and caudal), height of table above the floor, range of table travel in both the longitudinal and transverse directions, degree of table extension as a function of angulation, ability to tilt and drive the table at the same time, type and speed of table drive, range of movement of the Bucky mechanism within the table, whether the table is flat or curved, distance from tabletop to the plane of the image receptor, types of automatic stepping features, and the forces required for the various motions. For x-ray tube suspensions, the type of locks and suspension control, range of travel within the room, provision for automatic detents, range of tube angulation and the degree of column rotation should be considered. Similar considerations would be appropriate for suspension systems employed for image intensifier fluoroscopic systems. For spot film/image intensifier support assemblies, the size(s) of spot film cassettes which can be accommodated should be reviewed, as well as the available formats. Also important are provisions for and the type of myelographic stops, radiation protection interlocks, range of vertical travel of the spot film device, range of travel of the spot film device with respect to table center (longitudinal and transverse), location of spot film controls, provision for power assist, and available lock controls.

State and Federal Regulations

Many aspects of the operation and performance of radiologic equipment are subject to state and federal regulations. State regulations usually relate to radiation safety considerations and may vary widely from state to state. To determine the exact requirements in a given locale, the local health department should be contacted. General guidance may also be found in a document of the Conference of Radiation Program Control Directors entitled "Suggested Rules and Regulations Pertaining to Radiation Control." The major federal regulations related to radiological equipment are included in the document "Regulations for the Administration of the Radiation Control for Health and Safety Act of 1968," available from the Center for Devices and Radiological Health. These regulations apply to manufacturers and establish certain minimum levels of performance for equipment that releases ionizing radiation.

ROENTGENOGRAPHY

Performance specifications for conventional roentgenographic equipment that are common to all imaging modes (radiographic, fluoroscopic, and tomographic) include those for the x-ray generators, x-ray tubes, beam restriction systems, grids, and automatic exposure controls.

Typical performance levels that should be achievable by most modern x-ray units are presented in Tables 4.1 to 4.7. These performance levels are derived from experience with clinically installed equipment and are simply guidelines that may require modification for any specific application. Methods to evaluate equipment performance to de-

Table 4.1
Performance Specifications for X-Ray Generators

Exposure Time: The difference between the measured exposure time and indicated exposure time shall not exceed ±5% of the indicated exposure time for exposure times of 20 msec or longer and shall not exceed the manufacturer's specified percentage of exposure times of less than 10 msec. The exposure time shall be reproducible to within ± 5%.

kVp: The difference between the measured kVp and the indicated kVp shall not exceed ±5% of the indicated kVp. The kVp shall be reproducible to within ±5%. Overshoots associated with precontacting and/or load changes shall be less than 5 kVp. The difference between cathode voltage with respect to ground and anode voltage with respect to ground shall not exceed ±3 kVp. The rms value of the high voltage shall not vary during the time of exposure by more than 5% for exposure times of 1 sec or less.

mA/mAs: The difference between the measured mA/mAs and the indicated mA/mAs shall not exceed ±5% of the indicated mA/mAs. The mA/mAs shall be reproducible to within ±5%. For constant load systems, the mA shall not vary during the time of exposure by more than 5% for exposure times of 1 sec or less.

Tube Protection Circuitry: The x-ray tube protective circuitry shall prevent exposure techniques in excess of those allowed for the x-ray tube but shall not underrate the x-ray tube by more than 30% with respect to the maximum load for single radiographic exposures.

termine compliance with the performance specifications are presented in Chapter 7.

NUCLEAR MEDICINE

In this section, the scintillation camera is used as a vehicle to review issues to be addressed in a performance specifications document for nuclear medicine. The scintillation camera is assumed to be fully equipped with most available options (not necessarily available from a single vendor), including whole body scanning and single photon emission computed tomography (SPECT). A brief review that considers camera mobility has been included in the section. Guidelines are provided for both general and specific equipment requirements

defined by the clinical needs and financial constraints of the institution.

In the introduction to performance specifications, ground rules should be established for the vendor's response to the solicitation for bid. For example, an individual response may be desired from each vendor for each item of requested equipment, even though a particular vendor may not manufacture all of the items (e.g., phantoms, flood sources, computer software, testing equipment, and imaging tables). Clinical site or factory visits may be required between the time bids are received and an award is made. It may also be desirable to invite bid responses based on demonstration or prototype units. If separate prices for some components or for special design engineering are necessary, these should be established in the introduction. Special time constraints dictated by construction might also be included in the introduction, as well as consequences if a vendor fails to meet specifications or the delivery schedule.

General Equipment Requirements

Often it is helpful to describe the institution's present configuration of equipment, including the number and types of cameras and detectors, the types of studies performed, and any major anticipated changes in work load. A specific listing of the different isotopic studies and their frequencies may help identify the need for some camera options or configurations. A general description of the major components of the system to be purchased should also be included to give an overview of what the purchase is to include. This description may include the camera and all collimators required for the studies previously mentioned, an x-y-z imaging table, multiformat camera, EKG gate or monitor, phantoms, sources, software for tomography, training, delivery, installation, insurance, and warranty.

If an existing computer is to be interfaced to the new camera, the responsibility for the interfacing should be defined. The addition of a new camera with tomographic capability will require careful definition of software and hardware requirements for the resident computer. In the introduction, all equipment descriptions are fairly general, but they should cover the entire system.

Table 4.2
Performance Specifications for X-Ray Tubes

Focal Spot Size: The measured size of the focal spot shall meet the following criteria:

$$f_{nominal} \leq f_{measured} < 1.5\, f_{nominal} \text{ for } f_{nominal} \leq 0.8 \text{ mm}$$

$$f_{nominal} \leq f_{measured} < 1.4\, f_{nominal} \text{ for } 0.8 \text{ mm} \leq f_{nominal}\, 2.0 \text{ mm}$$

Focal Spot Size Variation: The variation in the focal spot size shall not exceed ±40% with respect to the measured size of the focal spot at one-half the maximum rated tube potential and one-half the maximum rate tube current at this potential at the highest anode rotational speed for a 0.1-sec exposure:

Leakage Radiation: The maximum leakage radiation shall not exceed 100 mR in 1 hr at 1 m when the tube is operated at its leakage technique factors.

Exposure: At 80 kVp the exposure shall be between 15 and 25 mR/mAs at 61 cm from the focal spot.

Exposure Reproducibility: For any fixed technique setting within the ratings of the x-ray tube/ generator combination, the variation in exposure shall be such that

$$\frac{\sigma}{\bar{X}} \leq 0.05$$

where $\bar{X}$ is the mean of successive exposure measurements and σ is the standard deviation.

Exposure Linearity: The linearity of exposure over the available rated range of the x-ray tube/ generator combination shall be such that

$$\frac{(mR/mAs)_{max} - (mR/mAs)_{min}}{(mR/mAs)_{max} + (mR/mAs)_{min}} \leq 0.10$$

where $(mR/mAs)_{max,min}$ are the maximum and minimum exposures per indicated *mAs*.

Beam Quality: The beam quality shall be equal to or greater than that specified by Title 21, CFR, Part 1020.30 mm, but shall not exceed these values by more than 40%.

Table 4.3
Performance Specifications for Beam Restriction System

Source to Image Receptor Distance (SID) Indicator: The indicated source to image receptor distance shall agree with the measured source to image receptor distance to within ±1% of the indicated SID.

Minimum Source to Patient Entrance Surface Distance: The minimum source to patient entrance surface distance shall be greater than or equal to 38 cm for fixed undertable fluoroscopic units and at least 30 cm for mobile fluoroscopic units.

Light Localizer Intensity: The intensity of the light localizer shall be at least 160 lux.

Light Localizer Contrast Ratio: The light localizer shall provide a contrast ratio of at least 4:1.

Coincidence of Radiation Field Center/Image Receptor Center: The center of the radiation field and the center of the image receptor (or selected portion thereof) shall coincide to within ±1% of the SID.

Congruence of Radiation Field Edges and Visually Defined Field Edges: The congruence of the radiation field edges and light (visual) field edges shall be such that misalignment along either the length or width shall not exceed 2.0% of the source to image receptor distance and that the sum of the misalignments along the length and width without regard to sign shall not exceed 3.5% of the source to image receptor distance.

Correspondence of Radiation Field Size/Image Receptor Size: The congruence of the radiation field size and image receptor size shall be such that the size difference along either length or width shall not exceed 2.0% of the source to image receptor distance and that the sum of the differences along length and width without regard to sign shall not exceed 3.5% of the source to image receptor distance.

Correspondence of Radiation Field Size/Numerically Indicated Field Size: The correspondence of the radiation field size and numerically indicated field size shall be such that the size difference along either length or width shall not exceed 2.0% of the source to image receptor distance and that the sum of the differences along length and width without regard to sign shall not exceed 3.5% of the source to image receptor distance.

Minimum Field Size: The minimum field size at the maximum source to image receptor distance or 100 cm, whichever is less, shall be less than or equal to 5 cm × 5 cm.

Table 4.4
Performance Specifications for Antiscatter Grids

Artifacts: The grid(s) shall be free of artifacts and nonuniformities.

Alignment: The grid(s) shall be aligned to the radiation field so that the centers coincide to within ½ inch.

Table 4.5
Performance Specifications for Intensified Fluoroscopic Imaging Systems

High Contrast Resolution: The high contrast performance of the intensified fluoroscopic imaging system shall permit the following mesh values to be resolvable over the entire field when the mesh pattern is located in close proximity to the image intensifier extrance plane with the grid removed at low kVp.

Intensifer input diameter (inch)	Visible mesh pattern recording/viewing mode	
	TV	Film
9–14	24	34
6–8	34	40
4–5	40	50

Contrast Sensitivity: The contrast sensitivity of the intensified fluoroscopic imaging system shall permit the visualization of a 3-mm hole in a 2% thickness penatrameter located midway between the x-ray source and image intensifier entrance plane with a grid in place at 80 kVp.

Exposure/Exposure Rate Control: The exposure/exposure rate control system shall maintain the exposure/exposure rate at the entrance plane of the image intensifier to a constant value (within the energy response of the input phosphor) over the range of 60 to 120 kVp and attenuator thicknesses of 2 to 12 inches of acrylic, except in those cases in which the maximum tabletop exposure rate is reached or in which the maximum allowed mAs is reached. The brightness of the displaced fluoroscopic image is expected to remain constant over the same range of conditions.

Maximum Patient Entrance Surface Exposure Rate: The maximum patient entrance surface exposure rate at the point where the beam enters the patient shall not exceed 10 R/min for systems equipped with automatic exposure rate/brightness control and shall not exceed 5 R/min for manual systems.

Table 4.6
Performance Specifications for Automatic Exposure Control Systems

Field Selection Wiring: Proper connection of the automatic exposure control (AEC) fields will be demonstrated by the normal termination of exposures corresponding to the selected field.

Reproducibility: With respect to reproducibility, the performance of the AEC system(s) shall be such that for attenuator thicknesses from 4 to 10 inches, kVp's from 60 to 120 and exposure times greater than 15 msec (or mAs values greater than 5)

$$\frac{\sigma}{\overline{X}} \leq 0.05$$

where $\overline{X}$ is the mean and σ is the standard deviation of ten consecutive exposure measurements at a given technique.

Field Matching: With respect to sensitivity matching, the performance of the AEC system(s) shall be such that all fields are matched to within ±10% unless otherwise specified by the manufacturer.

Field Size Compensation: With respect to compensation for variation in field size, the performance of the AEC system(s) shall be such that the variation in film density does not exceed ±0.3 optical density (OD) units.

Performance Capability: With respect to response capability, the performance of the AEC system(s) shall be such that the maximum variation in density does not exceed 0.6 density units.

AEC Backup Timer: The performance of the AEC system(s) shall prevent exposures greater than 60 kilowatt-seconds (kWs) and/or 600 mAs for kVp's greater than 50.

Specific Requirements

For scintillation cameras, many of the performance measurements for the detector have been documented by the National Electrical Manufacturers Association (NEMA) in Standards Publication No. NU-1-1980 (5). Use of this document for generation of performance specifications should be noted in the introduction to this section. Inclusion of NEMA test results obtained at the factory may also be required in the bid specifications; these results could include all NEMA measurements, even those designated as

Table 4.7
Performance Specifications for Tomographic Equipment

Tomographic Exposure Uniformity: The tomographic motion shall exhibit stability and uniformity over its geometrical path and shall correspond to the specified geometrical motion for the unit.

Tomographic Plane: The measured tomographic plane shall coincide with the machine-indicated tomographic plane to within ±0.25 cm.

Tomographic Angle: The measured exposure angle shall correspond to the machine-indicated exposure angle (if any) to within ±3°.

Flatness of Tomographic Plane: The measured flatness of the tomographic plane shall be in accordance with the manufacturer's specifield tolerance for plane flatness.

Tomographic Thickness: The measured section thickness shall be within ±50% of the section thickness specified by the manufacturer.

Tomographic Resolution: The measured tomographic resolution shall be in accordance with the manufacturer's specified tomographic resolution capabilities.

"class standards." Often there is a charge for including all of these measurements. If other definitions or measuring techniques arc to be used during acceptance testing, they should be noted in terms specific enough to allow their reproduction on the imaging equipment during testing in the factory. If an outside consultant will evaluate the camera during acceptance testing, then all definitions and testing methods should be supplied to the vendor to identify any variations from standard NEMA techniques. The vendor's response to the performance specifications document or published literature of the vendor at the time of bid response (whichever is better) should determine the performance required of the unit. All responses to the performance specifications document should become an integral part of the purchase order and should be so noted in the introduction.

Specific parts of the imaging system are considered in some detail below. Required system performance is first addressed, followed by examples of response forms that a vendor may use to describe the company's compliance with the required performance features and levels (Tables 4.8 through 4.14).

SCINTILLATION CAMERA

Physical Constraints

Vendors should be provided with the room dimensions available, or with the available area if a room is to be built to house the new equipment. A room diagram should be included that depicts door open-

ings, cabinets, existing power, and any other restricting architecture. The vendor should be asked to draw to exact scale the recommended setup for all equipment to be included in the room, including collimators, electronics, cabinets, service equipment, imaging tables, etc. Maximum allowable continuous noise levels should be specified. The minimum dimensions of all doorways from the receiving dock to the camera room should be specified, and the vendor should be asked to guarantee that delivery can be

Table 4.8
Specific Facilities Required for Scintigraphic System[a]

1. Number of dedicated 110-V, 20-A lines for the camera: _____
   Number of extra 110-V, 20-A lines for the accessories: _____
   Line regulation required: _____
2. Total power requirements for the camera: kW _____
                                    accessories: kW _____
3. Maximum room temperature for guaranteed reliable operation of the camera: °C _____

4. Air conditioning requirements: _____
5. Minimum room size for the camera, console, tomographic imaging table and photographic system:
   _____ ft × _____ ft and/or _____ sq ft
6. Noise level during operation of the camera and peripherals: _____ dB
7. Do all electronic components meet FCC class A RFI/EMI requirements?

   List exceptions:

[a] Tables 4.8 through 4.14 are typical vendor response forms for equipment acquisition. In a bid solicitation they are preceded by the desired or required components, features, and performance parameters of the scintigraphic system. The successful bidder response and any negotiated alterations should be incorporated into the purchase order. Some features and performance values are indicated in parentheses just before the response line as an indication of a desired or required item.

Table 4.9
Specific Physical Characteristics of the Scintillation Detector

1. Crystal thickness: _____ cm or _____ inch
2. Crystal diameter: _____ cm
3. UFOV: (39.0) _____ cm
4. CFOV: (29.25) _____ cm
5. Shape of field of view: _____
6. Number and type of photomultiplier tubes (PMTs): _____ — _____
7. Nominal PMT operating voltage: _____ V
8. Thickness of light pipe coupling PMTs to crystal (if any): _____ mm
9. Type of masking used: _____
   For 10 to 15—reference head movement relative to the crystal in a position parallel to and facing the floor.
10. Maximum head rotation in yoke: crystal toward observer: _____ °
                                    crystal away from observer: _____ °
11. Maximum yoke rotation: clockwise _____ ° counter clockwise _____ °
12. Maximum vertical height of crystal from floor: _____ cm
13. Minimum vertical height of crystal from floor: _____ cm
14. Maximum height of any support structure which is directly below the detector head: _____ cm
15. Type of locks employed on vertical travel: _____

Table 4.10
Specific Performance of the Scintillation Detector

1. Intrinsic spatial resolution in X or Y (average):

       UFOV   *CFOV*
    FWHM: (3.4) _____ mm FWHM: _____ mm
    FWTM: (4.5) _____ mm FWTM: _____ mm
    Maximum variance of X resolution from Y resolution:
    UFOV: _____ mm   CFOV: _____ mm

2. Intrinsic energy resolution in the UFOV:
    FWHM at 140 keV: _____ %
    FWHM at   80 keV: _____ %

3. Intrinsic flood field uniformity:
    With Correction

UFOV	CFOV	UFOV @ R ± 20%
Integral: _____ %	Integral: _____ %	Integral: _____ %
Differential: _____ %	Differential: _____ %	Differential: _____ %

    Without Correction

Integral: (11) _____ %	Integral: _____ %	Integral: _____ %
Differential: _____ %	Differential: _____ %	Differential: _____ %

4. Intrinsic spatial linearity:
    With Correction

UFOV	CFOV
Absolute: (.5) _____ mm	Absolute: _____ mm
Differential: _____ mm	Differential: _____ mm

    Without Correction

Absolute: (4) _____ mm	Absolute: _____ mm
Differential: _____ mm	Differential: _____ mm

5. Count rate performance over the UFOV with a 20% window at 140 keV:
    Maximum input count rate for 20% losses: (80,000) _____ cps
    System dead time without correction: _____ μsec
    System dead time with correction: _____ μsec
    UFOV intrinsic spatial resolution at 75,000 cps (observed):
        _____ mm FWHM
        _____ mm FWTM
    UFOV intrinsic integral flood field uniformity at 75,000 cps (observed):
        with correction: _____ %
        without correction: _____ %
    Intrinsic absolute spatial linearity at 75,000 cps (observed):
        with correction: _____ mm
        without correction: _____ mm

6. System sensitivity at 8 cm:
    for ^{99m}Tc with the high resolution collimator: _____ cpm/μCi
    for ^{99m}Tc with the general purpose collimator: _____ cpm/μCi

Please note method of measurement for all the values in this section if other than NEMA.

accomplished through existing doorways. If elevators must be used, weight restrictions should be considered in a similar fashion. Physical limitations on detector motion should also be specified, as should detector yoke rotation, vertical movement of the detector head, and the minimum detector height for under table imaging. Whole body scanning devices and noncircular orbit ECT cameras have an additional translational motion that should be specified.

Detector Configuration

Specifications for the detector head should include the desired useful field of view (UFOV) (8, 10, 12, 15, 19, or 21 inches) as determined by clinical needs, the number of photomultiplier tubes (i.e., 37 or 55 for standard design cameras or 61, 75, or 91 tubes for high resolution imaging), as influenced by the desired spatial resolution, the crystal thickness as determined by the work

Table 4.11
Specific Features and Operations of the Scintillation Camera

1. Maximum preset counts for study termination: _____ kcounts
   Maximum and minimum preset time for study termination:
   Max _____ sec
   Min _____ sec
   Can studies be terminated by counts or time whichever comes first? _____
2. Is there an audible indicator of study termination? _____
3. Number of predefined isotope selection buttons or switches: _____
4. Recommended period for reflood of correction circuitry:
   Uniformity _____ days, Energy _____ days, Linearity _____ days
   Average length of time required for reflood of correction circuitry:
   Uniformity _____ min, Energy _____ min, Linearity _____ min.
5. Number of channels in the MCA: _____
   Is the keV/channel variable? _____
   If it is variable, what is the range of energies which can be spread over all channels of the MCA? _____
   Can the MCA display be put on 8- × 10-inch film with the equipment as bid? _____
   Is the energy window width displayable on the MCA? _____
6. List all format possibilities for putting images on 8- × 10-inch film: _____
   What is the fastest framing rate possible for camera operation in the format closest to 16 on 1:
   _____ frames/sec
   Make and model of CRT to be employed in the analog imaging devices:
   _____ , _____ .
7. Collimator performance:
   General purpose low energy
       Foil or cast construction? _____
       Hole size, shape, and depth _____
       Number of holes/square inch _____
       Sensitivity _____ cpm/μCi
       Septal thickness (mil) _____ × 0.001 inch
       NEMA-system resolution at 8 cm   _____ mm FWHM
                                              _____ mm FWTM
   Medium energy
       Foil or cast construction? _____
       Hole size, shape, and depth _____
       Number of holes/square inch _____
       Sensitivity _____ cpm/μCi
       Septal thickness (mil) _____ × 0.001 inch
       NEMA-system resolution at 8 cm   _____ mm FWHM
                                              _____ mm FWTM
   High resolution low energy
       Foil or cast construction? _____
       Hole size, shape, and depth _____
       Number of holes/square inch _____
       Sensitivity _____ cpm/μCi
       Septal thickness (mil) _____ × 0.001 inch
       NEMA-system resolution at 8 cm   _____ mm FWHM
                                              _____ mm FWTM

load anticipated for high-energy photons, and the type of detector support desired (i.e., counterbalanced or motorized column support). The extent of radiation shielding should be specified to accommodate the highest energy photons to be imaged. Magnetic shielding of the phototubes may be important for conventional imaging at different orientations and especially for SPECT applications. The proximity of the camera to other devices such as an MR imaging unit or a high power hyperthermia therapy unit may require close attention to the electromagnetic shielding.

Intrinsic Detector Performance

Uniformity. Integral and differential uniformity requirements should be included for all camera configurations to be utilized. The

Table 4.12
Peripheral Components

1. ECG gate:
   a. Give make and model of the ECG synchronizer: _____ ,
      _____
   b. Maximum heart rate with less than 10% losses: _____ bpm
   c. Does it contain high frequency filters to remove muscular noise?
      _____
   d. Will the gate work reliably on patients under stress? _____
   e. Limits of delay on diastole trigger. _____ % of RR wave
   f. Limits of delay on systole trigger. _____ % of RR wave
   g. Is there any capability for arrhythmia rejection _____
   h. Is there any paper or CRT ECG output available _____
2. Accessories:
   a. Resolution phantom. State hole or bar spacings and sizes: An orthogonal hole phantom is preferred (CDRH test phantom).
      _____ mm center to center
      _____ mm hole or bar diameter
      Useful diameter of the phantom: _____ cm
   b. Imaging table:
      1. Maximum unextended length: _____ cm
      2. Maximum unextended width: _____ cm
      3. Height (or height range) of tabletop from floor: _____ cm
      4. Tabletop material: _____
         Attenuation coefficient at 140 keV: _____
         Thickness: _____
   c. An attachable lead mask to reproduce exactly the UFOV as presented by a collimator is included _____ (Y/N).
   d. A NEMA resolution/linearity test pattern is included _____ (Y/N).
   e. An FP11A floating point processor for a PDP-11/34A computer is included _____ (Y/N). Manufacturer: _____
   f. Complete operating manuals and service diagrams for all components and peripherals of the system are included _____ (Y/N).

Table 4.13
Delivery, Installation, and Training

1. Estimated camera delivery: (90) _____ days ARO.
   Estimated time for camera installation: (5) _____ days.
2. Estimated computer software and peripheral delivery: (90) _____ days ARO.
   Estimated time for computer software and peripheral installation: (5) _____ days.
3. Vendors will be liable for late delivery and installation, 1% of the total system purchase price will be deducted from the total obligation for each week's delay beyond the dates and times stated in items 1 and 2 if the delay is not the fault of the purchaser. Is this acceptable _____ (Y/N).
4. Please describe computer software training which will be provided.
5. Will operator training for the entire system be provided? _____ (Y/N)
   Location of training: _____
   Number of participants to be included (3) _____
   Cost to hospital of training sessions outlined above: $ _____
   Cost to hospital for each additional participant: $ _____
6. Is system maintenance training available for hospital personnel? _____
   Cost of training program per participant: $ _____
   Location of training program: _____
   Length of training program: _____
7. Provide the names and phone numbers of three institutions with systems most similar to the system described in this bid document. Include names of physicians in charge, if possible. _____

Table 4.14
Warranty, Service, and Fiscal Terms

1. Scintillation camera warranty: (12) _____ months
   Warranty limitations, if any: _____
   Labor charge for warranty work provided outside of regular working hours: _____ . Regular
   working hours are: _____
2. Computer peripherals warranty: (12) _____ months
   Responsible vendor: _____
   Warranty limitations, if any: _____
3. Warranty for ECG synchronizer gate: (12) _____ months
   Responsible vendor: _____
4. Warranty for computer software: (12) _____ months
   Responsible vendor: _____
5. All warranty periods will be extended by 1 month for every contiguous 3-day period of
   "downtime" during the warranty or extended warranty period. Is this condition acceptable? ____
   (Y/N).
   Warranty shall begin at acceptance of installation. Acceptance of the installation shall succeed
   acceptance testing which shall be completed within 5 working days after installation of all
   components and accessories. In the event that acceptance testing defines areas of noncompliance
   with performance specifications defined in this document then the acceptance testing period shall
   be extended 5 days beyond the date of final adjustments to the system to yield acceptable
   performance.
6. Following the warranty period a service contract will be available for up to (4) _____ yr at a
   cost not to exceed (8) _____ % of the total purchase price of the system.
7. Preventive maintenance will be provided during the warranty and service contract periods and
   will consist of at least _____ hours/month.
8. List the names and locations of service personnel responsible for this installation. _____
   _____
9. Guaranteed response time (on site) during warranty and service contract period is (4) _____
   hr.
10. Fiscal terms
    Payment is required according to the following schedule:
    (20) _____ % at time order is placed.
    _____ % at delivery.
    (30) _____ % upon completion of installation.
    (50) _____ % upon formal acceptance.

technique for determining uniformity can be implemented on standard imaging computers and can be in strict compliance with NEMA. Uniformity at low count rates for the UFOV and central field of view (CFOV), both with and without any or all correction circuits engaged, are the usual NEMA values quoted. Additionally, uniformity values at observed count rates of 75,000 counts per second and at R − 20% (the observed rate at which 20% of the counts are not registered) may be specified or requested. All reported uniformity values must be independent of camera orientation. Uncorrected integral camera uniformity at low count rates may range from 10 to 15%. Corrected floods, on the other hand, will produce integral uniformity near 5%.

Point source sensitivity (another NEMA measurement) can be expected to be less than 5%. This parameter is a class standard specification by NEMA, but the measurement is easily accomplished in the field and should be guaranteed in a specific camera bid.

Energy Resolution. Intrinsic energy resolution for the detector is specified as a percentage of the 140 keV photopeak of ^{99m}Tc. A value on the order of 11% can be expected for a NaI(Tl) crystal. If the energy resolution is requested at any other energy, a special measurement would probably be required of the vendor. The useful energy range of the camera might also be specified. A range of 0 to 511 keV was available in older cameras; however, the detector head shielding has been decreased on many newer camera models for purposes of weight reduction, and the upper energy limit has been reduced accordingly. Low energies (<50 keV) are sometimes eliminated electrically because of interference by electronic noise in the amplifier circuitry.

Spatial Resolution. The required intrinsic spatial resolution should be specified in millimeters for all count rates and correction circuitry configurations measured for uniformity. The resolution refers to the full width at half maximum (FWHM) of the image of multiple 1-mm wide slits in a lead plate. According to NEMA, the resolution should be determined at 3-cm square grid locations over the UFOV, and the mean of these results should be reported as the resolution. These measurements can be made with a computer with 8-bit analog-digital converter (ADC) resolution. If this procedure is followed, however, only small areas of the detector can be measured, and the averaging of a much smaller number of measurements should be noted as a departure from the standard NEMA protocol (6). Full width at tenth maximum (FWTM) can also be specified for the imaged lines as an additional measure of camera resolution.

If resolution specifications are to be stated in terms of line pairs per inch or per centimeter, then images of a line pair phantom should be included in the vendor's response, since the observation of resolvable line pairs is a rather subjective determination.

Spatial Linearity. Spatial linearity specified in millimeters indicates the maximum deviation of any part of a straight line image from an "ideal line pattern" constructed to represent the actual line location in the test pattern. Any deviations from the NEMA-specified measuring techniques should be noted. Some compromises may be necessary if a standard departmental computer is used. If a NEMA type computer analysis is not feasible, then an analog image of the same NEMA phantom (or some other line patterned phantom) can be analyzed with film densitometry, and the nonlinearity can be defined similar to NEMA. Both NEMA integral and differential linearity should be specified for both the UFOV and the CFOV, since camera linearity often deteriorates rapidly near the periphery of the field of view. Linearity, like resolution, is more count rate dependent and, consequently, should be measured at all count rates and correction circuitry configurations used for measurement of uniformity (7). Nonlinearities near

1% of the field of view diameter are at the threshold of being visually noticeable and are therefore important for standard planar imaging. On the other hand, tomographic imaging is much more demanding of exact image symmetry to objects placed anywhere in the field of view. For tomography, nonlinearities are required to be in the 0.1% range or ±0.4 mm for large field of view cameras.

Count Rate Performance. Count rate performance is specified by four NEMA parameters: (1) the maximum count rate of the camera; (2) the camera deadtime (τ); (3) the count rate at which 20% of the valid events in the NaI(Tl) crystal are lost (this loss can be calculated from the deadtime); and (4), the observed vs the true count rate curve. All specifications should be made with and without correction circuitry and for both a 20% window and a maximum energy acceptance window. Source configuration and location are critical for these measurements, and any deviations from the NEMA source specifications should be described.

An additional count rate specification should be included from measurements with an Adams phantom as a scatter medium (8). This deadtime measurement resembles a clinical situation more closely, and the deadtime is more indicative of clinically achievable count rate performance.

System Performance

System Sensitivity. Decisions concerning which collimator to use for a particular study or which collimator to buy for a camera usually involve a balance between resolution and sensitivity. Hence, system sensitivity and system resolution values should be evaluated together. Both of these measurements are specified for each collimator. The system sensitivity can be measured by exact NEMA techniques and is reported in counts per minute per microcurie (counts/min-μCi).

System Resolution. Compared to intrinsic resolution, system resolution yields a more realistic indication of clinically achievable resolution. To measure this characteristic a scatter medium is employed much like the Adams phantom, and NEMA traceable analysis can parallel the method used for intrinsic resolution. Values should be specified in millimeters, just as for the intrinsic resolution.

Multiple Window Spatial Registration. To increase the detection efficiency for multiple photopeak isotopes, separate energy windows often are utilized. Each energy window (Z pulse) is utilized to normalize the x and y spatial coordinates of the image attributed to that window. Therefore, the amplifier gains for each energy window must be independently adjusted to provide exact overlap of images from the multiple photopeaks. The maximum allowable misregistration is specified in millimeters. There are some easier alternatives to the NEMA measurement of multiple window spatial misregistration; Chapman et al (9) describe the visual detection of doubly exposed edge packing images from multiple energy windows to determine misregistration errors. Since any detectable difference in registration between windows is unacceptable and field service adjustable, quantitation of the error seems unnecessary.

Required Camera Features

Camera components or features that do not require extensive specification should be listed for completeness. Some of these items might include:

1. Camera Start/Stop control by foot switch on 8-ft cable.
2. Persistence scope erasure by foot switch on 8-ft cable.
3. All x, y orientation controls available at the detector head.
4. Acquisition and termination predefined by time, counts, or information density.
5. Persistence scope mounted within 3 ft of the detector head/stand at a height of not more than 6 ft. A video or conventional persistence scope may be specified if there is a preference.
6. At least six predefined energy window selections for each energy channel.
7. Multichannel analyzer (MCA) with at least 256 channel resolution and display, background subtraction, peak integration, energy window indicators for all windows simultaneously, variable energy per channel adjustment, and individual channel number and content readout.
8. In magnification mode, a maximum magnification of at least ×3. The magnified area of the detector should be selectable from any portion of the detector. All intrinsic detector specifications should be maintained under magnification mode.
9. Uniformity, energy, and/or linearity correction circuitry, if available and if required to produce the desired intrinsic camera performance, must be included.
10. Digital display of each degree of freedom of the detector head, yoke, and camera base. Locking positions and/or interlock switches for collimator replacement positions of the detector head, if collimators are not intended to be changed manually, should also be included.
11. An analog multiformat imaging device with formats ranging from 1 on 1 to at least 64 on 1 on 8- × 10-inch film. CRT dot size and camera optics must be of sufficient quality to resolve any scintigraphic line bars in the 16 on 1 format that are resolvable on the 1 on 1 format. Automatic electronic methods must be provided for entering the counts and duration of the image on the film. A method to enter patient demographic data on the film also should be available. Multichannel analyzer (MCA) output must also be available as input to the photographic device. "Film cassette missing" and "dark slide in place" warning lights should be included on the camera. Manual frame advance controls must be available in addition to an automatic control activated by the Start/Stop signals of the scintillation camera.
12. A backup CRT with Polaroid photography should be included.
13. At least 12 film cassettes for the camera described in 11 (above) should be included.

Collimators

Collimator construction may be specified if strong preferences exist. Collimators often are supplied by independent sources, and a wide variety is available. Round, square, or hexagonal hole cores, foil or molded septa, septal thickness, core replacement, and full collimator types are all candidates for spec-ification. The performance of collimators can be evaluated as part of the camera system resolution and sensitivity tests described earlier. Requested collimators might include:

1. One low energy, 7 mil septa, general-purpose collimator.
2. One low energy, high resolution collimator.
3. One medium energy (up to 240 keV), general-purpose collimator.
4. One pinhole collimator for imaging below 240 keV.
5. A storage cabinet and cart or carts for all collimators. Total collimator storage space should be limited to a 4- × 4-ft area.
6. A lead ring with inside diameter equal to that of the collimator core. This ring must be the same weight as the collimators if the camera is of a counterbalanced design and if the collimator weight is necessary for counterbalancing during head rotation in any direction.

A statement concerning the uniformity of collimators would be appropriate; however, NEMA does not provide for such measurements. One approach would be to describe the camera uniformity utilizing NEMA intrinsic uniformity measuring methods, but employing a ^{57}Co flood source and a collimator rather than the point source specified by NEMA. It should be pointed out, however, that most flood sources are constructed to guaranteed uniformity of only ± 5%.

Accessories

For new departments in particular, it may be advantageous to include accessories with the camera purchase. Some examples of accessories include:

1. X, Y, Z imaging table with low Z surface for through table imaging. Desirable specifications include:
   - Total weight not to exceed 150 lbs.
   - Unextended length not to exceed 80 inches.
   - Unextended width not to exceed 32 inches.
   - Vertical extension range to meet or

exceed 24 to 36 inches, measured from the floor.
   - Ball bearing, 360° swivel, rubber-tired wheels in excess of 4-inch diameter on all four legs.
2. Test phantom as described by the Center for Devices and Radiological Health (10).
3. Adams deadtime scatter phantom (8).
4. NEMA linearity-resolution slit phantom (5).
5. Three complete sets of operator manuals covering all components of the system.
6. One complete set of engineering diagrams and documentation suitable for "in-house" service of all system components.

Mobile Cameras

Most mobile cameras are rather large and cumbersome. Accommodating the size is the major concern in specifying the appropriate mobile camera. Maximum allowable width and length are major concerns in considering the maneuverability in aisles and doorways. Some mobile cameras are built in a C-arm configuration; in this design, part of the camera must fit under the patient bed. Maximum allowable clearance of patient beds should be specified for such a system. For yoke-extension mobile cameras, the maximum extension of the detector head beyond the outside edge of the mobile vehicle will determine whether cross-bed imaging can be effectively accomplished. Total camera weight can present problems for some elevators. Wheel size and motor power may require specification if an elevator drops under weight or other small bumps or gaps have to be navigated. For power-driven mobile cameras, rugs and slopes must be considered as major obstacles, and the speed at which a camera moves over these obstacles is important. For these units, it is important to detemine how the unit can be moved in an emergency situation with a loss of power.

Other considerations include low battery indicators, the length of continuous battery operation of the detector, required warm-up times for the camera electronics and imaging oscilloscope, placement of emergency interrupts to suspend motion on collision, capacity of the on-board storage area for collimators, isotopes, film, and cassettes. Other, more exotic options include an on-board data acquisition and processing computer, an alternative device for data acquisition only, an EKG gate, and the future upgrading of any of these devices into the mobile unit if they are not already available. All necessary variations in system size and weight with these field upgradeable items should be established in the specification response. An alternative to on-board digital data acquisition is provided by cable networks back to a main computer (11). This may be a viable and less expensive alternative if only limited and nearby locations are involved. Specifications for such cabling should include limits on the acceptable degradation in camera performance after transmission (12).

Rotating Detector Single Photon Emission Computed Tomography (SPECT)

Specifications for the rotational performance of a camera should include limits on the accuracy of the rotation angle, the maximum rate of change or drift of the spatial coordinate registration of the detector, the maximum angular rotation in one direction, the minimum force applied normal to the axis of rotation of the detector that is required to stop rotation, the maximum and minimum radius of rotation, and the maximum clearance from the center of the detector head to the gantry when the collimator is at a 25-cm radius relative to the center of rotation. The availability and placement of emergency stop buttons, rotation control without a computer, noncircular motion capability, and methods for defining attenuation correction might also be specified. For some purchases, software may also be included; in these cases, the reconstruction times, matrix sizes, filters available, reorientation flexibility, and calibration and correction methods should all be established. For some installations additional computer hardware may also be required for an existing computer. These items may include floating point processors, array processors, interfacing and larger disk capacities. These items, and the party responsible for their installation, should be defined as part of the purchase specifications document.

In addition to the items specific to scintil-lation camera installation, the general concerns of on-site training, warranty, service contracts, shipping insurance, and installation should also be described. These specifications should be included in vendor response sheets similar to those shown in Tables 4.8 through 4.14. The specifications, vendor responses, and any negotiated exceptions should also be referenced as an integral part of the purchase order.

ULTRASOUND
Performance Specifications for an Articulated Arm Ultrasound B-Scanner

For pulse-echo ultrasound systems, a guide for preparing performance specifications is given in reference 13. Many of the major performance tests are similar to the routine quality control procedures (14) described in Chapter 8.

To illustrate the preparation of specific performance requirements for ultrasound equipment, a general purpose articulated arm B-scanner with gray scale display is considered. The imaging system should include a variety of single element pulse-echo transducer assemblies ranging in frequency, diameter, and internal focus from 3.5 to 7.5 MHz, 6 to 19 mm, and short (3.0 cm) to long (9.5 cm) focus, respectively. A broad band (temporally short) pulser should be included that permits the user to adjust the amplitude of the output excitation pulse used to drive the transducer assembly. The unit should have a broad band receiver with protective circuitry against the difference in voltage amplitude between the excitation pulse and the pulse-echo signals (e.g., 500 V vs 5 μV or 160 dB). A digital scan converter should permit some preprocessing of echo signals before storage and some postprocessing of stored information before video gray scale display. A multiformat camera is required for hard copy recording of the video image.

The articulated arm of the imaging system should faithfully register the two-dimensional scan plane in patient (or object) space onto the two-dimensional coordinate axes in image space. The registration should be presentable as an image on the display monitors. Selectable minification reduction factors (e.g., 2-cm patient space/1-cm image space, 4-cm patient space/1-cm image space, etc.) should be available. Most modern equipment provides a minification range from at least 2:1 to 4:1, with an operator-controlled Read Zoom (does not require rescanning) or Write Zoom (requires rescanning) switch available to magnify any part of the final stored image by a factor of 2 or 4. The zoom feature is useful primarily for the larger image/object factors.

Other desirable controls are calibrated electronic calipers with a digital readout; alphanumeric keyboards for labeling images; individual controls for initial gain, near gain, far gain, time (or depth) varied gain TVG (DVG) or time gain compensation (TGC), gain delay, overall receiver gain; individual selectable preprocessing and postprocessing transfer functions; machine-detachable foot switches and/or hand switch controls labeled Read, Write, Erase, Autocenter (of arm), CM Marker Dots, and Scan Plane Lateral Motion for obtaining serial planes; all required cables and interconnecting wiring; and all other standard accessories.

Specific Equipment Requirements

Specific performance requirements for an articulated arm static B-scanner are outlined below. The requirements are stated in a form to facilitate response by all potential vendors. In their responses, potential vendors would be expected to supply the most complete specifications (e.g., product data sheets) available. Where specific technical information is requested, vendors are expected to provide the requested information in a clear and concise manner; if the requested information cannot be provided, the potential vendor should explain the reason. In all cases, the purchaser should not assume anything regarding specific equipment or performance requirements. It should be made clear to the vendor exactly what is desired and to what degree of precision each parameter is to perform. An example of a specification list with performance tolerance is given in the next section.

Equipment Requirements

(One of each item, unless otherwise specified.)

1. Main unit consisting of:

a. Console with minimum 6-inch monitor suitable for Polaroid photography.
b. System base unit, with depth selectable amplifier/receiver in maximum of 2-cm adjustable increments; accurate to ±3 dB.
c. A-mode scope with maximum of 2-cm incremental depth selectable gain curve.
d. Mobile instrument console with remote control handle and remote control footswitch(s) for minimum of control over Read/Write, Erase, and Photography.
e. Minimum 10-inch video preview monitor.
f. Broad band pulser and receiver units capable for operating between about 1 MHz and 10 MHz with operator control of power emitted from transducer assembly.
g. Digital scan converter with minimum features as follows:
   (1) Set of digital calipers and 1-cm marker dots; accurate to ≥98%.
   (2) Gray scale postprocessing enhancement capability; minimum 4 bytes of memory, operator-selectable.
   (3) Echo signal amplitude preprocessing; minimum 4 bytes of memory, operator-selectable.
   (4) Write magnify feature.
   (5) Read Zoom or Write Zoom feature.
   (6) Gray scale wedge; minimum 16 shades of gray.
   (7) D/A converter, A/D converter.
   (8) External storage; computer interface data port.
   (9) Horizontal and vertical calibration (linearity); accurate to ≥97%.
h. Full alphanumeric data entry; built-in keyboard.
i. Mobile scanner assembly consisting of minimum of:
   (1) Mobile scanner stand.
   (2) Motorized patient transversing table.
   (3) Portascan head with electronic echoguard and transducer mount of male ultrahigh frequency (UHF) or TNC type.

(4) Articulated arm with B-mode registration; accurate to $\geq 95\%$.

2. High resolution, multiformat automatic camera with minimum of four cassettes suitable for camera with from 1 to 9 image format on 8-inch × 10-inch standard x-ray film.

3. Optional minimum of at least the following transducer:

   a. A focused 5.0-MHz, 13-mm diameter, 4- to 14-cm depth of focus multimatching layer or, if unavailable, $\frac{1}{4}$ λ B-scan transducer. In focal plane, axial resolution ≤ 1.0 mm; -20 dB pulse echo response beam width ≤ 0.08 F, where F is focal length in millimeters.

4. Two (2) complete operator's manuals and circuit diagrams.

5. Listing of the following acoustic output parameters and transducer labeling requirements as recommended in the AIUM/NEMA Safety Standard for Diagnostic Ultrasound Equipment (15) and required by the F.D.A. form 510 (k):

   a. Absolute maximum ultrasonic power.

   b. Absolute maximum spatial peak temporal average intensity (SPTA).

   c. Absolute maximum spatial peak pulse average intensity (SPPA).

   d. Pulse repetition frequency.

   e. Absolute maximum spatial average temporal average intensity (SATA) in the same plane and with the same control settings used to measure the absolute maximum spatial peak temporal average intensity. If different transducer assemblies are provided:

      (1) Fractional bandwidth of each transducer assembly.

      (2) Focal length, focal area, and depth of focus for each focused transducer assembly.

Prices quoted should be F.O.B. at hospital and include installation and demonstration of specifications; 25% of total cost will be paid upon delivery into the ultrasound area. A 2-month (60-day) side-by-side comparison with present compound scanners and complete acceptance testing by a qualified individual should be allowed before final acceptance is complete and the final 75% of cost is paid. Also, the equipment should carry a minimum 1 yr (12 months) warranty on all parts and labor. Following the warranty period, a service contract should be available. At all times, equipment service must be available within 24 hr after a problem is reported to an agreed upon service office.

Explanation of Specifications

EQUIPMENT REQUIREMENTS

These specifications are essentially self-explanatory. For entries 1.a, 1.b, 1.c., 1.e., 1.g., and 1.i., specifics are given on size or required precision of equipment variables (e.g., monitors, depth variable gain, calipers, calibration linearity, etc.).

TRANSDUCER ASSEMBLY

The number of transducers requested is the buyer's option. Usually the vendor supplies at least two transducers with the unit.

OPERATOR'S MANUALS

Two operator's manuals and sets of circuit diagrams should be specified, so that one can be kept with the unit while the second can be filed in the ultrasound clinic where other service manuals and quality assurance test tools are kept.

ACOUSTIC OUTPUT PARAMETERS AND TRANSDUCER ASSEMBLY LABELING

Since passage of the regulatory form 510 (k) by the Food and Drug Administration, based on the American Institute of Ultrasound in Medicine (AIUM)/National Electrical Manufacturers Association (NEMA) Recommended Safety Standard for Diagnostic Ultrasound Equipment (15), the possibility is recognized of potential risk at diagnostic intensity levels of pulsed ultrasound. To perform studies safely, purchaser and vendor should be aware of certain acoustic output parameters of the ultrasound systems.

The last paragraph clarifies to potential vendors the type of quotation desired, what the potential buyer will do before making final payment of the system, and the date from which the warranty agreement will commence. Of course, all necessary Federal regulations are assumed to be satisfied.

A similar approach to performance specifications should be taken for any real-time sector or electronic sequential linear array system. In this case, some of the important variables to cover are: the number of scan lines per image, the number of images per frame, the number of frames per second (frame rate), the depth of field, and the size of the sectoring angle. If the sonographic study is displayed at less than 10 to 12 frames/sec, image flicker will be apparent. At the other extreme, a frame rate of at least 30 to 33 frames/sec is required for good cardiographic studies. Since frame rate, scan lines per frame, and scan lines per second are interrelated and are ultimately limited by the speed of sound in the medium of interest, there may be a need for some trade-offs between these parameters (16).

The other major option to consider is whether a stationary (add-on for static gray scale scanner) or portable real-time system is desired. The patient load, hospital's or institution's bed size, and rooms available for diagnostic ultrasound procedures weigh heavily in this decision. One advantage of a portable real-time system is that it enables examination of patients who cannot be brought into the diagnostic ultrasound clinic.

COMPUTED TOMOGRAPHY SCANNER

This section on computed tomographic (CT) scanners is divided into three parts. The first is a general statement of performance specifications for a CT scanner; the second is a more specific outline of the requirements and characteristics of the scanner; and the third is a questionnaire that requests specific information concerning a variety of mechanical, electronic, and performance variables from the manufacturer. The questionnaire offers the manufacturer the opportunity to specify alternative specifications that may differ slightly from those requested in the first two parts.

At the time of acceptance testing, it is impractical to measure all performance variables at all possible techniques (kilovolt peak, dose, algorithms, etc.). For test purposes, a few techniques are selected that represent those used most frequently. Many of the variables are interrelated (e.g., dose and low contrast resolution), and scanner settings for optimization of one variable (e.g., high contrast resolution) may not be appropriate for another variable (e.g., low contrast resolution). Vendors should quote performance characteristics for each variable at the technique factors that produce the optimal value for that variable. To some extent, this is recognized in the request for technical information by asking for performance characteristics of specific "normally used" techniques, as well as at the "best" technique.

General Equipment Requirements

The general nature of this equipment shall be a head- and body-computed tomography (CT) scanner. The equipment shall include, but not necessarily be limited to, the following items:

1. Gantry with patient table, beam locating device, anatomical localization system, and patient positioning restraints.
2. High voltage power supply, including x-ray tube and cables.
3. Scan control console.
4. Image viewing and manipulation console (including CRT for image display).
5. Multiformat hard copy camera.
6. Necessary computer hardware for reconstructing, selecting, manipulating, transferring, displaying, and storing images.
7. Means for writing or transferring images or raw data files for archival storage (floppy disk and/or computer tape drive).
8. Necessary computer software for controlling the scanner, reconstructing images, presenting images on CRT, manipulating images and data, and storing images when required.
9. All necessary cables and interfaces
10. Instruction and maintenance manuals.

Specific Equipment Requirements

The specific performance requirements for a whole body CT scanner are outlined below. For head-only scanners, appropriate modifications may be made, and some requirements may be relaxed.

These specifications are presented in two sections. The first section is a statement of the required performance characteristics for all components. The second section is a questionnaire to be completed by the vendor. Potential vendors are requested to provide answers to the questionnaire to facilitate a feature by feature comparison of the various aspects of CT scanners.

X-RAY GENERATOR AND CONTROLLER

An x-ray generator capable of providing high voltage to the x-ray tube shall be provided. In addition, the cables necessary to convey the high voltage to the moving x-ray tube and to provide all auxiliary power to the x-ray tube (e.g., anode drive, cooling pumps, filament power) shall be provided. An x-ray generator controller that automatically initiates and terminates x-ray production and other tube functions at the proper sequence during the scan shall be included as part of the CT scanner. No specific wave form characteristics are specified.

X-RAY TUBE

X-ray tubes may be of the rotating or fixed anode type. A tube cooling system is desirable. If overheating of the anode is possible through a sequence of one or more successive scans at techniques available to the operator, then the system shall provide for an x-ray tube protective system when overheating is likely to occur. Automatic exclusion of exposure initiation with an audio or visual indication of overheating is preferred as a protective system.

The x-ray tube and housing shall conform to maximum x-ray leakage and other requirements of the United States Food and Drug Administration and applicable state agencies at the time of installation.

COLLIMATION SYSTEM

An adjustable collimation system that permits the operator to select x-ray beam width is required. The x-ray collimation system shall be designed to minimize patient dose in regions on either side of the scan section. A measure of patient dose known as the CT Dose Index (CTDI) (17), which usually is equivalent to the Multiple Scan Average Dose (MSAD), is preferred for specifying patient dose for several clinically utilized techniques. In some scanners, the x-ray beam width transversing the patient is substantially wider than the beam width incident on the detectors. The CTDI effectively "penalizes" these types of scanners by raising the value of the CTDI. However, the CTDI accurately represents the amount of radiation received by the patient undergoing a typical CT examination consisting of several contiguous slices.

GANTRY

The type of motion of the x-ray tube and detectors is not specified. However, the motion shall be such to allow completion of CT scans of the largest radius (e.g., a patient body) in less than 5 sec.

The gantry shall be capable of tilting at least ±15°, enabling CT scans of oblique sections of the patient. Alternatively, a tilting patient bed will be considered. The geometrical aperture of the gantry shall be a minimum of 50 cm (20 inches) in diameter, and the largest reconstruction diameter shall be a minimum of 48 cm (19 inches).

X-RAY BEAM LOCALIZER

A light or laser beam localizer visible on the patient and indicating the position of the x-ray beam shall be provided. The center of this light field along the axial direction and the center of the radiation field shall agree to 2 mm or less at the center of the aperture at all gantry orientations.

RADIOGRAPHIC LOCALIZATION SYSTEM

A means shall be provided for radiographing a patient using the x-ray tube and detector system held stationary and passing the patient through the x-ray beam. Subsequent to reconstructing this image, the system shall have the capability to relocate the patient and/or gantry orientation automatically to scan any plane that is chosen from the image. The accuracy of relocation shall be within 2 mm at the center of the gantry aperture. At least two projections (lateral and anteroposterior (AP)) of the patient shall be possible with this system.

BED CONTROL

The axial motion of the patient bed shall be controllable from either the control console or from bed controls positioned on the bed or gantry. Other motions of the bed (e.g., angulations) shall be controllable from the bedside. The position of the bed, relative to some reference location, shall be displayed near the bed and/or at the control console. It is desirable to indicate the bed position on the hard copy image and CRT monitor.

HEAD HOLDER

A device for conveniently immobilizing the patient's head shall be provided.

CONTROL CONSOLE

The control console shall provide, but shall not necessarily be limited to, an indication of and the updating capabilities for the following:

1. Patient data, including name, ID number, and scan number.
2. Scan technique, including kilovolt peak, milliamperage, scan time, scan width, and bed increment between scans.
3. Computer status and data storage device (disk) status.
4. Software, including algorithm type and radius of reconstruction (magnification).

As an optional feature, a CRT monitor suitable for displaying images shall be provided at the console. This monitor must be in such a location that the scanner operator can easily verify that the patient has been correctly positioned and that all components are functioning properly.

DISPLAY CONSOLE

The display console shall have a CRT monitor that is capable of displaying any CT image that exists on the data storage device (disk). The window width (contrast) and window level (brightness) shall be operator-controllable. Arbitrary settings of the width, level, and preset combinations of width and level are desirable. The following information shall be displayed or shall be available on the console or on the CRT monitor.

1. Patient name and ID number.
2. Bed position.
3. Right/left identification.
4. Scan number.

5. Kilovolt peak, milliamperage, scan time, scan thickness.
6. Algorithm type.
7. Window width and level.

MULTIFORMAT CAMERA

A camera for creating hard copy images shall be provided. Although a camera that creates images on transparency film is preferred, alternative devices that create high fidelity images on other media may be considered. The camera shall be capable of using 8 × 10-inch (or 11 × 14-inch or 14 × 17-inch) transparency film. The number of images per film may be fixed or selectable. Although no quantitative specifications are given for the fidelity of the photographed image referenced to the CRT image, the hard copy image shall be of high diagnostic quality. The distortion of this camera shall be such that if the image is projected to actual size and overlapped with the object, the measured separation of any two corresponding points on the image and object shall be less than 2 mm.

MAGNETIC STORAGE DEVICE

To accommodate archival storage of digital data, the CT scanner shall be equipped with a 9-track magnetic tape drive. The drive shall be capable of writing 1600 bytes per inch (BPI). The reel size shall be 12 inches. Software shall be furnished to transfer images from disk to tape, and vice versa. Alternatively, the CT scanner shall include a floppy disk drive with software that writes digital image data on floppy disks.

OTHER SOFTWARE FEATURES

In addition to the basic software for controlling the CT scanner, manipulating data, reconstructing images, and displaying images, the system is required to have other features.

Multiplanar Reconstruction

The CT scanner shall have the capability of reconstructing images not in the planes of the original scans. These images may be displayed in arbitrarily oriented planes. In particular, sagittal and coronal planes are required.

Region of Interest (ROI)

The software shall be able to display on the CRT image a geometrical area defined by the operator. An arbitrarily shaped ROI of variable size and location is preferred; however, a rectangular or elliptical area with selectable dimensions and location is acceptable. The following calculations shall be on that portion of the image inside the ROI:

1. The area of the ROI scaled to true object size.
2. The average (mean) CT number of all pixels within the ROI.
3. The standard deviation of CT numbers within the ROI.
4. A histogram showing the distribution of CT numbers within the ROI.

Length-Measuring Device

A means for determining the linear distance between two arbitrary points on the CRT image shall be provided. This device may consist of such schemes as the length of a vector line, distance between two points, or an overlaid grid pattern. The dimensions presented must be scaled automatically to actual object size and shall be accurate to within 1 mm of actual size.

Reconstruction Magnification

The CT scanner software shall be capable of reconstructing a magnified image. This feature is *not* a simple geometrical magnification of the reconstructed image with interpolation.

Other Software Features

Vendors are invited to list in the following section other useful standard and optional software features included on their scanner. These items are not required but may contribute to the desirability of a particular CT scanner.

WARRANTY

For the CT scanner, the minimum acceptable warranty period shall be 12 months. The vendor shall provide all labor during the normal work week (8 AM to 5 PM, Monday through Friday) and all parts except x-ray tubes at no cost to the institution. Provision of replacement x-ray tubes at no cost

to the institution is desirable, but not required.

TRAINING

The vendor shall provide a training program at the institution for up to eight institutional representatives. The training program will emphasize the operation, clinical functioning, and maintenance of the CT scanner. It will be directed toward radiation technologists, radiologists, and physicists at the institution. All costs associated with this training shall be borne by the vendor.

RADIATION THERAPY
Treatment Unit

In specifying the capabilities of a radiation treatment unit, one must keep in mind the anticipated use of the unit (18, 19). This analysis should consider the expected patient characteristics for both the present and the future, and the goals of the physicians using the unit. For example, a department which requires an additional unit to handle a large number of palliative cases would find its needs more effectively met with a low energy photon beam unit than with a complex, high-energy, multiple modality unit.

The desired beam modalities must first be selected, as many other equipment characteristics are directly affected by this decision. Many modern treatment units provide beams of either photons or electrons, and a radiation therapy department may be interested in these types of unit. Some large research institutions may be interested in a machine that produces pions, neutrons, or heavy charged particles; the purchase procedure is considerably different when such exotic equipment is considered. This chapter is addressed to departments considering the purchase of more conventional equipment.

The selection of modality is dictated by the patient mix, the expected types of treatment, and the facilities available. The intention to treat superficial disease suggests the use of electron beams, while high-energy photons are desirable for treatment of deep-seated tumors. A unit with electron beam capability is necessarily complex and demands a commitment to physics and engineering support services. In addition, high-energy photon beams require substantial room shielding (including neutron shielding

Technical Information for CT Scanner

The following section should be submitted to the vendor so that he can provide the information requested in the table.

The vendor should return the completed form along with the price quotation to the institution.

1. Power Requirements

A. Electrical power sources required for operation of CT scanner system.

Voltage	Phase	kVA	Equipment To Be Powered (e.g., generator gantry, computer, etc.)
(1)			
(2)			
(3)			
(4)			
(5)			
(6)			
(7)			
(8)			

B. Required line regulation _____ %.

2. Air Conditioning Requirements

Control Area	_____ BTU/hr.
Diagnostic Area	_____ BTU/hr.
Computer Room	_____ BTU/hr.
Equipment Room	_____ BTU/hr.
Gantry Area	_____ BTU/hr.

(2)

Other	_____ BTU/hr.
Other	_____ BTU/hr.

List areas where raised "computer floor" may be required: _____

Humidity Requirements: _____

3. Mechanical (Floor Stress)

A. Total weight of equipment = _____ lbs (kg)

Gantry:	_____ lbs (kg)
Control Console:	_____ lbs (kg)
Display Console:	_____ lbs (kg)
HV Generator:	_____ lbs (kg)
HV Controller:	_____ lbs (kg)
Other _____:	_____ lbs (kg)
Other _____:	_____ lbs (kg)

B. Suggested Floor Space: _____ sq. ft. (sq. meters)

4. Plumbing

Location of Tap and Drain (e.g., Gantry, Equipment Room, etc.)	Amount of Water Required (gal/min)	Temperature °F
(1)		
(2)		
(3)		
(4)		

(7)

Highest kVp available _____ kVp

Number of intermediate stations _____ kVp

(b) X-ray Beam Filtrations Available (list type)

(1) _____

(2) _____

(3) _____

(4) _____

(c) Available mA Techniques

Lowest mA station _____ mA

Highest mA station _____ mA

Number of intermediate stations _____ mA

8. Available Scan Speeds

List all available scan times, starting with fastest scan.

Scan Speed		Mode (e.g., partial scan, small scan diameter, full head, etc.)
(1)	_____ sec	_____
(2)	_____ sec	_____
(3)	_____ sec	_____
(4)	_____ sec	_____
(5)	_____ sec	_____
(6)	_____ sec	_____
(7)	_____ sec	_____

---

5. Under-Floor Cable Runways

From Equipment (e.g., Gantry)	To Equipment (e.g., Control Console)	Approximate Size Of Runway
(1)		
(2)		
(3)		
(4)		
(5)		
(6)		

6. X-ray Generator

(a) Voltage waveform _____

(b) Continuous [____] Pulsed [____]

7. Scanning Techniques

Information regarding techniques in this section should be provided only for those techniques that may be operator-selected for routine clinical operation of the CT scanner. Techniques at which the scanner is not normally calibrated (e.g., for research purposes) should be excluded from the following section.

(a) kVp Techniques

Lowest kVp available _____ kVp

(10.) (c) Nominal focal spot size: _____ mm x _____ mm

(d) Type of cooling system: _____

(e) Anode heat storage capacity (cold): _____ HU

(f) Housing heat storage capacity: _____ HU

Housing cooling rate: _____ HU/min.

(g) Overload protection system?: Yes [ ] No [ ]

Type: _____

11. Collimation System

(a) Adjustable collimators in axial dimension (beam width)?

Yes [ ] No [ ]

If yes, minimum slice thickness: _____ mm

Maximum slice thickness: _____ mm

List other intermediate slice thicknesses available: _____

_____

_____

(b) Transaxial (angular width of fan beam) collimation possible?

Yes [ ] No [ ]

If yes, minimum size available at center of gantry: _____

Maximum size available: _____

---

(8)

(8) _____ sec

(9) _____ sec

(10) _____ sec

(11) _____ sec

(12) _____ sec

9. Reconstruction Time

List reconstruction times and corresponding modes (e.g., matrix size, number of data samples, with or without calibration, etc).

Begin with mode that is usually employed for routine head scans.

Reconstruction Time	Mode
(1) _____ sec	_____
(2) _____ sec	
(3) _____ sec	
(4) _____ sec	
(5) _____ sec	
(6) _____ sec	
(7) _____ sec	
(8) _____ sec	

10. X-ray Tube Type

(a) Rotating anode [ ]   Stationary anode [ ]

(b) Anode material: Tungsten [ ]   Other _____

12.) (e) Data Sampling

Scan Time	No. of Views	Ray Samples/View	Total Number of Ray Samples
_____ sec (fastest)	_____	_____	_____
_____ sec	_____	_____	_____
_____ sec	_____	_____	_____
_____ sec (slowest)	_____	_____	_____

(f) Gantry Tilt (or Bed Tilt)

Gantry Tilt [ ]   Bed Tilt [ ]

Maximum "forward" tilt: _____°
(Top of gantry toward patient's feet)

Maximum "backward" tilt: _____°
(Top of gantry away from patient's feet)

13. Localization System

Localization system available?

[ ] Yes, no additional cost.

[ ] Yes, as option. Cost: $_____

[ ] No.

Localization projections available:

[ ] AP

[ ] Lateral

[ ] Arbitrarily chosen angle

(11.) If scanner is of translate/rotate type, can translation motion be limited for small regions of anatomy?

Yes [ ]   No [ ]

12. Gantry

(a) Type of Scan Motion

Fan beam, translate/rotate: [ ]

Fan beam, rotating detectors: [ ]

Fan beam, stationary detectors: [ ]

Other _____: [ ]

(b) Does x-ray tube shift to closer and farther positions from scan center, depending on scan diameter?

Yes [ ]   No [ ]

Do detectors shift to closer and farther positions from scan center, depending on scan diameter?

Yes [ ]   No [ ]

(c) Detectors

Detector Type: _____

Number of Detectors: _____

(d) Gantry Aperature

Physical Diameter of Gantry Aperature: _____ cm

Maximum Diameter of Scan: _____ cm

(13.) Maximum length (along patient axis) of projected region: _____ cm

Maximum width (transverse to patient axis) of projected region: _____ cm

Time required for largest localization scan (not including reconstruction): _____ sec

Time required for reconstruction of largest localization scan: _____ sec

14. Light-Field Localizers and Positioning Aids

(a) Light-field beams have the following geometry:

    [ ] Trans-axial

    [ ] Sagittal

    [ ] Coronal

(b) Trans-axial light field:

    [ ] In gantry

    [ ] External to gantry

(c) Accuracy:

    Center of light field (trans-axial) coincides with center of x-ray field to within _____ mm.

15. Bed

(a) Maximum in/out bed motion ("full out" to "full in"): _____ cm.

(b) Vertical bed motion range: _____ cm.

(15.) (c) In/out motion accuracy (with patient on bed):

    Incrementing accuracy: _____ mm

    Maximum backlash: _____ mm

    Reproducibility: _____ mm

(d) Bed position indicated on:

    [ ] Gantry

    [ ] Bed

    [ ] Control Console

    [ ] Image

(e) Bed detachable from gantry:

    [ ] Yes, standard feature.

    [ ] Yes, optional feature. Cost: $_____

    Cost of extra beds: $_____

    [ ] No.

(f) Bed tilting features:

    Up/down tilt? Yes [ ] No [ ]

    Right/left tilt? Yes [ ] No [ ]

(g) Other features available:

    Head holder:

    [ ] Standard

    [ ] Optional Cost: $_____

    [ ] Not available

(15.) (g)

Pediatric holder:

[ ] Standard

[ ] Optional   Cost: $_____

[ ] Not available

Flat "therapy" patient bed:

[ ] Standard

[ ] Optional   Cost: $_____

[ ] Not available

(h) Manual bed controls located on:

[ ] Gantry

[ ] Bed

[ ] Control Console

16. Control Console/Diagnostic Console Layout

The configuration of the control console and the diagnostic console is described by one or more of the following:

[ ] The control console and diagnostic console are side by side within a single cabinet, although the controls are relatively independent.

[ ] The diagnostic console occupies a separate cabinet from the control console and can be operated relatively independently.

(16.) [ ] An independent diagnostic console is available as an option at a cost of $_____.

Images are communicated to this console by:

[ ] Magnetic tape

[ ] Floppy disk

[ ] "Hard" wiring to system disk

[ ] Other

[ ] Other configurations (describe): _____

17. Control Console

(a) Can scan be initiated while reconstruction is in progress?

Yes [ ]   No [ ]

(b) Control console matrix size(s):

_____ Pixels x _____ Pixels

_____ Pixels x _____ Pixels

[ ] No image CRT on control console.

(c) Control console image controls:

Window level adjust?   Yes [ ]   No [ ]

Window width adjust?   Yes [ ]   No [ ]

Ability to display any image on disk?

Yes [ ]   No [ ]

CRT size: _____

Number of raster lines on control console CRT: _____

18. Diagnostic Console

(a) Which of the following data are displayed on the diagnostic console?

Patient name:	Yes ☐	No ☐
Patient identification:	Yes ☐	No ☐
Date of scan:	Yes ☐	No ☐
Time of examination:	Yes ☐	No ☐
Scan number:	Yes ☐	No ☐
Scan width:	Yes ☐	No ☐
Bed position:	Yes ☐	No ☐
Bed increment:	Yes ☐	No ☐
Algorithm type:	Yes ☐	No ☐
Gantry tilt:	Yes ☐	No ☐
Right/Left identification:	Yes ☐	No ☐
Magnification factor:	Yes ☐	No ☐
Window level:	Yes ☐	No ☐
Window width:	Yes ☐	No ☐

(b) Diagnostic console matrix size(s):

_____ Pixels x _____ Pixels

_____ Pixels x _____ Pixels

(c) CRT size:

Number of raster lines on diagnostic console CRT:

(18.) (d) Images accessed from:

System disk ☐

Floppy disk ☐

Magnetic tape ☐

(e) Can images be accessed and manipulated during a scan?

Yes ☐ No ☐

(f) Can images be accessed and manipulated while other images are being reconstructed?

Yes ☐ No ☐

19. Additional Software Features

(a) The following features are available (at time of delivery):

	Yes (Standard)	No	Optional:------Cost
Square region of interest (ROI)	☐	☐	☐ -- $
Rectangular ROI	☐	☐	☐ -- $
Elliptical ROI	☐	☐	☐ -- $
Arbitrarily shaped ROI	☐	☐	☐ -- $
Average CT number within ROI	☐	☐	☐ -- $
Standard deviation of CT number within ROI	☐	☐	☐ -- $
Histogram of CT numbers within ROI	☐	☐	☐ -- $
Distance measuring mechanism	☐	☐	☐ -- $
Accuracy: _____ mm			
Grid overlay	☐	☐	☐ -- $
Plot of CT numbers along a line segment	☐	☐	☐ -- $
Visual indication of pixels within CT number range	☐	☐	☐ -- $
Multiple images displayed simultaneously	☐	☐	☐ -- $
Image inversion (black to white)	☐	☐	☐ -- $
Image inversion (left to right)	☐	☐	☐ -- $

(19.) (a)

	Yes (Standard)	No	Optional:------Cost
Subtraction of two images	☐	☐	☐ -- $
Multi-planar reconstruction:			
Sagittal	☐	☐	☐ -- $
Coronal	☐	☐	☐ -- $
Arbitrary plane	☐	☐	☐ -- $
Other: _____	☐	☐	☐ -- $
Reconstruction magnification	☐	☐	☐ -- $
Geometric Magnification	☐	☐	☐ -- $
High density artifact removal	☐	☐	☐ -- $
Radiation treatment planning	☐	☐	☐ -- $
Patient directory	☐	☐	☐ -- $
Patient billing	☐	☐	☐ -- $
Inventory of supplies	☐	☐	☐ -- $
High level language (e.g., Fortran) user-accessible compilers, interpreters, editors, etc.			☐ -- $
			☐ -- $
			☐ -- $
			☐ -- $

20. Reconstruction Algorithms

(a) Total number of reconstruction algorithms avail-

able: _____

NAME	CHARACTERISTICS (e.g., high spatial resolution, pediatric heads, etc.)
1. _____	_____
2. _____	_____
3. _____	_____
4. _____	_____
5. _____	_____
6. _____	_____
7. _____	_____
8. _____	_____
9. _____	_____
10. _____	_____

21. Dynamic Scanning Capabilities

(a) Does CT scanner have physiologic (e.g., cardiac) gating

capabilities as an "off-the-shelf" feature?

Yes [/]   No [/]

Optional [/]   Cost $ _____

(b) Is software available that reconstructs images according

to phase of physiologic cycle?

Yes [/]   No [/]

(21.) (c) Minimum delay between successive scans: _____ sec

(d) Maximum number of closely spaced scans possible before

x-ray tube heat capacity attained (at usual body tech-

nique): _____ scans

(e) Number of images that can be reconstructed from a

single scan: _____ images

(f) In part (e) above, what fraction of the data from a scan

is used to reconstruct one of the images and what is the

minimum time elapsed during the data collection for this

image? _____

_____

(g) Other dynamic capabilities: _____

_____

_____

_____

22. Performance Data

(a) Low contrast resolution (e.g., low contrast pins or holes). Contrast = 0.5% or state contrast and how measured: _____.

TECHNIQUE

	(1) Head Technique Normally Used	(2) Head Technique Best For Low Contrast	(3) Body Technique Normally Used	(4) Body Technique Best For Low Contrast
kVp				
mA				
Scan Time (sec)				
Scan Diameter (cm)				
Beam Width (mm)				
Algorithm				
Dose, MSAD (rad)				
Smallest Pin or Hole Perceivable (mm)				

22. (b) High Contrast Resolution (Contrast $\geq$ 10%)

Type of Test Pattern   Diameter Of Phantom

- Round hole phantom   _____ cm
- Square hole phantom (e.g., AAPM type)   _____ cm
- Bar/plate phantom   _____ cm
- Star pattern   _____ cm
- MTF from LSF (cutoff at _____ % on MTF curve)   _____ cm
- MTF from ERF (cutoff at _____ % on MTF curve)   _____ cm
- Other: _____ cm

	(1) Head Technique Normally Used (same as 22a)	(2) Head Technique Best For Low Contrast	(3) Body Technique Normally Used (same as 22a)	(4) Body Technique Best For Low Contrast
Result (mm or lp/mm)				

Append MTF curves, if desired.

These results are valid: [ ] Center of image   [ ] Throughout entire image.

(22) (d) CT Number vs. Phantom Size Dependence (Water Phantoms):

WATER PHANTOM SIZE

	Adult Body (30 cm)	Adult Head (20 cm)	Pediatric Head (15 cm)	Premie Head (5 cm)
kVp				
mA				
Scan Time (sec)				
Scan Diameter (cm)				
Algorithm				
Average CT Number in Center of Phantom				

22. (c) Patient Dosimetry

Type of measurement reported:

[ ] Multiple Scan Average Dose[17]
[ ] Single Slice Peak Dose

Phantom diameter: _____ cm

Phantom thickness (length): _____ cm

Location in Phantom	(1) Head Technique Normally Used (same as 22a)	(2) Head Technique Best For Low Contrast (same as 22a)	(3) Body Technique Normally Used (same as 22a)	(4) Body Technique Best For Low Contrast (same as 22a)
Anterior	rad	rad	rad	rad
Posterior	rad	rad	rad	rad
Left	rad	rad	rad	rad
Right	rad	rad	rad	rad
Center	rad	rad	rad	rad
Other	rad	rad	rad	rad

(22) (e) CT Number Flatness

Measured CT number averaged over approximately 100 contiguous pixels.

Define: Range of CT numbers = (maximum average CT number anywhere in phantom) - (minimum average CT number anywhere in phantom).

Range in head phantom (20 cm) = _____ CT numbers.

Range in body phantom (30 cm) = _____ CT numbers.

23. Image Storage Devices

(a) Standard image storage device (short term):

[ ] Floppy disk: Capacity: _____ bytes

Capacity: _____ images for _____ x _____ .
matrix size of

[ ] Hard disk: Capacity: _____ bytes

Capacity: _____ images for _____ x _____ .
matrix size of

Capable of storing "raw" (unreconstructed) data?

Yes [ ] No [ ]

(23) (b) Archival Storage Devices

	Standard	Available	Optional Cost	Approximate Capacity (no. of images)
9 Track magnetic tape drive	[ ]	[ ]	$_____	_____
Floppy disk drive Type: _____	[ ]	[ ]	$_____	_____
Magnetic tape cassette drive	[ ]	[ ]	$_____	_____
Other: _____				

Right column for matrix size: _____ x _____

24. Hard Copy Images

(a) Multi-format camera:

Standard model camera (manufacturer/model): _____

Does camera CRT have a "gamma correction" or device that matches output of CRT phosphor to sensitivity curve of film?

Yes [ ] No [ ]

25. Training Program

Recommended number of personnel (technologists, radiologists, physicists, etc.) in training program: _____

Length of training program: _____

Cost to institution? [ ] Yes Cost: $ _____
                     [ ] No

26. Payment

Payment required according to the following schedule:

_____ % at time order is placed

_____ % upon delivery

_____ % upon completion of installation

_____ % upon formal acceptance

_____ %

27. Warranty

The warranty includes all parts and labor costs for a period of _____ months after formal acceptance.

The warranty: [ ] includes x-ray tubes
              [ ] does not include x-ray tubes

State normal service hours during warranty: _____

---

(24) (a)

Film Sizes Available	Format of Images on Film
____ x ____	____ x ____
	____ x ____
	____ x ____
	____ x ____
	____ x ____
	____ x ____
	____ x ____
	____ x ____
____ x ____	____ x ____

(b) Polaroid Camera

Polaroic camera is:

[ ] Standard

[ ] Not Available

[ ] Optional Cost: $ _____

(c) Other hard copy imaging devices available:

Device	Cost
_____	$ _____
_____	$ _____
_____	$ _____

(27) The warranty period will be extended by _____ days for every day of "down time" during the warranty period.

A preventive maintenance period of

_____ hrs. per week

_____ hrs. every two weeks

_____ hrs. per month

is required during the warranty period.

28. (a) Service Contract

Following the warranty period, service will be offered at the annual rates listed below. Service is required from 8:00 A.M. to 5:00 P.M., five days per week. After hours and weekend service may be charged to the institution at a "premium" rate. All parts (except x-ray tubes) and labor are to be included.

Year (following warranty period)	Cost	
1	$ _____	(firm)
2	$ _____	(approx.)
3	$ _____	(approx.)
4	$ _____	(approx.)
5	$ _____	(approx.)

(28) (a) Can you guarantee a response time during normal working hours?

[   ] Yes, _____ minutes

[   ] No, because: _____

What is the average number of CT units per field service engineer maintained by your service organization?: _____

(b) If not included in service contract, state cost of x-ray tube (exchange) during the following service periods:

Year (following installation)	Cost		Prorated Life (No. of Scans)	Cost/Scan
1	$ _____	(firm)	_____	$ _____
2	$ _____	(approx.)	_____	$ _____
3	$ _____	(approx.)	_____	$ _____
4	$ _____	(approx.)	_____	$ _____
5	$ _____	(approx.)	_____	$ _____

(c) Premium Time Service

"Premium" time is the time that a serviceman spends outside of the normal service period.

Premium time rate charged to customer: $ _____ /hr.

Minimum: $ _____

29. Delivery

Delivery time: _____ months ARO.

Installation time: _____ weeks after delivery.

Will manufacturer deduct from purchase price a late delivery/installation penalty of 0.5% of the total purchase price for each week past the above stated delivery and installation periods?

Yes [   ]   No [   ]

30. Other Features

Describe other features of this CT Scanner that are relevant, useful, and/or unique to this scanner.

31. Other Users

List other institutions that have purchased a CT Scanner similar to the one described in this bid. Where possible, list names, addresses, and telephone numbers of radiologists and physicists associated with the scanner.

1. _____

_____

2. _____

_____

3. _____

_____

4. _____

_____

5. _____

_____

32. Price

Please offer price on an attached formal quotation. The price is to be FOB at this institution for the CT scanner installed, fully operational, and capable of meeting the specifications listed above (Sections 1 through 30).

Manufacturer: _____

Model: _____

This information and bid was prepared by:

Name: _____

Title: _____

Address: _____

_____

_____

_____

Phone: (___) _____

Signature: _____

Date: _____

in some cases), and installation of a treatment unit with this capability requires additional space for the shielding.

The choice of beam energy depends upon the clinical needs and capabilities of the department. For example, a department planning to install only a single unit (or replacing an existing simple unit) should consider the reliability, as well as the capability, of the unit. Excessive downtime may offset any benefit derived from an advanced treatment capability. Low energy photon beam units (4 to 6 million volts (MV)) have demonstrated superior reliability and should be the foremost contender for a single unit department.

Departments with two or more treatment units in place or proposed might consider a higher energy photon beam for its increased penetration. Electron beam capability may also be desired for treatment of superficial lesions with simultaneous protection of deeper tissues.

Photon energy frequently is specified as the energy of the electron beam incident upon the x-ray target. The resulting beam of bremsstrahlung x-rays will have a maximum energy equal to the electron energy and a mean energy of approximately one-third the maximum.

Electron beam energy is most conveniently specified at the entrance surface of a patient or phantom. The beam energy at this location generally is lower by perhaps 1 MeV than the energy of the beam as it exits from the accelerator guide. This decrease reflects the energy lost by the beam as it traverses a bending magnet, a scattering foil, and a distance of typically 1 m to the patient. While some manufacturers specify the beam energy at the exit window of the accelerator, this location is inaccessible to the user. In practice, the energy of the electron beam at the treatment distance is determined from the range of the beam in water. Procedures have been described for determining the most probable energy and the mean energy (20–23). Therefore, it is logical to specify the energy at the patient surface. An alternative to specifying electron beam energy is to specify the beam characteristics in a water phantom. Often, one specifies the depth on the central axis at which the dose falls to 80% of the dose at the depth of maximum dose (d_{max}).

The energy spectrum of the electron beam as it impinges upon the phantom surface defines the shape of the depth dose curve. For an electron beam of stated energy, a narrow energy spectrum produces a decreased surface dose, a greater depth of maximum dose, and a steeper fall-off at depths past d_{max}. The maximum dose rate from a betatron is usually lower than that from an accelerator, so that treatment times are longer (24).

Some accelerators are equipped with scanning electron beams rather than scattering foils, with the advantage that the electron beam loses less energy in traversing a scanning electromagnet system than a scattering foil. However, dosimetry of scanning-beam accelerators is considerably more difficult because very high instantaneous dose rates are encountered by measuring equipment. The hazard imposed by a faulty scanning mechanism requires safety monitoring devices.

The dose rate required for a treatment unit should be specified in detail. For convenience and consistency, dose rate is usually specified at the isocenter or at the nominal SSD, in a 10-cm square field, at the depth of maximum dose in a phantom. A dose rate of between 200 and 300 rad/min is acceptable for most routine work. Higher dose rate capability may be desirable for treatments at large distances (e.g., total body irradiation). The use of beam modifiers such as wedges and compensators reduces the dose rate incident on the patient surface. Extensive use of these devices may warrant higher dose rate capabilities.

The variation in dose rate with field size should not exceed approximately ±10% in photon beams over the normal range of field sizes. On the other hand, this variation may be considerably greater with electron beams, depending upon the type of treatment unit.

Control of the dose rate of an accelerator by the operator is generally provided, and may permit continuous variation from some minimum to the maximum dose rate available. Many accelerators, however, provide an incremental adjustment of dose rate. This method of control may be sufficient for most circumstances. Only in situations requiring unusually high or low dose rates is greater control desirable.

The maximum and minimum field dimensions should be specified to ensure that sufficiently large fields are available without having to resort to extended treatment distances. For acceptance testing and routine quality assurance, it is convenient to be able to close the collimator completely, even though this capability has no clinical value. Some newer accelerators permit independent movement of each collimator jaw to allow asymmetrical setups. This capability may be useful in some situations but clearly increases the complexity of the unit. The wide variation in unusual field shapes and sizes greatly increases the number of measurements required to fully characterize the treatment unit.

Some collimators reveal rounded corners at large field sizes. If this is undesirable, square corners up to the maximum field size should be specified. The purchase specifications should indicate whether motorized control of the collimator is required and, if so, where the controls should be located. The specifications should also state whether single speed motors are acceptable or if two speed or variable speed motors are required.

All accelerators provide separate collimation systems for use with electron beams. Most often these collimators are cones of fixed sizes that are mechanically attached to the treatment unit. There is considerable variation in the design of the cones, their weight, the range and number of sizes available, and the ability to attach additional field-shaping devices. Electron cones of variable size are available, but the specifications should be examined closely to ensure that the resulting beams are controlled adequately. A wide variety of field shapes and sizes is possible with variable electron cones, and full characterization of the electron beams can be extensive and time-consuming.

It is useful to specify the field flatness and symmetry desired of the radiation beam (25). Most manufacturers publish their own specifications, and it is unreasonable to expect them to agree willingly to alterations. However, the purchaser should identify the degree of nonuniformity and asymmetry that can be tolerated. Recommended levels of flatness and symmetry have been developed by the International Electrotechnical Commission (IEC) (26).

Whether arc therapy capability is desired should be stated, even though such capability is standard on many units. Aspects of the unit's arc therapy performance should be characterized, such as the range of permissible angular dose rates (in rads per degree) and the manner and precision with which the dose rate is selected. The accuracy and uniformity of this parameter should be specified, as well as the speed and consistency of gantry rotation. The method of regulation should be investigated; some accelerators vary gantry rotation speed while holding the dose rate constant, while others modulate the beam to deliver a precise dose as the gantry moves through each increment of arc.

The purchaser should investigate the source of radiation utilized by each piece of equipment under consideration. If an isotope source is desired, the choices are few, and the decision is simple. If an accelerator is being considered, several aspects of operation must be investigated. For example, the source of RF energy used to accelerate electrons in a linear accelerator may be either a klystron or a magnetron. Because of the difference in power capability between the two devices, a klystron is probably preferable for higher energy units. The magnetron is inherently a simpler device and is preferable for use with low energy accelerators. Whether the accelerator employs bending magnets has a significant impact on its reliability and simplicity. In all but the lowest energy accelerators (4 to 6 MV), bending magnets are required because the accelerating structure is too long to be mounted colinearly with the treatment beam. The use of achromatic bending magnets provides greater stability and is a desirable feature. Such considerations have no bearing on the selection of a betatron.

An important factor in the design of an accelerator is the operation of the dosimetry system. It is critical that the dosimetry circuitry not only measure the delivery of dose accurately and reliably, but also monitor beam symmetry and flatness in the case of bent-beam accelerators. The design of dosimetry systems varies from one manufacturer to another. To reduce the degradation and scattering of electron beams, at least one manufacturer substitutes a separate mesh-walled ion chamber system when the electron beam mode is selected. The design of the chamber requires that it remain open to the atmosphere. This design requires the use of additional sensors and circuitry to compensate for temperature and pressure fluctuations. Some variation in response still may be observed (27).

Some of the mechanical requirements (such as an isocentric vs stand-mounted mechanical support system) of the treatment unit can be established early in the specification process. Other aspects may be specified later in the process. For example, some treatment units are provided with fixed beam stoppers, retractable beam stoppers, or counterweights. Most users prefer a counterweight-equipped unit, because the absence of a beam stopper permits easier access to the patient and greater flexibility in treatment setup. Deletion of a beam stopper is not always practical, however, since substantially thicker walls are required for adequate shielding. The range and speed of motor-driven motion should be specified, as should the accuracy of scales or digital displays of position. For example, the minimum distance above the floor to which the treatment couch may be lowered should be specified, since this will affect routine operation. The speed of motor-driven motions is important; if they are too slow, the operators may become impatient or frustrated; if they are too fast, the risk of a collision or injury is increased.

For most purchasers, the size, distribution, and appearance of the components of the piece of equipment play some role in the purchase decision. From a patient's viewpoint, as well as that of an administrator, appearance is rather important. The customer rarely has any input into the design of steel or fiberglass covers, but the arrangement of the various components and the means by which pipes and cables are routed may be specified.

The characteristics of the devices to position the patient for treatment should be specified. These devices include a front pointer, an optical distance indicator, a field-defining light, and wall and ceiling positioning lights. Aspects to be specified might include light intensity, agreement of the light field with the radiation field and with the distance from a reference point on the treatment unit. A backpointer is a useful item and is not always provided. Additional capabilities to be specified might include control over the room lights from the treatment unit console, capability to open the collimator automatically for port films with a safety interlock to limit the dose and, possibly, provision for port filming at a lower photon energy than the standard treatment beam.

The maximum tolerable leakage radiation should be specified and should include such items as head leakage, beam stopper transmission, and other radiation-producing components such as a klystron. Such emission must conform to state and Federal requirements. For high-energy units, the resulting photoneutron production must be considered in light of up-to-date requirements and regulations.

The purchaser should consider aspects of routine operation and safety. It may be useful to specify a preference for modality and energy selection, desired safety interlocks, the design of dosimetry interlocks and their redundancy, and the presence and protection against electrical, thermal, and optical hazards.

An important feature of the purchase specifications package is the part that deals with assurance of proper operation following installation. This part includes consideration of features such as the warranty, service contract, availability of services, operator training, and a list of satisfied users. These features are similar to those described earlier for various imaging devices.

Simulator

As described in the appendix, a radiation therapy simulator is a combination of two pieces of equipment. In many cases, the simulator consists of a fairly standard radiographic and fluoroscopic x-ray imaging system, mounted on a mechanical structure designed to be similar to, and reproduce the motions of, a radiation therapy unit. Because of the complex nature of the design of a simulator, the preparation of purchase specifications must follow those of both a treatment unit and a radiographic system. As is the case with other pieces of equipment, the needs of the department must be kept in mind when specifying the capabilities desired. Initially, the overall purpose of the simulator must be determined. Will the simulator be used to develop, in an interactive fashion, an optimal treatment plan, or will the simulator be used simply to document the treatment plan already determined by a physician? The answer to this question will determine the complexity of the proposed piece of equipment.

These two components of the typical simulator, the radiographic system and the simulator mechanical frame, frequently are developed and supplied by different manufacturers. Therefore, it is logical to address each component separately and develop distinct performance specifications for each one.

Complete descriptions of simulators and comparisons between a number of available systems may be found in references 28 and 29.

The radiologic system consists of an x-ray generator, an x-ray tube, and, if necessary, a fluoroscopic imaging system. X-ray generators are available which operate either in single phase or three-phase mode, with secondary voltages of up to 150 kVp or more, and capacities of 600 mA or greater. Radiation therapy simulation is not as demanding on a radiologic system as many diagnostic imaging procedures, and these extremes in capability are not required. A single-phase generator is generally adequate, as long as the generator provides a capacity of 500 mA at 90 kVp. A maximum secondary voltage of 125 kVp should be acceptable. The generator should be provided with primary solid-state contacting, automatic line voltage regulation, and automatic kVp and space charge compensation. Tube and generator overload protective circuitry is highly desirable, as is the capability for high-speed rotation with rapid acceleration. An anode heat integrator is an extremely useful device and represents only a small increase in the total cost of the system.

The choice of an x-ray tube represents a compromise between the high resolution that may be obtained with small focal spots and the increased power rating and full coverage of the x-ray field available with larger focal spots. Dual focus tubes are most often specified, so that both high resolution and a high power rating may be available when

required. Useful focal spot sizes are in the range of 0.6 mm to 1.2 mm. A target angle should be specified which provides full coverage of a 45- × 45-cm field at 100 cm from the target, to match the largest field size available from the department's treatment units. The power rating of the x-ray tube should be chosen to match closely the available generator power over the range of available kilovoltage.

The fluoroscopic imaging system should include the following components: the image intensifier; an automatic brightness control; a TV chain, including a monitor; and a cassette holder. The characteristics of the fluoroscopic imaging system which are of greatest importance to the users of a simulator are the contrast and spatial resolution and the field coverage available. As a result, the construction of the devices is not crucial, provided these minimum capabilities are met. Naturally, the user would want to consider the history of reliability of each component, as well as the actual imaging characteristics. Frequent use will be made of the cassette holder, and its characteristics should not be neglected. It should be designed to accommodate cassettes up to 14 inches × 17 inches and should be rotatable. This last capability not only allows insertion of the cassette from any angle, which makes the technologist's job much easier, but also allows the dimensions of the cassette to be oriented with respect to the anatomy of interest.

The simulator frame consists of a gantry, which supports the x-ray tube, collimator, image intensifier, and a patient support couch. The gantry assembly must allow for a variable source-to-axis distance over a range which duplicates the treatment equipment available in the department. In addition, increased source-to-axis distance is often desirable to duplicate treatment at extended source to skin distances. Due to the presence of the image intensifier, the simulator couch often may not be moved to as low a setting as the treatment couch; therefore, to simulate extended source to skin distance treatment, the tube head must be raised a corresponding distance. The mechanical rigidity of the simulator frame is of paramount importance. The frame must support the x-ray tube and the image intensifier in a fashion which allows isocentric stability that is comparable to that of the treatment units. This isocentric stability should be maintained through all of the motions of the gantry.

The collimator also must duplicate the motions of the treatment units. Rotation of plus and minus 180° is desirable, although provided by only a few manufacturers. In practice, it is not necessary that the collimator rotate to any greater extent than the collimators of the treatment units. The collimator should be equipped with a beam-shaping platform which may be positioned at distances corresponding to those of the department's treatment units. The beam-shaping platform and the collimator bearings must be designed to support conventional lead and cerrobend blocks, since verification of blocks is an important function of a simulator. The purchaser should verify that the use of lead and cerrobend blocks will not affect the isocenter tolerances.

As is the case with the other equipment, the patient support couch should duplicate the couches provided with the treatment units. Important specifications that should be considered for the treatment couch include the range of motions available, the ability of the couch to support heavy patients, and the deflection of the couch top that would be experienced when a heavy patient is positioned for a treatment. The table top construction should not interfere with the radiologic imaging ability of the simulator. The range of couch motions should facilitate patient handling and positioning.

For ease of operation, the simulator control panel and control functions should be similar to those of the department's treatment units. Position displays should be provided for all motions and should be designed along the same angle and coordinate conventions as the treatment unit displays.

Certain safety features are desirable with a simulator. Emergency Off buttons which remove all power from the simulator and the x-ray system should be provided. Some state regulations require that a positive action be made by the operator to re-set the machine after operation of an emergency Off button. The simulator should include mechanical stops and electrical limits which prevent motions from exceeding reasonable limits. Motions which are equipped with mechanical stops should incorporate slip clutches in the drive mechanism. Collision detection or avoidance systems should be provided on the tube head, collimator, and the image intensifier. Anticollision devices should permit motion of the affected component in the direction away from the collision. Some simulators are equipped with microcomputers which continuously monitor the location of each component and modify the motions requested by the operator to avoid collisions. While such systems convey a sense of security and safety, the purchaser should verify that the system exhibits a reasonable level of reliability. It is important to recognize that a false sense of security can be encouraged by the use of such systems.

The purchase specifications should also identify the acceptance testing procedure that is proposed by the prospective purchaser. Some of the aspects of performance of radiologic imaging systems may be evaluated by a variety of acceptable techniques, which provide substantially different results. Therefore, it is prudent to seek the manufacturers agreement to the proposed test procedures before the equipment is purchased. References 30, 31, and 32 describe recommended test procedures suitable in many cases to simulators.

Treatment Planning Computer

The selection of a treatment planning computer is a rather personal endeavor. While the commercially available systems vary considerably in capabilities, hardware, and calculation algorithms, a very important criterion, and one which may determine just how often the computer is used, is the degree to which the operator feels comfortable with the system. A treatment planning computer which provides highly accurate treatment plans, but which is extremely difficult to use on a routine basis, is likely to be used only in unusual circumstances. On the other hand, it is important to guard against the purchase of a system which is very "user friendly," but which provides inaccurate dose distributions. Therefore, the prospective purchaser of a treatment planning system should, whenever possible, arrange to spend time at the keyboard of every system under consideration, performing treatment plans of the type frequently done in that institution. In this fashion, both the accuracy of the plans and the ease with which they are generated may be evaluated.

At the moment, treatment planning systems are available from at least 12 manufacturers. The differences between the systems are considerable, as are the prices. The recent availability of faster, more powerful computers, microprocessors, and array processors, makes the variation between systems, even those of a single manufacturer, even more pronounced. The choice of a suitable system represents a formidable task for the prospective purchaser, as it requires the consideration of a large number of variables (33).

For convenience, it is appropriate to divide the capabilities of the treatment planning computer into two categories: external beam dosimetry and implant dosimetry. External beam dosimetry may or may not include the dosimetry of irregularly shaped fields. Some manufacturers offer a separate set of programs for irregular field dosimetry.

It may be convenient, when specifying a treatment planning system, to consider separately the hardware and software. Once again, this is a rather personal decision, as the hardware selected by one user may be considered completely unacceptable by another user. For example, some users of com-

puter systems find certain display monitors uncomfortable to look at for extended periods. In addition, the hardware required will depend to some extent on the degree to which the user will become involved in the design and programming of the system. Some treatment planners have extensive computer experience and are interested in applying their own modifications to the software. (It should be noted that, in some cases, manufacturers discourage or actually prevent this practice.) In other institutions, the computer will be used not only for treatment planning, but for general purpose computer work. In such circumstances, additional hardware may be necessary to provide the user with the capabilities he desires. In any case, the computer must be provided with sufficient hardware to support all of the capabilities requested by the purchaser. This will include, at a minimum, devices for the entry of patient contours; the transfer of CT scans, if desired; the entry of data describing the users treatment units; a keyboard and monitor for user interaction with the system and possibly an additional monitor for displaying CT images and isodose curves; and a device for the hard copy output of the completed treatment plan. The prospective purchaser may be limited in his choices to some of these items to those provided by the

Table 4.15
External Beam Planning

1. *Field Sizes:* Minimum, maximum required for compatibility with treatment units.
2. *SSD and SAD:* Should be compatible with treatment units.
3. *Plane of Calculations:* Planes aligned with the central axis of the beams, planes parallel to the beam central axes, planes which are not parallel to the central axes of the beams, and planes parallel to the central axes, but representing collimator rotation.
4. *Normalization:* Desirable to normalize to the depth of maximum dose, the isocenter, or any other point selected by the user.
5. *Beam Data Entry:* Ability to enter measured beam data is desirable; however, the ability to generate beam data analytically provides greater convenience and flexibility for the user. Accurate representation of rectangular fields is required, as is modification of the beam by wedges and blocks.
6. *Corrections for Oblique Incidence and Heterogeneities:* Corrections should be suitably accurate and should be realistic for both photon and electron beams.
7. *Arc Therapy:* Capability for photon beams is essential; capability for electron beams may be desirable.
8. *Combination of Beams:* Combinations of SSD and isocentric photon beams, together with electron beams, is desirable.
9. *Accuracy:* The accuracy desired should be specified in both high dose gradient regions and low dose gradient regions. Accurate calculations in the buildup region may be desirable.
10. *Irregular Field Calculations:* The ability to decompose the dose calculation into contributions from primary and scattered radiation with the capability of drawing isodose curves is desirable.

Table 4.16
External Beam Planning—Implant Dosimetry

1. *Data Entry:* Entry of source locations should be from orthogonal or stereo films or by input of source coordinates through keyboard.
2. *Capacity:* Program should handle largest implant likely to be performed by institution.
3. *Source Entry:* Techniques for entering source locations should be as convenient and rapid as possible.
4. *Sources available:* A large variety of source data should be available to encompass all implants likely to be performed.
5. *Calculations:* Correction for tissue attenuation is desirable. Correction for heterogeneities may be desirable.
6. *Display:* Sufficient user interaction is required to allow orientation of implant in any plane.
7. *Normalization:* Dose distributions should be available in terms of dose rate at time of implant and total dose.

manufacturer, although in other cases the user may be able to specify certain pieces of hardware.

In selecting the treatment planning software, the prospective purchaser must consider the requirements of the department. Departments which routinely practice unusually complex and innovative treatment techniques will require treatment planning software with more extensive capabilities and greater flexibility for adapting to unusual situations. In exchange, these institutions will probably be willing to sacrifice some operator convenience.

Lists of items which users may wish to consider in selecting software are provided in Tables 4.15 and 4.16. These tables are intended not as exhaustive lists of important characteristics, but as a starting point for developing a list of items to consider.

References

1. Hendee WR, Rossi R P: Performance specifications for diagnostic radiological equipment—a delicate interface between purchaser and supplier. *Proceedings of the Society for Photooptical Instrumentation Engineers.* Bellingham, WA, Sept 1975, vol 70, pp 238–242.
2. Hendee WR, Rossi RP: Performance specifications for diagnostic x-ray equipment. *Proceedings of the Society for Photooptical Instrumentation Engineers.* Bellingham, WA, 1980, vol 233, pp 279–281.
3. Workshop in Purchase Specifications and Performance Evaluation of Radiological Imaging Equipment. Midwest Chapter AAPM, Chicago, May 12–13, 1978.
4. Hendee WR, Rossi RP: Performance specifications for diagnostic x-ray equipment. *Radiology* 120:409–412, 1976.
5. National Electrical Manufacturers Association (NEMA): *Performance Measurements of Scintillation Cameras.* Washington, DC, Standards Publication No. NU1-1980, 1980.
6. Raff U, Spitzer VM, Hendee WR: Practicality of NEMA performance specification measurements for user-based acceptance testing and routine quality assurance. *J Nucl Med* 25:679–687, 1984.
7. Strand S-E, Larsson I: Image artifacts at high fluence rates in single-crystal NaI(Tl) scintillation cameras. *J Nucl Med* 19:407–413, 1978.
8. Adams R, Hine GJ, Zimmerman CD: Deadtime measurements in scintillation cameras under scatter conditions simulating quantitative nuclear cardiography. *J Nucl Med* 19:538–543, 1978.
9. Chapman DR, Garcia EV, Waxman AD: Misalignment of multiple photopeak analyzer outputs: effects on imaging. *J Nucl Med* 21:872–874, 1980.
10. Paras P, Hine GJ, Adams R: BRH test pattern for the evaluation of gamma-camera performance. *J Nucl Med* 22:468–470, 1981.
11. Spiers EW, Feiglin DHI, Cocks NCF: A method for the remote acquisition of gated nuclear medicine images. *Radiology* 145:548–550, 1982.
12. Harris CL: Transmission of gamma camera signals over long coaxial cables. *Radiology* 142:525–527, 1982.
13. Carson PL, Zagzebski JA (eds): *Pulse Echo Ultrasound Imaging Systems: Performance Tests and Criteria,* American Association of Physicists in Medicine, Report 8. New York, American Institute of Physics, 1981.
14. Goldstein A: *Quality Assurance in Routine Preventive Maintenance in Clinics and Diagnostic Ultrasound. New Techniques and Instrumentation.* New York, Churchill Livingstone, 1981, vol 5.
15. National Electrical Manufacturers Association (NEMA): *Safety Standard for Diagnostic Ultrasound Equipment.* AIUM/NEMA Standards Publication No. UL1-1981. Washington, DC, American Institute of Ultrasound in Medicine. 1981.
16. Dick DE, Carson PL: Principles of autoscan ultrasound instrumentation. In Fullerton GD, Zagzebski, JA (eds): *Medical Physics of CT and Ultrasound: Tissue Imaging and Characterization.* New York, American Institute of Physics, No. 329. 1980.
17. Shope TB, Gagne RM, Johnson GC: A method for describing the doses delivered by transmission x-ray computed tomography. *Med Phys* 8:488–495, 1981.
18. Karzmark CJ, Pering NC: Electron linear accelerators for radiation therapy: history, principles, and

contemporary developments. *Phys Med Biol* 18:321–354, 1973.

19. Galvin JM: The physics of radiation therapy equipment. *Semin Oncol* 8:18–37, March 1981.
20. Radiation Therapy Committee, AAPM: A protocol for the determination of absorbed dose from high-energy photon and electron beams. Report of Task Group 21. *Med Phys* 10(6), Nov/Dec 1983.
21. Nordic Association of Clinical Physics: Procedures in external radiation therapy dosimetry with electron and photon beams with maximum energies between 1 and 50 MeV. *Acta Radiol Oncol* Suppl 20, 1981.
22. Markus B: Energibestimmung schneller elektronen aus tiefendosiskurven. *Strahlentherapie* 116:280, 1961. Beitrage zur entwicklung der dosimetrie schneller electronen. *Strahlentherapie* 124:33, 1964.
23. Almond PR: Radiation physics of electron beams. In Tapley N (ed): *Clinical Applications of the Electron Beam.* New York, Wiley, 1976.
24. Johns HE, Cunningham JR: *The Physics of Radiology,* ed 3. Springfield IL, Charles C Thomas, 1978.
25. Science Council of AAPM by Task Group 10 of the Radiation Therapy Committee (P. Wootton, Chairman): Code of practice for x-ray therapy linear accelerators. *Med Phys* 2:110–121, May/June 1975.
26. International Electrotechnical Commission: TC 62, Subcommittee 62 C.
27. Sharma C, Wilson DL, Jose B: Variation of output with atmospheric pressure and ambient temperature for Therac-20 linear accelerator. *Med Phys* 10:712, 1983.
28. British Institute of Radiology Working Party: *Treatment Simulators.* Special Report No. 10 on the Applications of Modern Technology in Radiotherapy.
29. McCullough EC, Earle JD: The selection, acceptance testing, and quality control of radiotherapy treatment simulators. *Radiology* 131:221–230, 1979.
30. Rauch PL, Block RW: Acceptance testing experience with fourteen new installations. *Proceedings of the Society for Photooptical Instrumentation Engineers.* Bellingham, WA, Sept 16–19, 1976.
31. Hendee WR, Rossi RP: *Quality Assurance for Radiographic X-Ray Units and Associated Equipment.* HEW Publication (FDA) 79-8094, August 1979.
32. Hendee WR, Rossi RP: *Quality Assurance for Fluoroscopic X-Ray Units and Associated Equipment.* HEW Publication (FDA) 80-8095, October 1979.
33. McCullough EC, Edmundson G, Kisrow K: *Selection of A Treatment Planning System.* Orlando, FL, ASTR Exhibit, October 1982.

CHAPTER FIVE

Development and Selection of a Bid

WILLIAM R. HENDEE, Ph.D.

INTRODUCTION

As part of the process of evaluating clinical needs and developing performance specifications for a particular item of radiologic equipment, a list is compiled of manufacturers who may be able to supply equipment compatible with the performance specifications. This list describes the potential vendors who should receive the institution's request to bid on the desired equipment. The request for bid contains three items. The first item is a cover letter describing the desired equipment in rather general terms, a deadline for bid submission, and dates for the pre-bid conference and formal bid opening. Also included is the name of the individual to be contacted if some aspect of the bid request is unclear. The second item in the bid request is the compilation of performance specifications, prepared as described in Chapter 4. The third part is the description of acceptance test methods and the criteria for acceptable performance, as described in Chapter 7. All three documents are distributed in a package that constitutes the bid request, and the potential vendors are asked to respond to the request as a package, since the information in all three documents ultimately will be referenced in the purchase order.

Often it is useful to conduct a pre-bid conference a week or two after the bid requests have been distributed. All potential vendors are invited to this conference with instructions to raise any questions they may have about the bid request. In this manner, all potential vendors are assured of receiving the same information if they attend the pre-bid conference. This conference often also reduces the time required to respond to questions received from potential vendors on an individual basis.

Once the pre-bid conference has been held, the purchasing institution usually can await the receipt of bids without further disturbance. The deadline for receipt of bids must be stated explicitly in the bid request, and no exceptions should ever be made to this deadline. The bids are to be submitted in sealed envelopes and should be opened at an appointed time. Some institutions invite the potential vendors to the bid opening; others feel that this is an unnecessary formality.

Once the bids have been opened, the successful vendor should be chosen, and all vendors should be notified of the decision concerning their bid proposals. These actions should be conducted as expeditiously as possible. In cases where the successful vendor is not the lowest bidder, a written justification for vendor selection may be required as institutional policy. With a detailed set of performance specifications, justification of the successful vendor should present few difficulties. As an example, Table 5.1 presents a summary of the justification of the successful vendor for a film-screen x-ray mammographic unit.

For the unsuccessful bidders, a letter informing them that the successful bidder is another vendor usually is sufficient. For the successful bidder, on the other hand, notification usually includes a purchase order specifying the equipment desired. It is very important that the purchase order include the bid proposal by reference, as well as the performance specifications and acceptance tests prepared by the purchaser and agreed to by the vendor. An example of a purchase order written in the recommended fashion is reproduced in Figure 5.1. By appropriate referencing, the performance specifications, bid proposal, and acceptance test criteria are included in the purchase order and are considered a formal contract between purchaser and vendor. Upon equipment installation, any noncompliance with the performance specifications and acceptance test criteria,

Table 5.1
Justification of Vendor Selection for a Film-Screen X-Ray Mammographic Unit

Vendor	Cost	Exclusions	Delivery date	Focal spot size	Terms
A	$72,000	No automatic exposure control (list price: $5,500) No viewing table (list price: $6,600) No automatic compression device (not available).	90–120 days from receipt of order.	0.09 mm/0.45 mm	10% on order; 80% on delivery; 10% on first clinical use.
B	$82,000	None	60 days from receipt of order.	0.2 mm/0.6 mm	10% on order; 70% on delivery; 20% on first clinical use.
C	$68,032	No dual focal spot capabilities (not available).	Nine months from receipt of order.	0.2 mm × 0.3 mm to 0.4 mm × 0.4 mm	10% on order; 80% on delivery; 10% on first clinical use.

UNIVERSITY OF COLORADO MEDICAL CENTER

PURCHASE REQUEST

ACCT. NO. TO BE CHGD. 2-5-35002 — CLASS / / / / / / /

NAME OF ACCT. TO BE CHGD. Radiology Equipment

DEPARTMENT RADIOLOGY - Diagnostic Radiology

DELIVER TO Diagnostic Radiology — ROOM NO. 2203

DATE OF REQUEST April 15, 1983 — MAIL BOX NO. ---

PURCHASING DIV. F.O.B. / / / / / / / — VIA / / / / / / / / / / — CASH TERMS / / / / / / / / / — BUYER / / / / / — DATE / / / / /

QUANTITY	UNIT	DESCRIPTION OF MATERIAL (COMPLETE SPECIFICATIONS PREVENT ERROR.)	PURCH. DEPT. ONLY	ESTIMATED COST
1	ea	Diagnostic Mammographic Unit as per bid proposal equipment requirements, performance specifications and acceptance test procedures as specified on attached 12 pages.	$	82,000

REQUESTED BY / / / / / / / — EXTENSION NO. / / / / / / / — SUGGESTED VENDORS Vendor B

APPPROVED BY DEPT. HEAD / — / / / / / / / / / / / / / /

APPROVED BY FINANCE / — / / / / / / / / / / / / / /

FORM 2 — PLEASE MAKE OUT A SEPARATE PURCHASE REQUEST FOR EACH CLASS OF ITEM.

Figure 5.1. Example of a Purchase order.

and their modifications in the vendor's bid, become a breach of contract which has a straightforward legal interpretation should events progress to that point.

Once the purchase order is delivered to the vendor and accepted according to the terms of the bid response, a period of waiting ensues while the vendor prepares to deliver the desired equipment. The purchasing institution uses this time to prepare a site for eventual installation of the equipment. Site preparation is covered in the next chapter.

CHAPTER SIX

Facility Preparation and Planning

RAYMOND P. ROSSI, M.S.

INTRODUCTION

In this chapter, general guidance is offered in the area of facility preparation and planning for diagnostic medical imaging systems. Primary emphasis is given to aspects of project management and general facility requirements, rather than to detailed specifications such as square footage requirements for different types of imaging facilities and equipment configurations; extensive discussion of these aspects of facility design is available in numerous publications (1–5). A project management tool known as the critical path method is illustrated by its application to a general purpose radiographic/fluoroscopic suite.

Goals of Facility Preparation and Planning

When planning the construction of a new facility or the renovation of an existing facility to accommodate one or more diagnostic medical imaging systems, it is essential that the planning and preparation be carried out with several important goals in mind. The goals include minimizing the: (1) time required to prepare the facility to accept the equipment; (2) time required to install the equipment; (3) interruptions to clinical service; and (4), cost associated with the specific project. Achievement of these goals is desirable whether dealing with a completely new facility or with the renovation of an existing facility. Achievement of these goals depends largely on how well the project is planned initially and how well it is supervised and monitored during its evaluation. This chapter presents some approaches to project management which have been found to be particularly useful in achieving the goals outlined above.

General Considerations in Facility Planning and Preparation

In the following discussion of facility planning and preparation, it is assumed that the equipment to be installed has been selected, the clinical requirements and performance specifications for the equipment have been determined, and the successful vendor has been identified.

PURCHASE ORDER

The first element in facility planning and preparation is proper wording of the purchase order for the equipment. There are several issues that the purchase order should address to expedite the planning process.

1. The purchase order should reference the vendor's specific quotation number for the desired equipment. This reference ensures that no confusion should arise regarding the specifics of the desired equipment.
2. The purchase order should reference the bid document associated with the equipment. This reference is particularly important because performance specifications and acceptance testing methods have been delineated in the bid document.
3. The purchase order should specify who is responsible for each phase of facility construction and renovation. In general, this responsibility will be shared between equipment purchaser and vendor. Usually the purchaser is responsible for the actual construction and renovation of the facility, and the vendor is responsible for providing detailed drawings and the mechanical, electrical, and plumbing specifications required for the equipment. Occasionally the equipment vendor may act as the general contractor; in this case, the responsibilities as general contractor should be specified. It is also useful to identify the responsibility for union labor costs associated with equipment installation, if only union labor is available for installation of the equipment.
4. The purchase order should identify the

responsibility for removing existing equipment when the project involves an existing facility. When old equipment is traded in, the vendor normally removes the equipment as part of the quoted price. For leased equipment, on the other hand, it may be necessary to budget separately for removal costs.

5. The purchase order should describe the schedule for delivery and installation of the equipment. In general, delivery and installation schedules should be referenced to the date of "receipt of order" by the vendor. Specification of delivery and installation schedules is especially important when penalty clauses have been incorporated as part of the bid document; otherwise, questions can arise regarding nonconformance to the schedules.

6. The purchase order should state that the vendor is responsible for site acceptance once the construction and renovation have been completed. Once the site is accepted, any changes requested by the vendor are provided at the vendor's cost.

7. If performance specifications are delineated in the bid document and acceptance testing is to be performed, the purchase order should clearly reference the agreed upon performance levels and the methods by which acceptable performance will be determined.

8. The purchase order should specify the dates when working and final drawings of the facility construction and renovation requirements will be provided to the facility by the vendor.

9. The purchase order should clearly state that the equipment is to be "free on board" (f.o.b.) at the purchaser's site; in this manner, costs associated with shipping do not become an additional expense to the purchasing institution.

Attention to the proper wording of the purchase order will assist in the proper planning and preparation of a facility for new equipment.

Specific Considerations in Facility Planning

In planning a facility for radiological imaging equipment there are several important factors that require detailed consideration. These factors include (1) electrical power requirements; (2) mechanical requirements; and (3) other utility requirements.

ELECTRICAL REQUIREMENTS

These requirements may be separated into primary and secondary requirements.

Primary Requirements

All radiological imaging systems require one or more sources of electrical power for their operation. The exact requirements for the power sources depend on the type of equipment and range from a standard 110 volts ac (VAC) line to a dedicated 480 VAC line with high current capacity. For radiological imaging equipment it is generally considered good practice to use power sources dedicated to the specific piece of equipment, rather than those already in use. Dedicated lines eliminate potential problems caused by excessive line loading. Radiological imaging equipment often places heavy loads on a power source for relatively short periods (e.g., a radiographic unit during exposure). It is essential that the power source have the capacity to provide the required power under maximum load; otherwise, the performance of the equipment may be compromised. All manufacturers provide specifications for the power source; these specifications must be followed.

Secondary Requirements

Secondary power sources also are frequently required for functions such as table motion, tilt, and drive for a radiographic-fluoroscopic (R-F) unit, etc. These sources must be provided as specified by the vendor. It is frequently desirable to have a separate circuit breaker for the secondary power sources to facilitate servicing of the equipment. With the increasing use of computer systems in medical imaging, isolated power sources with protection from transient voltages and noise are becoming increasingly important.

MECHANICAL REQUIREMENTS

Mechanical requirements depend on the type of equipment and vary from extremely simple to quite complex. In the past, facilities have frequently been designed to accommodate a specific vendor's equipment; replacement of the equipment often requires time-consuming and costly renovations. This problem has been particularly prevalent with radiographic/fluoroscopic equipment. Several methods are available to overcome the problem. When planning new or renovated facilities, as much information as possible should be obtained from different vendors regarding the facility requirements for their equipment. By combining the information, it often is possible to develop a facility design that incorporates a universal approach to facility requirements. Particular attention should be given to electrical conduit and troughing runs, as these are likely to exhibit the greatest variance among different vendors. Ceiling support structures are accommodated best by the use of a universal ceiling grid using components, such as Unistrut, that permit the installation of any component that must be suspended overhead. A similar approach can be used for floors by installation of computer style flooring that provides an open space of 6 inches or so below its surface. Interconnect cabling can be run in this space.

The siting of major components of the system such as high voltage transformers and power units should be given special consideration from the point of service access. In particular, those components should not be installed in locations where access is difficult. Lighting requirements for the facility should be carefully planned. It is not uncommon to find procedure suites where poor illumination makes work difficult and tiresome. Satisfactory lighting often involves the use of both incandescent and fluorescent lights. The fluorescent lighting is operated by a standard "On-Off" switch, and the incandescent lighting is controlled by a dimmer switch. When properly designed, this configuration provides any desired level of room illumination.

OTHER UTILITY REQUIREMENTS

Some imaging equipment requires water and special ventilation (e.g., equipment with dedicated film processors); these requirements must be considered in planning the facility.

Environmental control of the facility should also be thought out. Not only is the temperature and humidity of the facility important to the comfort of the staff, but also the increasing use of computers in medical imaging necessitates very rigid control of the environment.

Steps in Facility Planning and Preparation

Execution of the process of planning and preparing a site for installation of medical imaging equipment is achieved best by following specific steps.

1. As discussed previously, the first step is issuance of the purchase order.
2. The next step is obtaining a set of working drawings from the vendor that provide a detailed layout of the equipment in the room, along with the electrical, mechanical, and environmental specifications for the equipment. Ideally, these drawings should be available within 30 days following the issuance of a purchase order.
3. These drawings should be provided to the general contractor who is to handle the construction and renovation of the facility. Representatives of the facility and the equipment vendor should meet with the general contractor to review the drawings and make any modifications necessary for installation of the equipment.
4. A set of final drawings should then be prepared. These drawings will guide the actual construction and renovation of the facility. The final drawings should be reviewed and signed by all parties involved in the project.
5. Following acceptance of the final drawings, the actual construction and renovation of the facility may commence. Where equipment must be removed from an existing facility, the removal should be scheduled so that the new equipment will arrive when the renovation is just completed. In this manner, the disruption of clinical services can be minimized along with the storage time for the replacement equipment.
6. Once the facility has been completed and the equipment delivered, installation of the equipment can begin. A representative of the facility should carefully monitor the equipment in-

stallation to ensure that it is conducted properly and that nothing compromises the ultimate clinical utility of the equipment.

7. Following installation of the equipment and prior to its first clinical use, the equipment should be subjected to acceptance testing to verify conformance to the specifications which have been delineated in the purchase contract. Any deficiencies found during acceptance testing should be communicated to the vendor in writing for corrective action. After the equipment has been found acceptable, a letter of formal acceptance should be sent to the vendor. Operator training should then be provided and the equipment placed into clinical service. It is frequently useful to limit utilization of the equipment to certain operators and normal working hours during the first month or so of clinical use, as this will help distinguish between equipment problems and problems associated with operator unfamiliarity with the equipment.

The Critical Path Method of Planning*

The critical path method is a management tool used in the planning, scheduling, and controlling of a wide spectrum of engineering projects (6). It is a quantitative technique to determine project duration and to identify potential problems. The critical path method has been employed for several years in industrial construction and has achieved substantial success in reducing project completion times and costs (7–9).

Application of the critical path method has two requirements: (1) planning the project (i.e., identifying what is to be done), and (2) scheduling the project (i.e., determining when various phases must be completed).

To implement a critical path method of planning, a diagram is prepared that depicts all operations in the project and the order in which the operations relate to each other. An operation is any activity that consumes time and may affect completion of the project. On the critical path method diagram,

each operation is represented by an arrow that depicts its beginning and end and is pointed in the direction of project completion.

To identify the time relationships among operations, each operation is evaluated with the knowledge that:

1. It must precede some operations.
2. It must follow some operations.
3. It may occur simultaneously with some operations.

Suppose that three operations, A, B, and C, must be performed. (1) A is the first operation; (2) A and B can be done concurrently; and (3) C follows B but can be initiated only after A has been completed. In this example, the dependence of operation C on the completion of A is indicated by a dashed arrow called a dummy. A dummy is merely a device to identify a dependence among operations. To facilitate an understanding of a critical path method diagram (or arrow network), common diagrams and an explanation of the logic they represent are presented in Figure 6.1. An example of a portion of an actual critical path method diagram is shown in Figure 6.2.

Once the operations and their time dependence are identified, the computation of project duration can commence and a critical path can be identified. Numbers are assigned to each operational arrow reflecting the sequence of operations. These are termed node numbers and usually are placed in circles at the junction of the arrows. Although the first node in the critical path method diagram usually is assigned a value of unity, node numbers need not be consecutive.

Once node numbers are assigned, the duration of each operation in the project is estimated and noted near the center of the appropriate arrow. It also is convenient to prepare a table in which operation name, number, duration, and sequence can be listed together with other variables. With such a diagram and listing, important project characteristics can be identified:

1. The length of time required to complete the entire project.
2. Operations which control the completion time for the project (the critical path).

* This section is extracted from Rossi RP, Hendee WR: New equipment for room 2210: the critical path method, with permission from *American Journal of Roentgenography* 134:1084–1088, 1980.

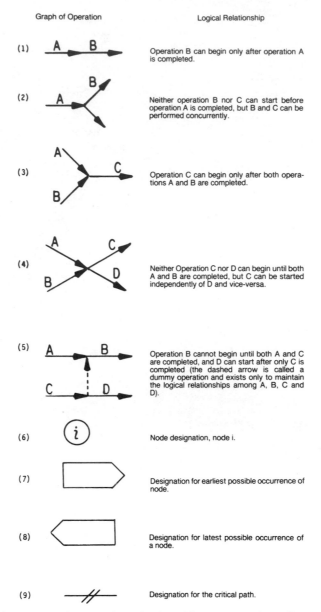

Figure 6.1. Operations and logical relationships in critical path method diagrams. (From Rossi RP, Hendee WR: New equipment for room 2210: the critical path method. *AJR* 134:1084–1088, 1980.)

3. The latitude that can be tolerated in operations which are outside the critical path (i.e., do not control the project completion time).

To accomplish this identification, nodes are considered as points in time with zero (0) assigned to the first node and designated by the symbol ▭▷ next to the node. For each node, the earliest possible occurrence is the earliest point in time for starting all operations (arrows) that originate at the node. The earliest finish time of a node is the sum of the node's earliest possible occurrence plus the duration of the operation. For any particular node, the earliest possible occurrence is the maximum value of earliest finish times for all operations that precede it. The earliest finish time of the final node is the earliest possible completion time for the entire project. Computations involving earliest possible occurrences and earliest fin-

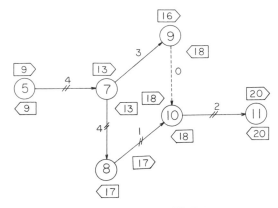

EARLIEST POSSIBLE OCCURRENCE OF NODE
LATEST POSSIBLE OCCURRENCE OF NODE
// DENOTES CRITICAL PATH

Figure 6.2. Selected portion of critical path method diagram presented in Figure 6.3, demonstrating the logical relationships presented in Figure 6.1. Consider the operations 7, 8; 7, 9; 8, 10; and 9, 10. The operation 7, 8 is represented by the *arrow* connecting nodes 7 and 8. The duration of operation 7, 8 is 4 days, and this operation lies on the critical path as denoted by "//." Operation 7, 9 can be carried out at the same time as operations 7, 8 and 8, 10; however, operation 10, 11 cannot begin until operations 7, 8; 8, 10; and 7, 9 have been completed. This interdependence is denoted by the dummy operation 9, 10 represented by the *dashed arrow* and requiring no time. The node 9 has an earliest possible occurrence of 16 and a latest possible occurrence of 18. Thus, its free float is 2, and it is not on the critical path.

ish times are diagrammed with symbols and proceed from left to right on the critical path method network.

Associated with each operation in a project is a certain amount of time referred to as free float. This is the difference between the earliest finish time of an operation and the earliest possible occurrence of the node of the next operation. The free float represents the amount of time that the operation can be delayed without affecting the earliest possible occurrence of any successive operation. Operations with a finite free float cannot influence the duration of the project so long as the free float is not exceeded. Operations for which free float equals zero are known as "critical operations." Critical operations which form a continuous path from the first to the last nodes in the network constitute the project's critical path. In crit-

ical path method diagrams, the critical path commonly is designated with the symbol "//" at the center of each operational arrow.

While the procedure described above is sufficient to satisfy most requirements for project planning, it is possible by additional processes to gain further insight into a project and to identify the critical path in a different way. The latest possible occurrence of a node is the latest possible time that all operations terminating at the node can be completed without extending the project beyond the time originally computed with earliest possible occurrences and earliest finish times. The latest start time of an operation is the latest possible occurrence of the node at which the operation terminates, minus the duration of the operation. The latest possible occurrence of a node is the minimum value of the latest start times of the operations that originate at the node. In this manner, the latest possible occurrence of each node is computed by proceeding from right to left through the critical path method graph and is denoted by ⊲ on the critical path method chart. The latest possible occurrence of the final node on the chart is equal to its earliest possible occurrence.

If the earliest possible occurrence and latest possible occurrence of a node are identical, the latest possible time for the node to occur is also the earliest possible time it can occur. Such nodes connect two critical operations, and this series of nodes constitute the critical path.

The final computation to be performed is determination of the total float. Total float is the length of time that a particular operation can be delayed or extended in time without affecting the completion time for the overall project. The total float is equal to the latest start time minus the earliest start time of an operation. Operations for which the total float equals zero define the critical path.

It should be noted that a critical path method diagram can be updated at any time during a project if unpreventable problems and delays occur. The updated critical path method diagram yields a new estimate of project completion time.

Application of this approach to installation of a radiograpic-fluoroscopic installation is presented in Table 6.1 and Figure 6.3. The critical path method should be ap-

Table 6.1
Critical Path Method Computation Table for Arrow Network Shown in Figure 6.3

Operation name	Operation number	Duration	Earliest		Latest		Float	
			Start	Finish	Start	Finish	Total	Free
Close room and remove old equipment	1, 2	2	0	2	0	2	0	0
Remove old ceiling, electrical fixtures, wiring and cabinets, etc.	2, 3	3	2	5	2	5	0	0
Install unistruct framework for ceiling and transformer platform	3, 4	2	5	7	5	7	0	0
Channel walls	4, 5	2	7	9	7	9	0	0
Install new power lines	4, 6	4	7	11	30	34	23	23
Install conduit and pull boxes	5, 7	4	9	13	9	13	0	0
Dummy	6, 22	0	11	11	34	34	23	23
Pull electrical wiring	7, 8	4	13	17	13	17	0	0
Plaster and tile walls	7, 9	3	13	16	15	18	3	2
Install wall cabinets and shelves	8, 10	1	17	18	17	18	0	0
Dummy	9, 10	0	16	16	18	18	2	2
Paint room	10, 11	2	18	20	18	20	0	0
Vendor review and accept site	11, 12	1	20	21	20	21	0	0
Release shipment for delivery	12, 13	1	21	22	21	22	0	0
Deliver shipment to site	13, 14	2	22	24	22	24	0	0
Receive and inventory shipment	14, 15	1	24	25	24	25	0	0
Identify and order missing or damaged parts	15, 16	1	25	26	25	26	0	0
Install overhead bridge suspensions	16, 17	4	26	30	26	30	0	0
Install transformer and power unit	16, 18	1	26	27	26	32	0	5
Install RARC and collimator module	16, 19	1	26	27	26	31	0	4
Await, receive, and install missing/damaged parts	16, 24	10	26	36	26	39	0	3
Install table	17, 21	2	30	32	30	32	0	0
Dummy	18, 21	0	27	27	32	32	5	5
Install vertical wall board	19, 20	1	27	28	31	32	4	4
Install x-ray tubes, collimators, and image intensifier assembly	19, 21	2	27	29	30	32	3	3
Dummy	20, 21	0	28	28	32	32	4	4
Pull and route interconnecting cable	21, 22	2	32	34	32	34	0	0
Complete electrical wiring	22, 23	2	34	36	34	36	0	0
Complete mechanical assembly and adjustment	23, 24	3	36	39	36	39	0	0
Low voltage checkout	24, 25	3	39	42	39	42	0	0
High voltage checkout	25, 26	2	42	44	42	44	0	0
Install special modifications	26, 27	1	44	45	44	45	0	0
Complete final mechanical and electrical calibration	27, 28	2	45	47	45	47	0	0
HEW certification	28, 29	2	47	49	47	49	0	0
Install ceiling tile and touch up paint	29, 30	2	49	51	49	51	0	0
Room cleanup and release for testing	30, 31	1	51	52	51	52	0	0

Table 6.1—*continued*

Operation name	Operation number	Duration	Earliest		Latest		Float	
			Start	Finish	Start	Finish	Total	Free
Equipment acceptance testing	31, 32	15	52	67	52	67	0	0
Operator instruction	32, 34	2	67	69	67	69	0	0
Review acceptance testing results	32, 33	1	67	68	67	69	0	1
Dummy	33, 34	0	68	68	69	69	0	1
Formal acceptance and release for clinical use	34, 35	1	69	70	69	70	0	0

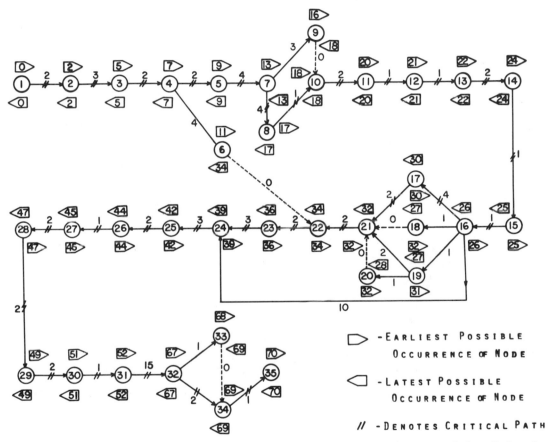

Figure 6.3. Critical path method diagram for the pediatric radiographic/fluoroscopic installation. In developing this critical path schedule, it was assumed that the project began with removal of old equipment, even though certain events occurred prior to this. Among these were selection of the successful vendor, issuance of a purchase order, development of architectural plans by the vendor and remodeling contractor, and shipment of the equipment to the institution, etc. These and other operations could have been incorporated into a more extended critical path method diagram. For purposes of illustration, only the installation phase is depicted in this figure.

plied under the close supervision of a radiological physicist, radiologic engineer, radiologic administrator, or other individual knowledgeable about and interested in the details of the installation. This individual must work closely with construction personnel and with the vendor's installation team to prove that the project follows the procedural and time constraints of the critical path method plan. Designation of an individual to coordinate the overall effort should reflect the individual's familiarity with equipment installation and performance and his or her comprehension of architectural drawings and space allocations. During installation the individual should become familiar with the equipment and well acquainted with the vendor's service personnel. He should assist the installation team in verifying that the equipment is installed within the space constraints of the room to realize maximum versatility. He should verify that the unit performs according to the specifications outlined in the purchase contract. For certain calibration procedures, the supervisory individual might recommend alternate test methods that yield more reliable data. All of these tasks are included in the critical path method (CPM) plan for the laboratory.

During installation of the equipment, certain operational characteristics of the equipment might be modified under the CPM supervisor's direction to enhance the reliability and clinical utility of the equipment. As examples, these might include: (1) blocking of unnecessary generator controls in pediatric applications, thereby reducing potential operator error; (2) digital display of exposure time for automatically controlled exposures, thereby facilitating identification of under- or overexposed films prior to processing; (3) digital display under the television monitor of the cumulative fluoroscopic exposure time and number of spot films to encourage reduction of fluoroscopic time and number of spot films by radiologists in training; and (4) development of a fluoroscopic imaging system capable of providing reduced patient exposure (10). Inclusion of modifications such as these in the critical path method not only ensures their early identification to the equipment vendor, but also facilitates their completion at an appropriate time in the renovation.

Discussion

The critical path method for installation of radiological equipment has proven useful in a variety of settings. At the University of Colorado Health Sciences Center, typical installation problems that occurred with earlier installations and that could have been prevented by the critical path method approach include the following.

INADEQUATE ELECTRICAL SPECIFICATIONS PROVIDED BY THE VENDOR

During installation of a new automatic chest x-ray unit, specifications provided by the vendor indicated that all electrical wiring to be delivered to a wall junction box between the generator control and high voltage transformer was to be terminated on terminal strips in the box. When the x-ray equipment was installed, it was determined that the specifications were incorrect and that the wires should not have been terminated but instead should have been extended 6 ft out of the junction box. This misinformation resulted in an installation delay of 1 week and could have been detected by review of the specifications by the vendor, the installation team, and the electrical contractor at an early state in the critical path method.

INADEQUATE FUNDING FOR FACILITY RENOVATION

In one x-ray installation, planning for facility renovation was initiated approximately 3 months prior to equipment delivery. At that time facility renovation costs were estimated at $17,000 per room, far in excess of available funding and previous rough estimates. This budgeting error caused an installation delay of approximately 4 months and could have been prevented by use of the critical path method plan which called for renovation costs estimated by an earlier date.

MECHANICAL INTERFERENCES

During final installation of a general purpose radiographic-fluoroscopic room, inadequate clearance was discovered for the motion of the image intensifier support bridge with respect to the overhead radiographic bridge and cable take-up trough. In addition, the image intensifier could not be parked in a location which was safe from collision with the examination table. The problem was corrected by repositioning the bridge suspension, cable take-up trough and examination table, at a cost of 5 additional days installation time.

During the same installation, it was discovered that the general contractor had neglected the position of the overhead suspension stationary rails as denoted on the room layout and had installed the room lighting fixtures in locations where replacement of light bulbs was impossible. This was corrected at a cost of 4 days installation time.

These problems could have been resolved without delay of installation if a properly constructed critical path method plan had been followed. These types of problems have largely been circumvented since initiation of the critical path method for facility renovation and equipment installation. However, the approach requires a manpower commitment to an area that traditionally has been outside the purview of the institution. This commitment is more than compensated by savings in time and effort during the installation, as well as by extra income generated as a result of reduced downtime. For example, a modest workload of 20 examinations/day at an average professional charge of $20 per examination constitutes a loss of $400 in professional income for each day of downtime. Recovery of this income by reduced downtime more than compensates for the commitment of a supervisory individual to the critical path method planning effort.

Prestating of Imaging Equipment in Relationship to Facility Planning

The prestaging of radiological imaging systems represents an approach by a few equipment vendors to overcome some of the more common problems associated with equipment installation. With the prestaging approach, the components of an imaging system are not shipped directly from the factory to the installation site; instead, they are sent first to a prestaging facility where they are assembled and tested as a fully operating system. At the prestaging facility all of the major components of the system are assembled and tested. The shipment is checked for correctness and completeness and is then assembled in special staging bays in the prestaging facility. Interconnecting cabling is pre-cut and preterminated for the actual installation site.

During the prestaging process the equipment is completely calibrated and tested for all operation aspects by highly trained technicians. Any deficiencies can be readily corrected at the prestaging facility prior to shipment of the equipment to the purchaser. In principle, once the equipment arrives at the installation site it should be possible to accomplish installation in a very short period of time with a minimum of mechanical and

electrical adjustments. Also, since the equipment has already been tested as a system, enhanced reliability and performance might be expected.

Prestaged x-ray systems can help enhance system performance and reliability. Installation time can be reduced to as little as 4 weeks for a typical radiographic-fluoroscopic facility, provided that the facility is ready to accept the equipment on delivery. Similar results might be obtainable with x-ray equipment that has been thoroughly tested on a subcomponent level and precabled for a particular site, provided that the installation is done with care and by experienced service personnel. All too frequently, however, these criteria are not satisfied. Prestaging is not without certain problems of its own; overall, however, it appears that the advantages of prestaging outweigh the disadvantages, and that prestaging should be considered as an integral part of facility planning and preparation.

References

1. Tuddenham WJ (ed): *Planning Guide for Radiologic Installations.* American College of Radiology, Chicago, Chicago Inst; Fascicle 1: Radiation Therapy Installations, 1978; Fascicle 2: Mammographic, Thermographic and Ultrasonic Installations, 1976; Fascicle 3: Computerized Tomographic Facilities, 1976; Fascicle 4: Basic Concepts: Layout Considerations, 1977; Fascicle 4A: Basic Concepts: Layout Considerations, 1977; Fascicle 5: Pediatric Facilities, 1977.
2. Fischer HW: *Radiology Departments: Planning, Operation, and Management.* Ann Arbor, MI, Edwards Bros, 1982.
3. National Council on Radiation Protection: *Medical X-Ray and Gamma-Ray Protection for Energies up to 10 MEV—Equipment Design and Use.* NCRP Report No. 33, Bethesda, MD, 1968.
4. National Council on Radiation Protection: *Structural Shielding Design and Evaluation for Medical Use of X-Rays and Gamma Rays of Energies up to 10 MEV.* NCRP Report No. 49, Bethesda, MD, 1976.
5. Braestrup CB, Wyckoff HO: Shielding design levels for radiology departments. *Radiology* 107:445–447, 1973.
6. Shaffer LR, Ritter JB, Meyer WI: *The Critical Path Method.* New York, McGraw-Hill, 1965.
7. Berman H: The critical path method for project planning and control. *Constructor* 43:24–29, 1961.
8. Pocock JW: PERT as an analytical aid for program planning—its payoff and problems. *Operations Res* 10:893–904, 1961.
9. Smith ME: *A Discussion of Action Planning and Control Technique.* Carlsbad, NM, International Minerals and Chemical Corp, 1961.
10. Rossi RP, Wesenberg RL, Hendee WR: A variable aperture fluoroscopic unit for reduced patient exposure. *Radiology* 129:799–802, 1978.

CHAPTER SEVEN

Acceptance Testing

WILLIAM R. HENDEE, Ph.D., RAYMOND P. ROSSI, M.S.,
VICTOR M. SPITZER, Ph.D., ROBERT K. CACAK, PhD.,
ANN L. SCHERZINGER, Ph.D., and STEVEN R. WILKINS, Ph.D.

INTRODUCTION

Following installation, a radiologic system should be evaluated thoroughly by the process of acceptance testing (1, 2). This process verifies that the radiologic equipment satisfies the performance specifications described in the purchase contract, manufacturer's specification sheets, and applicable state and federal regulations. Under ideal circumstances, the acceptance testing process is conducted by an individual who is not associated with the vendor of the installed equipment and who is experienced in the use of the required instrumentation and protocols for acceptance testing. When such an individual is unavailable, the acceptance testing process can be conducted by an employee of the vendor; however, testing results should be analyzed by a physician, technologist, or other representative of the host institution.

In any acceptance testing process, a complete inventory of the radiologic system should be conducted first to verify that each component is identical to that described in the purchase contract and the vendor's packing list for shipment. All information such as operator's manuals, service manuals, circuit diagrams, and parts lists should be present, as should all auxiliary devices ordered with the equipment.

Following the inventory, an inspection of the radiologic system should be performed to verify that its mechanical integrity is satisfactory. For example, all motion locks, mechanical detents and stops, power drives, and cable troughs should be checked for proper function and smoothness of operation. To verify that forces associated with various mechanical functions are at proper levels, spring scales are very useful. Moving parts of the radiologic system should be examined to ensure that no limitations in movement have been caused by improper installation. The electrical cabling of the unit should be inspected to verify that cables are properly channeled and seated and that no cable damage or interference with equipment motion is present. Appropriate tests for electrical safety (e.g., measurements of leakage currents and stray electrical fields) also should be conducted as part of the preliminary process of equipment evaluation.

Most imaging systems are sensitive to major fluctuations in voltage of the incoming power line. For proper operation of an imaging system, the incoming power line must provide the proper voltage and current capacity and must yield a minimal power loss under load. For multiphasic power sources, voltages and loading of all phases should be balanced.

The voltage regulation of the power line is defined (3) as

$$\frac{v_\eta - v_\ell}{v_\eta} \times 100$$

where v_η = line voltage with no load, and v_ℓ = line voltage with full load. The voltage regulation should be within the specifications of the equipment vendor. Evaluation of the incoming power line usually is conducted by the vendor during equipment installation, and reproducing these measurements should be unnecessary provided that the vendor signs a statement of acceptance of the power line. Measurements may be necessary only if equipment problems develop that may be attributable to the incoming power line.

ROENTGENOGRAPHY

In the following discussion, procedures for acceptance testing of roentgenographic equipment will be discussed. The procedures described are those which might be applicable to a general purpose radiographic-fluoroscopic unit with tomographic capability (4–6).

X-Ray Generators

Parameters of equipment performance associated with x-ray generators include the voltage applied to the x-ray tube (kVp), the current flowing through the x-ray tube (the tube current or mA), the duration of the applied tube voltage and current (exposure time), and the integrity of circuitry employed to protect the x-ray tube from thermal damage (7, 8). The evaluation of these parameters for acceptance testing purposes requires the use of invasive measurement techniques which must be carried out with caution. These techniques utilize a high voltage divider and storage oscilloscope for measurement of kilovoltage wave forms and exposure times.

Installation of a high voltage divider may be accomplished by either of the methods illustrated in Figure 7.1. In Figure 7.1A the high voltage divider is connected in-line with the x-ray tube by use of short jumper cables either at the x-ray tube or at the high voltage transformer. This method must be utilized on x-ray generators that employ rotary high voltage switching for multiple tube selection. Several disadvantages are associated with this technique. Frequently, it is difficult to gain convenient access to under table x-ray tubes to connect the high voltage divider. The presence of the jumper cable on the cathode side of the x-ray tube will produce some perturbation of tube current; this perturbation must be accounted for (9, 10). With grid bias tubes frequently encountered in fluoroscopic applications, a special adapter box (11) is required to interface the normal three-conductor high voltage cables to the four-conductor cables required for grid bias operation.

The method illustrated in Figure 7.1B overcomes these difficulties and is recommended for x-ray generators that employ parallel high voltage switching and that have available an unused set of high voltage receptacles. In this method, the high voltage divider is installed at the high voltage trans-

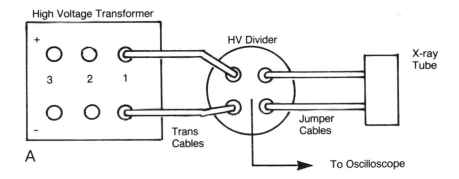

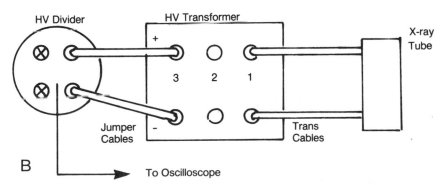

Figure 7.1. Arrangement of high voltage divider for kVp measurement. (*A*) divider inserted between high voltage transformer and x-ray tube (required for rotary-switched generators). (*B*) Divider inserted in auxiliary ports of high voltage transformer and placed in parallel with tube under test.

former in the unused set of high voltage receptacles. These receptacles are then placed in parallel with those of the x-ray tube under evaluation so that the voltage to the x-ray tube is also applied to the high voltage divider for recording by the storage oscilloscope. Regardless of the method employed, care must be taken to ensure that all high voltage connections are properly made, suitable insulating oil or grease is used, and grounding rings are present at the high voltage cable ends if required. The storage oscilloscope should always be floated with respect to ground when any measurements associated with the secondary side of the high voltage circuit are made.

The order in which the various aspects of x-ray generator performance are conducted is to some extent a matter of personal preference. However, the sequence described below has been found to be an efficient approach.

TUBE PROTECTIVE CIRCUITRY

The evaluation of the tube protective circuitry of an x-ray generator requires the use of rating charts for the particular x-ray tube installed on the imaging system. These charts are used to determine the maximum allowed exposure time for a specific kilovoltage peak, focal spot size, tube current, high voltage wave form, and anode rotation speed. Once this exposure time is determined from the charts, it is selected on the generator along with the corresponding kilovoltage peak, milliamperage, focal spot size, and anode rotation speed. If the tube protective circuit is functioning properly, no indication of exposure inhibition should be obtained. Increasing the exposure time to a value greater than the maximum allowed should result in an indication of exposure inhibition. With some x-ray generators, an indication that the technique exceeds the allowed maximum may occur upon technique selection or upon initiation of exposure. In some generators the time stations available may not coincide exactly with the maximum allowed time. In these cases, exposures should be permitted at the nearest time station below the allowed maximum and inhibited at the nearest time station above the maximum. Complete evaluation of the tube protective circuitry is performed

by repeating this test at multiple kilovoltage peak selections for all tube currents, focal spot sizes, and anode rotation speeds. In some cases substantial damage of an x-ray tube may occur due to the design of the tube protective circuitry. The circuitry may assume that all focal spots are the same size or may be unable to accommodate x-ray tubes that have greatly different characteristics. The exact capabilities and limitations of the tube protective circuitry should be determined from the manufacturer during the equipment acquisition process.

EXPOSURE TIME

The capability of the x-ray generator to control the duration of exposure in an accurate and reproducible manner is evaluated with a high voltage divider and storage oscilloscope. Interpretation of the recorded high voltage wave forms to determine exposure time depends on the form of the secondary voltage applied to the x-ray tube. For single phase full wave rectified equipment, the exposure time is defined simply as the number of recorded pulses times 8.3 msec per pulse. For three phase equipment, exposure time is normally defined as the width of the high voltage pulse at a given percentage of the peak value, with 75 to 80% specified by the majority of manufacturers. At low tube loadings, cable capacitance may produce a relatively slow decay of the high voltage wave form following exposure termination; hence, it is necessary to use sufficiently high tube loadings (e.g., 300 mA) to prevent this effect. This point is illustrated in Figure 7.2, demonstrating high voltage wave forms obtained at the same nominal exposure time but at substantially different tube loadings. The importance of measuring exposure time as the width of the high voltage pulse at a specified percentage of peak value is illustrated in Figure 7.3. For exposure times of approximately 50 msec or greater, the high voltage pulse approaches a square wave, and its width is relatively independent of the peak percentage where it is measured.

For cinefluorographic systems, exposure time usually is taken as the time between removal and reapplication of grid bias, as indicated in Figure 7.4.

Exposure times are determined from oscilloscope recordings of the displayed wave

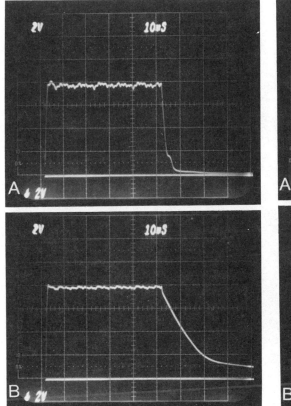

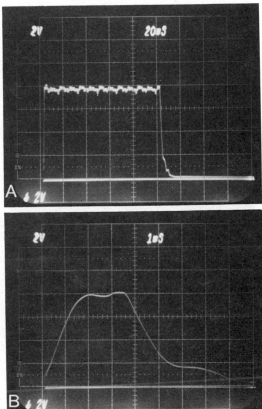

Figure 7.2. Effect of cable capacitance on measured exposure time. (*A*) 300 mA. (*B*) 10 mA. Nominal exposure time of 50 msec.

Figure 7.3. Influence of specified percent of peak on exposure time. (*A*) 100-msec exposure. (*B*) 5-msec exposure. Both at 80 kVp, 300 mA.

forms and compared to indicated exposure times to determine accuracy. Determination of exposure time reproducibility is accomplished by calculating the coefficient of variation of replicate measurements at a given exposure time. Performance testing is performed over the range of exposure times anticipated for clinical use.

KILOVOLTAGE

The kilovoltage performance of an x-ray generator should be evaluated by symmetry of the voltage wave form applied from anode to ground and from cathode to ground. Additional evaluations include reproducibility, accuracy of actual kilovoltage peak with respect to indicated kilovoltage peak, and independence of kilovoltage peak with tube current. Evaluation should be conducted for all tubes connected to the generator and for all modes of system operation over the working range of the generator.

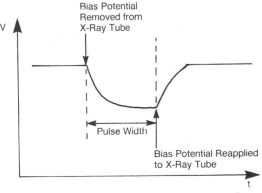

Figure 7.4. Diagram illustrating meaning of exposure time in grid bias (cine) systems.

Kilovoltage symmetry is evaluated by recording the anode to ground and cathode to ground high voltage wave forms at several different tube loadings at a midrange kilovoltage peak, such as 80 kVp. Typical wave forms are illustrated in Figure 7.5. The wave

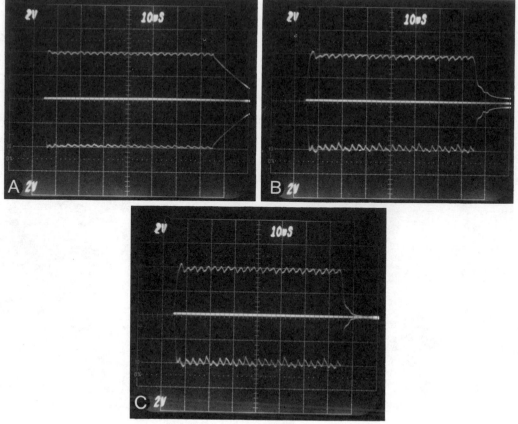

Figure 7.5. Wave forms for determining symmetry for high voltage applied to x-ray tube. (*A*) 10 mA. (*B*) 300 mA. (*C*) 800 mA. All measurements at 80 kVp.

forms should demonstrate equal kilovoltage peaks from anode to ground and cathode to ground and a proper phase relationship between anode and cathode kilovoltage peaks. Accuracy of measured to indicated kilovoltage peak should be evaluated over the typical working range of the generator (e.g., 50–150 kVp) and at all tube loadings consistent with the ratings of the x-ray generator and tube. In performing these tests exposure times of 100 msec typically are used, with the wave forms recorded at 10 to 20 kVp increments. Representative wave forms are illustrated in Figure 7.6. In analysis of the wave forms, particular attention should be paid to kilovoltage peak overshoots and wave form roundings at the initiation of exposure, unusual appearances in the shape of the high voltage wave form ripple, which may indicate phase imbalance, and uniformity of the kilovoltage over the duration of exposure. Replicate measurements are made

to determine reproducibility of kilovoltage peak.

Interpretation of kilovoltage peak from recorded wave forms is relatively straightforward for single and three phase systems (12–16) but can present some problems for systems such as cinefluoroscopic units, that employ a grid-biased x-ray tube. One satisfactory method of estimating kilovoltage peak for such systems is illustrated in Figure 7.7.

TUBE CURRENT

The tube current performance of an x-ray generator should be evaluated for reproducibility, accuracy with regard to indicated tube current, and independnce from tube kilovoltage. Evaluation should be carried out for each x-ray tube connected to the generator, for each operational mode and at each focal spot size, and for each tube current available over the working range of the generator within the x-ray generator and tube ratings, at 10 to 20 increments in kilovoltage peak.

Tube current can be measured by a number of methods. Direct measurements can be obtained by inserting a digital multimeter operated in the direct current milliamperage (DCmA) mode in series with the midsecondary of the high voltage transformer. This technique is suitable for the fluoroscopic mode of operation, although it may be influenced by secondary winding currents which do not contribute to actual tube current. The technique is unsuitable for the radiographic mode of operation because of the higher tube currents, limited recommended exposure times, and long response times of most measuring instruments.

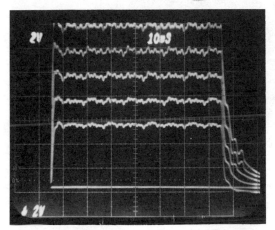

Figure 7.6. Typical wave forms used to determine kVp calibration. 60, 80, 100, 120, 140 kVp at 300 mA, 70 msec exposure.

Tube currents may be inferred from measurements of milliampere seconds with a direct reading milliampere-second meter connected in series with the midsecondary of the x-ray generator. The measured milliampere seconds are divided by the known exposure duration to determine tube current. This method must be employed for x-ray generators (e.g., falling load generators) that do not allow independent control of milliamperage and time. However, the method has certain limitations. The milliampere second meter integrates all current flowing during the exposure, including that due to cable charging at the initiation of exposure and cable discharge upon exposure termination. These limitations affect the accuracy of the technique, particularly at low tube currents and short exposure times. Also, the actual duration of exposure must be accurately established.

As an alternative technique (15), a 10-Ω, 50-W, 1% precision resistor may be inserted in series with the ground return lead of the x-ray generator midsecondary. Proper connection points for the resistor are usually available within the control console or at the high voltage transformer. The milliamperage can be inferred from the voltage drop measured with a storage oscilloscope placed across the resistor during exposure. For the specified resistance, 100 mA will be equivalent to 1 V. A typical milliampere wave form obtained by this technique is illustrated in Figure 7.8A. Note that substantial "ripple" is exhibited, making it difficult to determine the true DCmA value. To overcome this

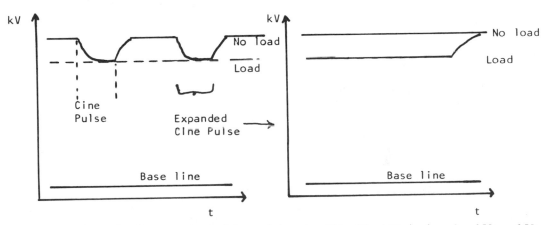

Figure 7.7. Example of one method of determining cine kVp. The kVp is given by: kVp = kVp (load) −0.33 (kVp [no load] −kVp [load]).

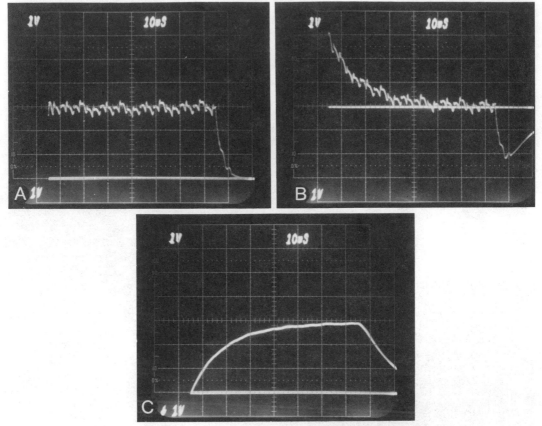

Figure 7.8. Illustrations of tube current wave forms. (*A*) Voltage signal developed across resistor, *V*(*A*); (*B*) Voltage signal developed across resistor and capacitively filtered, *V*(*B*); (*C*) Voltage signal resulting from algebraic addition of *V*(*A*) and *V*(*B*).

problem, the circuit illustrated in Figure 7.9 may be used. The voltage signal developed across the resistor is applied directly to channel 1 (Fig. 7.8*A*) of the measuring oscilloscope. This same signal is also applied to channel 2 (Fig. 7.8*B*) of the oscilloscope after capacitive filtering. Channel 2 is inverted and algebraically added to channel 1; the resultant wave form is illustrated in Figure 7.8*C*. As illustrated in the figure, interpretation of milliamperage is much easier in Figure 7.8*C* than in Figure 7.8*A*. For this technique, exposure times in the range of 70 to 100 msec usually are utilized.

Many x-ray generators include milliampere calibration resistors that may be utilized for testing. Interpretation of the *DCmA* value from recorded wave forms for three phase (3-φ) equipment is straightforward, as illustrated in Figure 7.10. For single phase full wave rectified equipment, the *DCmA* is

related to the peak voltage developed across a 10-Ω resistor by the expression:

$$mA = \text{(Recorded peak voltage)}$$
$$\times \text{(100 mA/V)} \times \text{(0.637).}$$

In analyzing the milliampere wave forms, one should look for unusual spiking or overshoots at the beginning of exposure (other than cable charging) which may arise from improper adjustments of the milliampere stabilizer, and variations in milliamperage over the course of exposure caused by electron cooling in the x-ray tube (16).

A few commercially available high voltage dividers provide a direct readout of milliamperage or milliampere seconds (as well as other x-ray generator parameters) when connected in the configuration of Figure 7.1*A*. While such dividers can be used to advantage, caution must be exercised because ex-

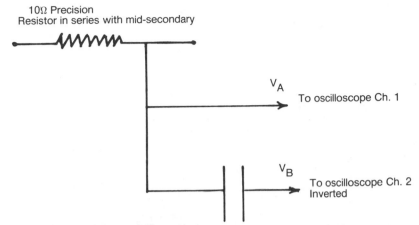

Figure 7.9. Use of a precision resistor for measurement of tube current.

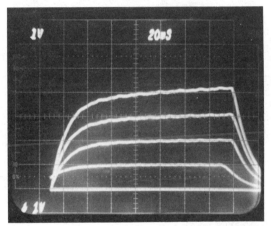

Figure 7.10. Examples of wave forms from which mA calibration is determined. 100, 200, 300, and 400 mA at 80 kVp.

cessive reliance on digital display data can be misleading. The manufacturer's instruction manual for the test device must be read carefully to ensure proper use of the device. In actuality, no substitute exists for the visual inspection of wave forms during testing.

DATA RECORDING/ DOCUMENTATION

The results of all measurements taken during initial acceptance testing of the x-ray generator should be carefully documented. Retention of actual oscilloscope recordings of wave forms may be useful for comparison at a later date. Abnormal measurements should most definitely be documented. Results of testing may be summarized as shown

in Table 7.1. The test instrumentation employed, along with a brief description of the test procedures, should be included in the documentation.

CAUTIONS/PITFALLS

In the previous sections procedures for initial acceptance testing of an x-ray generator have been provided that may be performed with little difficulty. However, several points should be kept in mind to ensure efficient testing and reliable results. One must always have a good working knowledge of the equipment being tested. Study of vendor's manuals and working with vendor personnel during installation are valuable. Test instrumentation should be selected carefully and calibrated properly. Caution must be exercised in connecting and using test instrumentation to preclude equipment damage and operator hazard.

Care should be used in making and interpreting tube current measurements. When a high voltage divider is placed in a system as illustrated in Figure 7.1A, the insertion impedence of the cathode jumper cable may produce changes in milliamperage by as much as 20 to 25%. This effect can be minimized, but still must be accounted for, by using the shortest practical jumper cables (5 ft). Compensation for insertion impedance can be achieved by calibrating the x-ray generator (kVp/mA) with the cathode jumper in place and then removing the cathode and readjusting milliamperage as required to the desired value.

The x-ray tube and system electronic com-

Table 7.1
Example of a Tabular Summary of Kilovoltage Peak/Milliamperage Results Obtained during Acceptance Testing

Nominal mA / kVp	25(S)	50(S)	100(S)	200(S)	300(L)	400(L)	500(L)	600(L)
60	60 / 25	58 / 50	60 / 100	57 / 210	60 / 320	61 / 410	61 / 500	62 / 600
80	80 / 24	81 / 49	80 / 105	78 / 210	80 / 315	81 / 405	82 / 500	80 / 600
100	101 / 24	101 / 49	100 / 100	98 / 207	99 / 305	100 / 410	101 / 500	99 / 610
120	122 / 25	121 / 49	121 / 100	118 / 210	118 / 315	120 / 415	119 / 510	118 / 620
140	143 / 24	141 / 49	140 / 100	138 / 210	138 / 315	140 / 420	139 / 515	138 / 630

ponents should be kept in a thermal condition similar to that encountered clinically. Tube current varies between a cold and hot x-ray tube, and thermal drift in electronic components ("covers" on vs "covers" off) of the x-ray generator control can exert a definite influence on measurements.

Multiple tube installations in which the x-ray tubes have substantially different filament characteristics may not achieve the desired level of performance unless special dissimilar tube kits are installed to extend the range of operation of the filament space charge transformer.

X-Ray Tubes/Source Assemblies

Performance parameters associated with x-ray tubes and source assemblies include leakage radiation, focal spot size and growth, exposure, exposure reproducibility, exposure linearity, and beam quality.

LEAKAGE RADIATION

Radiation that exits the x-ray tube and source assembly in directions other than the useful x-ray beam is known as leakage radiation. It is defined as the exposure (milliroentgens (mr)) produced in any 1 hr at 1 m from the focal spot when the tube is operated at the leakage technique factors specified by the manufacturer. Leakage technique factors are typically in the range of 125 to 150 kVp and 3 to 7 mA. The exit port of the x-ray tube and source assembly must be blocked with a thickness of lead equal to at least 10 half value layers at an energy in kiloelectron volts equal to the peak operating potential of the tube. An ionization chamber of suit-

able energy response and sensitivity is positioned 1 m from the x-ray target in a variety of locations on an imaginary sphere around the x-ray tube and source assembly, and measurements are made. Leakage radiation is difficult to measure on clinically installed x-ray units. Proper positioning of an ionization chamber is difficult, particularly for under table fluoroscopic tubes. Continuous operation at the leakage technique factors usually cannot be achieved; instead, the tube usually is operated at an elevated milliampere setting for short exposure times, with the leakage radiation inferred by linear scaling from the higher milliampere setting. Usually, x-ray tube manufacturers can supply data regarding leakage radiation measured as part of the production process. However, if a leakage problem is suspected, leakage measurements should be made.

FOCAL SPOT SIZE

The size of the x-ray focal spot can be measured by either a pinhole camera (17) or a star pattern technique (16, 17). When a pinhole camera is used, a magnified image of the focal spot is recorded on high resolution film. This image is similar to that shown in Figure 7.11 and represents the intensity distribution of the radiation emitted from the focal spot. To determine the size of the focal spot, the dimensions of the image are measured with an optical reticule, and the size of the focal spot is computed. The dimensions are normally determined as parallel and perpendicular to the anode-cathode axis of the x-ray tube. Technique factors for imaging are chosen to be 50% of the maximum rated peak tube potential and 50% of the maximum rated tube current at this potential for a 0.1-sec exposure during high-speed rotation. The actual exposure time used is determined by that required to produce an acceptable image density. Source to pinhole and pinhole to film distances are generally chosen to yield an image magnification of $(1 + 1/f)$ where f is the nominal size of the focal spot in millimeters.

While long used as the standard method for measuring focal spots, the pinhole technique has a number of disadvantages. Geometrical alignment is difficult, and long exposures are required to produce an acceptable image because of the extremely small size of the pinhole. The star pattern technique (18) overcomes these difficulties and is generally preferred for acceptance testing. The star pattern technique utilizes a radial pattern of alternating radioopaque and radiolucent material typically arranged in four quadrants. The spokes of the star constitute a bar pattern of continuously varying spatial frequency. For focal spot measurements, the star pattern is arranged with the spokes parallel and perpendicular to the anode-cathode axis of the x-ray tube. The resultant image, recorded on high resolution film, is shown in Figure 7.12. Moving from the outside towards the center of the star pattern image, a region is encountered where the radial spokes are blurred. This region of resolution loss is associated with the geometrical unsharpness of the focal spot. If the focal spot has a homogeneous intensity distribution, the size f of the focal spot is related to the diameter of the region of resolution loss according to the relationship

$$f_{\perp(11)} = \frac{\theta \pi d_{11(\perp)}}{180(M - 1)}$$

where $f_{\perp(11)}$ is the size of the focal spot perpendicular and parallel to the anode-cathode axis, respectively (in millimeters). θ is the spoke angle of the star in degrees, and $d_{11(\perp)}$ are the diameters of region of resolution losses parallel and perpendicular to the anode-cathode axis, respectively (in millimeters). M is the magnification factor.

The size of the focal spot measured by a star pattern is not the same as the physical

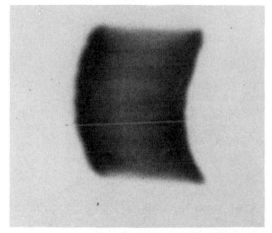

Figure 7.11. Example of a focal spot image obtained with a pinhole camera.

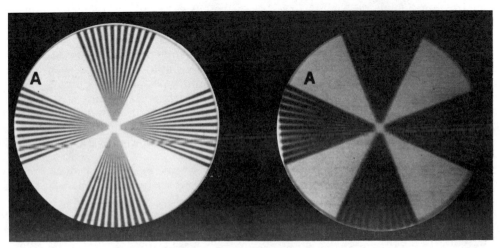

Figure 7.12. Example of a focal spot image obtained with a star test pattern.

size measured by the pinhole technique. The star pattern measurement indicates the size of a focal spot of uniform intensity distribution with resolution capabilities equivalent to the measured focal spot (18). For unusual distributions of focal spot intensity (e.g., a Gaussian intensity distribution) the star pattern may yield unsatisfactory results. In the majority of uses, however, the star pattern method has been found to be satisfactory (19–22).

Exposure requirements for imaging star patterns are much less than those for the pinhole technique. Accurate geometrical alignment is possible with special test fixtures. Kilovoltage and tube currents used for focal spot determinations with a star pattern are the same as those used with a pinhole camera. Comparative measurements with the pinhole camera and the star pattern on a variety of x-ray tubes with different focal spot sizes have shown that the focal spot measured by a pinhole camera can be related to that measured by the star pattern according to the relationship

$$f_\perp{}^{pinhole} = 0.93 f_\perp{}^{star}$$
$$f_{11}{}^{pinhole} = 0.83 f_{11}{}^{star}.$$

For acceptance testing, therefore, the star pattern technique may be used to estimate the size of the focal spot that would be measured with a pinhole camera.

FOCAL SPOT SIZE VARIATION

The variation in focal spot size as a function of imaging technique factors may be evaluated by the star pattern technique over the entire range of kilovoltage peaks and milliamperages of interest. For each kilovoltage peak and milliamperage setting, the focal spot size is determined, and the relative focal spot size is computed by normalizing to the technique factors used for the initial measurement of focal spot size. That is, the relative focal spot size f_{Rel} is:

$$f_{Rel} = \frac{f(kVp^i, mA^i)}{f\left(\dfrac{kVp\ max}{2} \cdot \dfrac{mA\ max \cdot HS,\ 0.1\ sec}{2}\right)}.$$

HS, high speed rotations. Measurements normally are made over the entire range of kilovoltage peaks and milliamperages, con-

sistent with thermal and space charge limitations of the focal spot. Usually the focal spot will increase rapidly in size with increasing milliamperage at fixed kilovoltage peak and decrease slowly in size with increasing kilovoltage peak at fixed milliamperage (23).

Exposure, Exposure Reproducibility, Exposure Linearity, Beam Quality

The exposure, exposure reproducibility, exposure linearity, and beam quality of the x-ray tube/source assembly x-ray generator combination are important characteristics of an imaging system. Measurement of these parameters requires an ion chamber and electrometer of suitable characteristics. Characteristics of the ion chamber include an ion chamber with a sensitivity between 10^9 and 10^{10} roentgens/coulomb (R/C) at 22°C and 760 mm Hg; a variation in sensitivity of less than ±5% between 20 keV and 150 keV; absolute accuracy of better than 95%; and a collection efficiency of better than 95% at instantaneous exposure rates of 2000 R/min. Measurements should be conducted in air under conditions of good geometry.

EXPOSURE

The exposure of an x-ray tube and source assembly (x-ray tube and collimator) is usually expressed as milliroentgens per milliampere second (mR/mAs) at a specified distance from the focal spot. This parameter is dependent on the high voltage applied to the x-ray tube, the high voltage wave form, the tube current, and the total filtration of the source assembly.

Illustrated in Table 7.2 are typical values of milliroentgens per milliampere second as a function of kilovoltage peak for 1-ϕ and 3-ϕ equipment as determined from extensive measurements on clinical systems known to be well calibrated. Also presented in this table are the half value layers (HVLs) associated with the various kilovoltage peaks. New x-ray systems often have excessive filtration, resulting in reduced exposure, increased beam quality, and excessive tube loading. Older x-ray tubes also occasionally exhibit reduced exposure and increased beam quality caused by tungsten deposition on the glass envelope of the x-ray tube.

Several inferences can be drawn from ex-

Table 7.2
Example of a Tabular Summary of Kilovoltage Peak/Milliamperage Results Obtained during Acceptance Testing[a]

kVp	mR/mAs	HVL (mm Al)
Single phase, full wave rectified		
50.00	5.13	1.90
60.00	7.54	2.26
70.00	10.46	2.62
80.00	13.87	2.99
90.00	17.80	3.35
100.00	22.25	3.71
110.00	27.22	4.07
120.00	32.73	4.44
130.00	38.77	4.80
140.00	45.36	5.16
Three phase, 6 and 12 pulse		
50.00	5.76	1.98
60.00	8.38	2.39
70.00	11.52	2.80
80.00	15.16	3.21
90.00	19.32	3.62
100.00	24.00	4.04
110.00	29.20	4.45
120.00	34.93	4.86
130.00	41.19	5.27
140.00	47.98	5.68

[a] Representative values for exposure per milliampere second at 24 inches from the source and first half value layer thickness for single phase and three phase equipment.

posure measurements. For example, high exposures with low to normal HVLs may indicate inadequate filtration or tube current miscalibration. High exposures with normal to high HVLs may indicate tube current or kilovoltage miscalibration. Low outputs with low to normal HVLs may indicate tube current or kilovoltage miscalibration, and low outputs with normal to high HVLs may indicate kilovoltage miscalibration or excessive filtration. Care should be exercised in interpreting these data, however, and the interpretations should be verified by primary measurements of kilovoltage peak and milliamperage.

EXPOSURE REPRODUCIBILITY

Sequential exposures at a fixed set of technique parameters (kilovoltage peak, milliamperage, and time) yield an evaluation of exposure reproducibility. Each technique parameter should be changed from the value at which the measurement is made and then returned to the value for the next exposure.

The number of measurements in the sequence should be 5 to 10. Exposure reproducibility is quantified in terms of the coefficient of variation for the sequence of exposures (3, 24, 25).

EXPOSURE LINEARITY

Exposure linearity may be evaluated from exposure measurements obtained over the working milliampere per milliampere second range of the generator consistent with the thermal rating of the x-ray tube and power ratings of the x-ray generator. At a given kilovoltage peak, milliamperage and time are varied reciprocally to yield approximately the same milliampere seconds for constant load generators; milliampere seconds are varied for falling load generators. The resultant data are used to calculate milliroentgens per milliampere second as a function of milliamperage or milliampere seconds. Ideally, this parameter should be constant.

Exposure linearity can be quantified by several methods. The first method defines exposure linearity as (3, 24, 25):

$$L = \frac{|mr/mAs_i - mr/mAs_{(i+1)}|}{mr/mAs_i + mr/mAs_{(i+1)}}$$

where mr/mAs_i and mr/mAs_{i+1} are the milliroentgens per milliampere second values obtained between two adjacent milliampere (milliampere second) stations differing by less than a factor of two. Performance is considered to be acceptable if this value is ≤ 0.1. The second method, which is more relevant to clinical systems, defines exposure linearity as:

$$L = \frac{mr/mAs_{max} - mr/mAs_{min}}{mr/mAs_{max} + mr/mAs_{min}}$$

where mr/mAs_{max} and mr/mAs_{min} represent the maximum and minimum milliroentgens per milliampere second values obtained over all milliampere (milliampere second) stations at a particular kilovoltage peak. Performance is considered acceptable if this value is ≤ 0.1.

A third approach defines exposure linearity as:

$$\sigma_{(mr/mAs)}/\overline{(mr/mAs)}$$

where $\overline{mr/mAs}$ is the average milliroentgens per milliampere second value over all milliampere (milliampere second) stations at the selected kilovoltage peak, and $\sigma_{(mr/mAs)}$ is its associated estimated standard deviation. Performance is considered acceptable if the value is ≤ 0.05.

Usually, exposure linearity is evaluated by varying milliamperage and time in a reciprocal fashion to maintain approximately the same milliampere seconds. Exposure linearity may also be evaluated by keeping the milliamperage constant and varying exposure time. For primary contacted generators, results will be identical for exposure times above about 5 msec. Below 5 msec it is not unusual to find that the milliroentgens per milliampere second increases with increasing exposure time. The increase is due to the nonideal shapes of the high voltage and tube current wave forms at short exposure times. An evaluation of this type provides useful information concerning potential clinical limitations of the x-ray system.

BEAM QUALITY

Measurements of beam quality (HVL) of x-ray tubes and source assemblies are important to verify that adequate filtration is present in the x-ray beam. Minimum values for total filtration and beam quality have been established by regulatory agencies (3). Several approaches exist for determination of beam quality. Measurements always should be made under conditions of good geometry with aluminum attenuators of high purity (type 1100).

The first approach to HVL measurement is determination of attenuation curves at each kilovoltage peak to at least the 40% transmission level. The resultant data are graphed and the HVL determined. A second method uses measurements of attenuation by three thicknesses of attenuator chosen to yield transmissions of approximately 60, 50, and 40% at each kilovoltage peak. Typical attenuation thicknesses are given in Table 7.3.

A third approach may be used if it is desired only to determine if the HVL is at least equal to the minimum required value. With this approach, an exposure is made with no attenuator in the beam. Then an attenuator of thickness equal to the minimum required HVL at the given kilovoltage peak is inserted in the beam and a second

Table 7.3
Typical Aluminum Thickness Required to Yield 60, 50, and 40% Transmission for Various Kilovoltage Peaks

kVp	mm Al thickness required to obtain approximate transmissions of		
	60%	50%	40%
60	1.3	2.3	3.8
80	2.0	3.1	4.6
100	3.0	4.0	5.8
120	4.0	5.0	6.2

exposure made. The ratio of exposures for the unattenuated and attenuated beam will be ≤ 2 if the HVL is at least equal to the minimum required value.

Beam Restriction System

In radiographic and fluoroscopic imaging systems, beam restriction systems (collimators) are used to confine the x-ray beam to the anatomical area of interest.

RADIOGRAPHIC BEAM RESTRICTION SYSTEMS

Features of the radiographic beam restriction system which should be evaluated during acceptance testing include the accuracy of the source to image receptor distance (SID) indicator, the alignment of the centers of the radiation field and the image receptor, congruence of the edges of the light and radiation fields, correspondence of the radiation field with the image receptor, correspondence of the radiation field size to the numerically indicated field size, minimum field size, minimum source to skin distance, intensity and contrast ratio of the light localizer, and function of the beam restriction system in the positive beam limitation mode.

Since many techniques are available for the evaluation of radiographic beam restriction systems, only general concepts are discussed here. Details of test methods may be found in the literature (4, 24–27).

The accuracy of the source to image receptor distance indicator may be evaluated by radiographing an object of known dimensions positioned at a known distance from the image receptor. The size of the image is measured, and the source to image receptor distance is calculated from the expression for image magnification. The size of the object and its distance from the image plane should be chosen to minimize errors, and the small focal spot should be used for the exposure.

Alignment of the center of the image receptor with the center of the radiation field may be evaluated by radiographing a special cassette in the image receptor holder. The center of the special cassette is delineated with a radioopaque marker. The x-ray tube is positioned at the usual source to image receptor distance and centered to the image receptor in the conventional manner. The field size should be smaller than the image receptor. A film exposed in the special cassette reveals the center of the image receptor as an image of the radioopaque object. The center of the radiation field is determined by drawing diagonal lines between the corners of the exposed area on the film. Displacement of the two centers suggests that misalignment is present.

Congruence of the visually defined field (i.e., collimator light field) and the radiation field may be evaluated from a radiograph exposed in the plane of the image receptor (or in a plane parallel to it) in which the edges of the visual field are delineated by radioopaque markers. In the image the displacement can be measured between the radiation field and the visually defined field as indicated by the opaque markers.

Correspondence of the numerically indicated field size with the radiation field can be determined from a radiograph exposed in the plane of the image receptor for the field size indicated for the SID. The radiation field size measured on the radiograph should agree with the numerically indicated values.

To evaluate the correspondence between the radiation field size and the size of the image receptor, a film may be exposed in a plane parallel to the image receptor at a known distance from the source. The radiation field size measured in this plane is projected geometrically onto the plane of the image receptor, and its correspondence with the size of the image receptor is evaluated.

The minimum field size may be determined by closing the collimators as completely as possible and exposing a film in the

plane of the image receptor. The image reveals the minimum field size at the SID at which the film was exposed.

Proper delineation of the visual field requires that the light localizer provide sufficient intensity and contrast with respect to the surroundings. The illumination and contrast provided by the light localizer may be evaluated by using small area photometers to determine the brightness level of the light field and the surrounding area.

For a radiographic beam restriction system that operates in a positive beam limitation (PBL) mode, all of the tests described above should be performed in both the PBL and the manual mode. In addition, in the PBL mode the system should automatically restrict the field size to the size of the image receptor or should inhibit exposure until the field size is manually adjusted.

FLUOROSCOPIC BEAM RESTRICTION SYSTEMS

For fluoroscopic beam restriction systems, performance characteristics include minimum source to skin distance, radiation field center-image receptor center alignment, and radiation field size-image receptor size correspondence. These characteristics are evaluated with approaches similar to those described for radiographic beam restriction systems (5, 24, 25, 27, 28). The evaluation should be conducted for both spot film and fluoroscopic modes of operation.

Grids

Antiscatter grids should be evaluated to verify that no grid damage is present that might produce artifacts and that the grid is aligned to the center of the radiation field.

The physical condition of a grid may be evaluated by low kilovoltage peak radiography with a high resolution direct exposure film. The x-ray source should be positioned at the focal distance for the grid. The resultant image should exhibit uniform density and be free of artifacts.

The alignment of the grid and radiation field centers may be determined by placing a fine radioopaque wire on the grid center line parallel to the grid axis. An x-ray film is exposed in a standard cassette with the radiation field restricted to a size smaller than the image receptor. The exposure time

should be sufficient to permit complete re-
ciprocation if a moving grid is employed.
For stationary grids the image will reveal the
center of the grid by the image of the radioopaque wire. Any differences are easily noted
between the grid center, image receptor center, and radiation field center. For reciprocating grids, the radioopaque line will be
imaged as a blurred area which should be
symmetrical with the centers of the image
receptor and radiation field. In analyzing the
images, care must be exercised not to interpret misalignment between the image receptor and radiation field as a problem of grid
alignment.

Fluoroscopic Imaging Systems

The fluoroscopic imaging chain is a complex assemblage of components that must
be carefully adjusted for optimal performance (29–37). Comprehensive investigation
of the fluoroscopic imaging chain requires
evaluation of the following performance parameters: automatic exposure and brightness
control function; image intensifier input
plane exposures and exposure rates, mode
tracking and consistency; patient entrance
exposure rates; TV system performance;
magnification ratio; distortion; contrast ratio; conversion factor; high contrast resolution; and low contrast performance.

Most fluoroscopic imaging chains employ
multiple image display and recording modes
(e.g., TV, photospot, cine). Performance of
a system should be evaluated for each mode.

AUTOMATIC BRIGHTNESS AND EXPOSURE CONTROL EVALUATION

The function of the automatic exposure
and brightness control (ABC) unit in a fluoroscopic imaging system is to maintain a
constant brightness at the output phosphor
for various image display and recording
modes, regardless of the imaging parameters
and patient variables. Constant brightness
usually is accomplished by sensing the
brightness of the output phosphor in some
manner to generate a signal that is compared
to a reference signal. The difference in the
signals is used to adjust the kilovoltage, tube
current, exposure duration, or some combination thereof. This adjustment alters the
exposure or exposure rate to the input phosphor to achieve the desired brightness on the

output phosphor. Many ABC systems can
be operated manually as well as automatically.

The most direct method to assess the performance of the ABC system is to measure
the exposure or exposure rate at the image
intensifier input plane. This measurement
may be accomplished with a pancake ion
chamber and suitable electrometer. The image intensifier is positioned approximately
12 inches above the table, a uniform attenuator is interposed in the beam, and the
system is operated in the automatic mode at
80 kVp. For systems that do not permit
independent control of the kilovoltage in the
automatic mode, the attenuator thickness
may be adjusted to provide a kilovoltage of
approximately 80. Exposure or exposure
rate values used by different manufacturers
vary somewhat. Typical ranges for a 9- to
10-inch image intensifier of modern design
are given in Table 7.4.

The performance of the ABC system may
be evaluated by measuring exposure rates at
the image intensifier input plane for a range
of kilovoltages and phantom thicknesses. In
a properly functioning system, the input
plane exposure rate will remain essentially
constant. A variation of ±20% or so might
be expected because of the energy dependence of the image intensifier input phosphor.

For multimode image intensifier systems
(e.g., 9/6/4.5) the exposure rate in the input
plane should increase approximately as the
reciprocal ratio of areas of the input field
size. In verifying this relationship, the attenuator thickness and kilovoltage remain
fixed, and the ion chamber is completely
irradiated.

Automatic exposure and brightness control system may be evaluated by exposure
rate measurements at locations other than
the input plane of the image intensifier; however, interpretation of the data is compli-

Table 7.4
**Representative Exposure Rates Measured at the
Input Plane during Automatic Brightness
Control Operation**[a]

Fluoroscopy	1.8–3.6 mR/min
Photospot (100/105 mm)	75–150 μR/frame
Cine (35 mm)	15–30 μR/frame

[a] The values are independent of the presence
of the grid.

cated by factors such as attenuation of the x-ray beam by the grid and changes in the amount of scatter radiation as a function of attenuator thickness for different chamber locations.

Automatic exposure and brightness control system performance can be inferred from measurements of exposure rates at the tabletop using the following guidelines:

1. For fluoroscopic imaging systems operated in manual mode, the tabletop exposure rate should increase with increasing kilovoltage peak at fixed milliamperage and with increasing milliamperage at fixed kilovoltage peak. Under no circumstances should the corrected exposure rate exceed 10 R/min during fluoroscopy.
2. If the phantom thickness is increased at constant kilovoltage peak, both the milliamperage and the exposure rate should increase.
3. If the phantom thickness is kept constant and the kilovoltage peak is increased, the exposure rate and milliamperage should decrease.
4. An increase in phantom thickness always should produce an increase in exposure rate. The exposure rate increase may be caused by an increase in milliamperage at constant kilovoltage peak, an increase in kilovoltage peak with a decrease in milliamperage, or an increase in both kilovoltage peak and milliamperage.
5. When a lead beam stop is placed on top of the phantom, the ABC will be driven to its maximum fluoroscopic technique factors and will yield the maximum exposure rate at tabletop.
6. For image intensifiers with multiple formats (i.e., dual or trifield tubes), a reduction in the size of the image intensifier field of view will produce an increase in exposure rate in approximately the ratio of the squares of the nominal intensifier diameters. For example, changing from the 9-inch to the 6-inch mode leads to an exposure rate increase of $(9/6)^2$ or 2.25. This relationship remains reasonably valid provided that the kilovoltage peak does not change.
7. The fluoroscopic image should maintain constant brightness regardless of phantom thickness, kilovoltage peak, or milliamperage. The only exception is when the lead beam stop is inserted in the beam; in this case no fluoroscopic image should be visible.

MAXIMUM PATIENT ENTRANCE EXPOSURE RATES

Regulatory and advisory groups have established maximum permissible patient entrance exposure rates for routine fluoroscopy. The point of measurement is 1 cm above the tabletop for conventional fluoroscopic units (undertable tube with overtable image intensifier), 30 cm above the tabletop with the source at minimum height for systems with overtable x-ray tube and undertable image intensifier, and 30 cm from the input plane of the image intensifier for C-arm units.

The maximum patient entrance exposure rate is 10 R/min for systems equipped with automatic brightness control (in either the automatic or manual mode), and 5 R/min for systems equipped with only manual brightness control. Exceptions to these limits are systems equipped with a high level mode for the fluoroscopic exposure rate. In these systems, the maximum exposure rate is 5 R/min unless the high level mode is activated, in which case no limit is specified. All of the preceding limits apply only during fluoroscopy and not during the recording of fluoroscopic images (i.e., photospot and cine).

MAGNIFICATION RATIO/ DISTORTION

Sometimes it is useful to know the degree of image magnification provided by the different operational modes of an image intensifier, and the degree of distortion present due to the electrooptical characteristics of the imaging chain. The magnification ratio can be determined with a test object containing a series of concentric circles of known spacing. The test object is imaged in each of the intensifier modes, and the ratios of magnification for each image are determined from the diameters of the circles in the image (38).

Distortion can be assessed by imaging a test pattern containing a 1-cm grid of fine wires placed as near as possible to the input plane. Comparison of the grid spacing at various locations in the field provides a measure of distortion (38).

CONTRAST RATIO AND CONVERSION FACTOR

Measurement of the conversion factor and contrast ratio is difficult on a clinically installed fluoroscopic system (39, 40). However, routine techniques are available to monitor the consistency of these parameters on a relative basis after they have been determined initially during acceptance testing.

Evaluation of the conversion factor requires the simultaneous measurement of exposure rates at the image intensifier entrance plane (input phosphor) and the corresponding brightness of the output phosphor (39, 40). Exposure rates are measured as discussed previously. The measurement of brightness requires a photometer with a suitable photometric response. The photometer can be mounted on the fluoroscopic system with a special adapter positioned at the location normally occupied by the TV camera. The conversion factor is the ratio of the output phosphor brightness in candela per square meter divided by the entrance plane exposure rate in mR/sec.

The contrast ratio can be measured for systems equipped with photospot recording mode (41). A series of photospot images is first obtained as a function of exposure measured at the entrance plane. Next, the central 10% of the image intensifier is blocked with a 100% attenuating disk, and a second sequence of images is obtained as a function of exposure. These images are obtained at exposure levels chosen to yield optical densities in the region of the disk that are approximately equal to those obtained without the disk.

The optical density versus exposure data for the two image sequences are used to determine the exposures for both nondisk and disk images yielding the same optical density. The contrast ratio is the disk to nondisk exposure.

All of the measurement procedures described above yield results for the total imaging chain and not simply the image intensifier alone.

HIGH CONTRAST RESOLUTION

The high contrast resolution performance of an intensified fluoroscopic imaging system may be evaluated by using either a lead line pair pattern containing spatial frequencies of 0.5 to 4 line pairs per millimeter (lp)/mm or a test pattern consisting of 25% open area mesh with mesh sizes from 8 to 80 mesh (number of wires per inch of wire cloth) (30, 36). The test pattern should be positioned as close as possible to the input plane of the image intensifier and should be imaged at a low kilovoltage with the small focal spot and with the grid removed, if possible. If the grid cannot be removed, the test pattern should be oriented at 45° with respect to the grid lines. The resolution performance for each image display and/or recording mode is documented.

LOW CONTRAST RESOLUTION

The low contrast sensitivity of an intensified fluoroscopic imaging system may be evaluated with a 2% thickness penetrameter (30, 36). This penetrameter usually consists of a $\frac{1}{32}$-inch aluminum plate contained between two $\frac{3}{4}$-inch aluminum plates. The penetrameter contains holes with diameters of $\frac{1}{4}$, $\frac{3}{16}$, $\frac{1}{8}$, $\frac{1}{16}$, and $\frac{1}{32}$ inch. The contrast penetrameter is positioned midway between the source and the image intensifier input plane, and the grid is left in place. With the penetrameter imaged at 80 kVp, the smallest visible hole size for each imaging display and/or recording mode is determined.

TV SYSTEMS

The television chain employed in intensified fluoroscopic systems is important to the overall performance of the system. The chain usually is not accessible for individual testing procedures during acceptance tests; however, it may be necessary at times to evaluate at least certain aspects of the performance of the television chain. In this event, a thorough understanding of the television chain is necessary if a meaningful evaluation is to be achieved (33, 35).

Automatic Exposure Control

The function of the automatic exposure control (AEC) is to maintain a constant optical density on film over a broad range of imaging techniques and patient variables (42–46). To evaluate the performance of the automatic exposure control, a variable thickness phantom is required to simulate the attenuating and scattering characteristics of patients. The phantom may be either water or acrylic; however, acrylic is easier to use. Performance is evaluated usually from exposure measurements or measurements of optical density on film. Exposure measurements are made on the beam entrance side of the phantom, whereas the film is exposed in the plane of the image receptor in the shadow of the active area(s) of the automatic exposure control pickup. Sensitometric evaluation may be required to separate density variations due to processing from those contributed by the automatic exposure control. Performance assessment should include field selection wiring, reproducibility, field matching, field size compensation, performance capability, and maximum allowed exposure duration. All evaluation procedures should be performed with the image receptor to be used clinically.

FIELD SELECTION WIRING

Proper selection of the AEC pickup fields may be verified by using lead to successively block all but the selected field and making an exposure. Proper wiring of the AEC fields is demonstrated by normal termination of exposure corresponding to the selected field.

REPRODUCIBILITY

The reproducibility of the AEC may be determined from analysis of multiple exposure measurements at various kilovoltage peaks and phantom thicknesses or from film density measurements. The coefficient of variation of the measurements serves as a criterion for acceptable performance.

FIELD MATCHING

The degree of sensitivity matching of multiple pickup fields in the AEC may be evaluated from analysis of multiple exposure measurements for each field at a fixed kilovoltage peak and phantom thickness or from film density measurements.

FIELD SIZE COMPENSATION

The variation in AEC performance with changes in field size can be determined from an analysis of film density measurements of radiographs exposed under identical conditions with the exception of field size. The field sizes employed for this evaluation should range across those employed clinically.

PERFORMANCE CAPABILITY

The capability of the AEC to provide constant film density over a broad range of kilovoltage peaks and patient thicknesses can be evaluated by analysis of film density over 60 to 120 kVp and phantom thicknesses of 2 to 10 inches of acrylic. Exposure times greater than 3 msec or milliampere second values greater than 5 should be used. Analysis of the resultant data as a function of kilovoltage peak and phantom thickness should demonstrate only small variations in film density.

BACK-UP TIMER

The maximum automatically controlled exposure may be determined by blocking the pickup fields with a ¼-inch thick lead plate and making an automatically controlled exposure. The measured exposure time or milliampere seconds during this exposure should be less than 60 kWs and/or 600 mAs for kilovoltage peaks greater than 50.

Tomographic Equipment

The following procedures are presented for evaluating the performance of analog tomographic equipment during initial acceptance testing. Included in the evaluation are the stability of motion, exposure uniformity, depth flatness and thickness of the tomographic section, exposure angle, and spatial resolution (6, 39, 47–50).

Tomography is the generally accepted term that specifies a class of radiologic procedures employing body section radiography. All tomographic units share the basic principle of motion between the x-ray source and image receptor or patient during exposure. Tomography can be conducted with a wide variety of geometrical motions including linear, circular, spiral, hypocycloidal, and random. The choice of motion usually is dictated by the anatomical structure to be imaged. The magnitude of the exposure angle can be varied to alter the thickness of the tomographic section; as the angle increases, the section thickness decreases.

The following nomenclature is used in discussing tomographic systems (39):

Fulcrum: A fixed axis around which the x-ray source and image receptor rotate.

Tomographic Scale: A means of indicating the height of the fulcrum above a reference plane (usually the plane of patient support). This scale indicates the location of the center of the tomographic section.
Objective Plane: The plane in which all points in the image will be sharply imaged in the image receptor; the plane of maximum focus; the central plane of the tomographic section.
Source-Image Receptor Distance: The distance between the x-ray source and image receptor.
Source-Plane Distance: The distance between the x-ray source and the objective plane.
Plane-Image Receptor Distance: The distance between the objective plane and image receptor.
Section Thickness: The effective thickness of a tomographic section.
Operative Angle: The angle through which the tomographic apparatus moves.
Exposure Angle: The angle through which the central ray moves during exposure.

By its very nature, tomography provides an image of apparently inferior quality compared to conventional radiography. It is essential to verify that the mechanical aspects of a tomographic system are optimized to ensure satisfactory clinical results. Hence, tests are necessary to determine the mechanical stability of tomographic motion, the uniformity of exposure during tomographic motion, the accuracy and linearity of the tomographic scale with respect to the objective plane, the flatness of the objective plane, the thickness of the tomographic section, the accuracy and symmetry of the exposure angle, and the resolution in the objective plane.
A variety of test objects (phantoms) are

available for assessment of tomographic equipment. A representative list of equipment required for a satisfactory evaluation of most analog tomographic units is given in Table 7.5.
Procedures for the evaluation of many aspects of radiologic imaging equipment are enerally agreed upon by the majority of users. The same cannot be said for the evaluation of tomographic equipment. The procedures outlined below are commonly encountered; however, several alternative methods of evaluation exist.

MECHANICAL STABILITY AND EXPOSURE UNIFORMITY

The most common method to evaluate the mechanical stability and exposure uniformity of a tomographic unit is to use a lead plate with a 3-mm beveled pinhole aperture. With the x-ray tube perpendicular to the image receptor, the aperture is positioned in the central ray approximately 12 cm above the objective plane (Fig. 7.13). Exposures are then obtained for the various tomographic motions, exposure angles, etc., available. For these exposures, technique factors should be used that yield an image density of approximately 1.2. As illustrated in Figure 7.14, the recorded image will describe the geometric form of the obscuring movement. In a properly functioning system, the density of the image should be uniform over the complete trajectory; for pluridirectional systems, proper closure of the geometric motion should be exhibited. Mechanical instabilities will be demonstrated as discontinuities in the recorded image, and incomplete exposures will be demonstrated as nonclosed trajectories. When evaluating 1-ϕ tomographic equipment, the pulsed nature of the x-ray beam will be apparent in the image. One should

Table 7.5
Test Instrumentation Required for the Evaluation of Geometrical Tomographic Equipment

Test object	Application
Aperture plate	Exposure uniformity, motion stability.
Inclined scale	Objective plane location, flatness of objective plane, exposure angle, thickness of cut.
Inclined mesh resolution pattern	System.

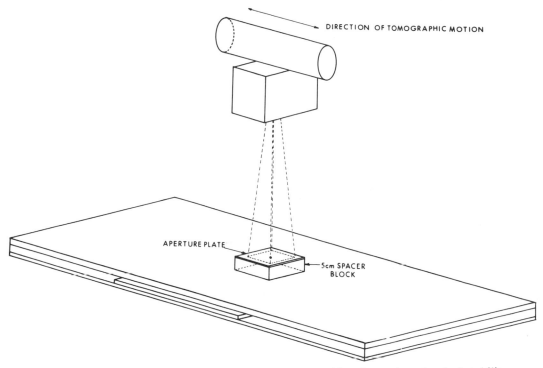

Figure 7.13. Arrangement for determining exposure uniformity and mechanical stability.

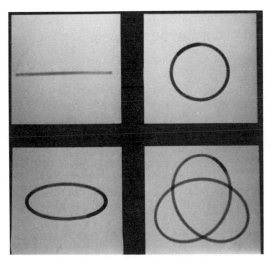

Figure 7.14. Typical test films for different tomographic motions from which uniformity of tomographic exposure and mechanical stability are determined. (*A*) Linear. (*B*) Circular. (*C*) Elliptical. (*D*) Hypocycloidal.

also verify that the exposure time set on the generator is longer than that required for the tomographic motion. If a spot exposure is superimposed on the film with the x-ray source in its perpendicular position, the re-sultant pinhole image will permit assessment of exposure angle.

TOMOGRAPHIC SCALE ACCURACY AND LINEARITY

The accuracy with which the tomographic scale indicates the level of the objective plane may be evaluated with a calibrated inclined wedge, as illustrated in Figure 7.15. For linear systems, the wedge should be oriented with the scale perpendicular to the direction of tomographic motion. Tomographic exposures are made for the various tomographic motions and speeds and at different settings of the tomographic scale (typically 5, 10, 15, and 20 cm). The location of the objective plane is readily determined from the image, as illustrated in Figure 7.16. The linearity of scale indication is determined by noting the correspondence of the measured location of the objective plane with that indicated by the tomographic scale.

FLATNESS OF OBJECTIVE PLANE

The flatness of the objective plane can be evaluated by the procedure used to determine the accuracy of the tomographic scale.

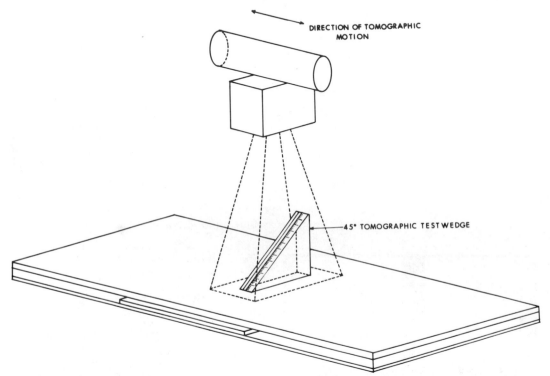

Figure 7.15. Arrangement for determining accuracy of tomographic scale with respect to objective plane.

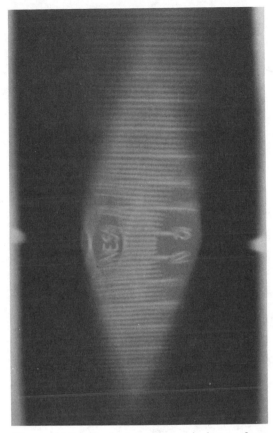

Figure 7.16. Typical tomographic image from which accuracy of tomographic scale is determined.

A series of tomographic exposures is obtained at each section level, with the inclined wedge positioned in different quadrants of the field during exposure. The images should indicate the same level of objective plane, regardless of the location of the wedge. A large coarse wire mesh positioned in the objective plane may also be used for these measurements.

THICKNESS OF THE TOMOGRAPHIC SECTION

The thickness of the tomographic section is inversely related to exposure angle. The section thickness is evaluated with the inclined wedge, as illustrated in Figure 7.17, with resultant images similar to those shown in Figure 7.18 for various exposure angles. The section thickness is defined as the region over which the scale on the inclined wedge is in sharper focus. Determination of the

limits of this region is somewhat subjective. For linear systems, the inclined wedge should be oriented parallel to the direction of tomographic motion.

Section thickness can also be determined with the test object shown in Figure 7.19 (39). This test object consists of a cylinder 7 cm in diameter and 12 cm long, wound with a coil of 1-mm diameter wire at a pitch of 1 cm. A wire also runs coaxillary to the cylinder. The cylinder is placed with its long axis perpendicular to the objective plane, with the objective plane bisecting the cylinder. A tomographic image will show some portion of the wire coil in focus. This portion yields a measure of the section thickness.

EXPOSURE ANGLE

The tomographic angle can be measured with the inclined wedge in the geometry shown in Figure 7.20. For linear systems, the wedge is oriented perpendicular to the direction of motion. The tomographic scale is set for an objective plane of approximately 12 cm, and tomographic exposures are made for various motions and exposure angles. An example of the resultant tomographic image and the necessary reconstructions to determine the exposure angle are shown in Figures 7.21A and B. For a wedge angle inclination of 45°,

$$\tan \beta_1 = c_{11}/b_1$$
$$\tan \beta_2 = c_{21}/b_1$$

for points above the objective plane, and

$$\tan \beta_1 = c_{12}/b_2$$
$$\tan \beta_2 = c_{22}/b_2$$

for points below the objective plane, where c and b are measured in the tomographic image using the same scale.

For the case in which the exposure angle is symmetrical, the exposure angle is given by:

$$\alpha = 2 \tan^{-1}(c/2h)$$

For the general case in which the exposure angle is not symmetrical,

$$\alpha = b_1 + b_2.$$

For points above the objective plane,

$$\tan \alpha = \frac{b_1 (c_{11} + c_{21})}{(b_1^2 - c_{11} c_{21})},$$

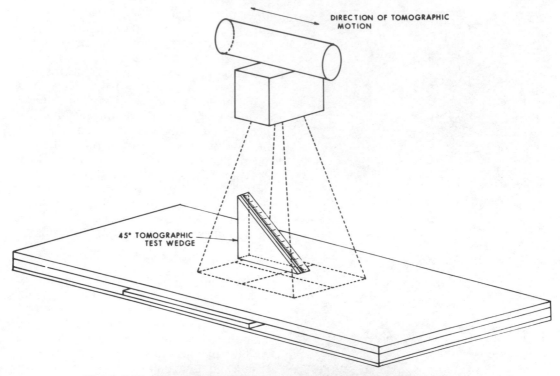

Figure 7.17. Arrangement for determining tomographic section thickness.

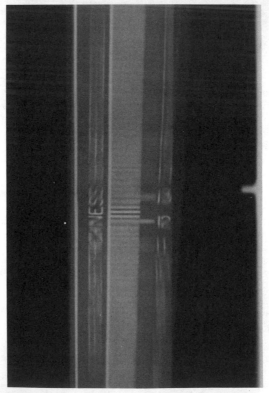

Figure 7.18. Typical tomographic image from which section thickness is determined.

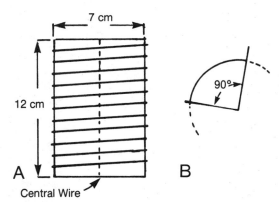

Figure 7.19. Test object (*A*) and reconstructed tomographic image (*B*) which may be used to determine section thickness.

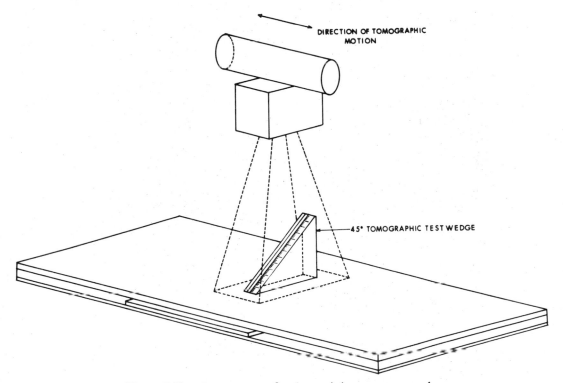

Figure 7.20. Arrangement for determining exposure angle.

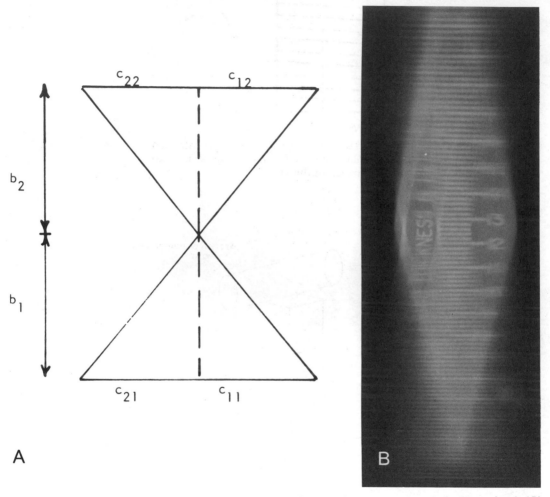

Figure 7.21. (*A*) Reconstructed tomographic image from which exposure angle is determined. (*B*) Exposure angle determined from tomographic image.

and for points below the objective plane,

$$\tan \alpha = \frac{b_2 (c_{11} + c_{21})}{(b_2{}^2 - c_{11} c_{12})}.$$

The exposure angle may also be determined with the test device illustrated in Figure 7.22 (39). This device is a 0.5-mm thick lead foil pitched at an angle of 45° and containing a narrow slit with radioopaque wires at 1-cm intervals. Also present is a horizontal lead foil containing a single hole in line with the slit. The x-ray tube is positioned with the central ray perpendicular to the objective plane. The test object is placed on the table with the hole in the horizontal lead foil in line with the central ray. A nontomographic exposure is made to record an image of the hole and slit. The x-ray tube is then moved to any angle, the hole is covered with lead, and a second nontomographic exposure is made. Finally, the slit is covered, the hole is uncovered, and a tomographic exposure is made. The resultant tomographic image will appear similar to those shown in Figure 7.23. These images may be used to determine the location of the objective plane. The exposure angle can be derived from the excursion of the image of the hole to each side of the central dot according to the relationships:

$$\tan \alpha_1 = (D - h) S_1/Ah$$
$$\tan \alpha_2 = (D - h) S_2/Ah$$

Another method of determining exposure angle uses the technique of recording an image of a narrow slit fixed to the collimator of the x-ray tube, together with a stationary film oriented at a slight angle with respect to the central ray. The exposure angle may be measured directly from the recorded image. Details of this procedure may be found elsewhere.

SPATIAL RESOLUTION

The ability of a tomographic unit to demonstrate anatomical detail depends not only on the mechanics of the system, but also upon the type of image receptor employed, the size of the x-ray tube focal spot, and the magnification employed to form the image. Tomographic resolution may be evaluated with the arrangement shown in Figure 7.24.

The test object consists of a resolution pattern that passes through the objective plane at a slight angle (e.g., 15°). The pattern may be either a series of wire meshes ranging from 10 to 50 mesh or a bar pattern of spatial frequencies from 0.5 to 5 lp/mm. When using a bar pattern with a linear tomographic unit, the bar groups should be oriented at right angles to the tomographic motion. The tomographic image will appear similar to that shown in Figure 7.25. The highest resolvable mesh or spatial frequency is the resolving capability of the system, including the influence of focal spot size, magnification, and image receptor.

In evaluating the performance of analog tomographic equipment for purposes of initial acceptance testing, the criteria for acceptable performance should be those agreed upon in the equipment purchase contract. Guidance as to realistic levels of performance to be expected are described in Chapter 4.

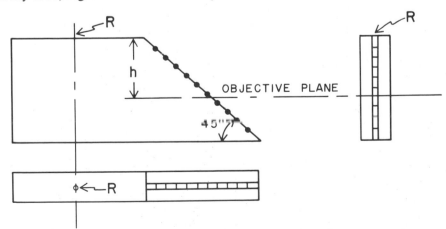

Figure 7.22. Alternate test object for determination of exposure angle.

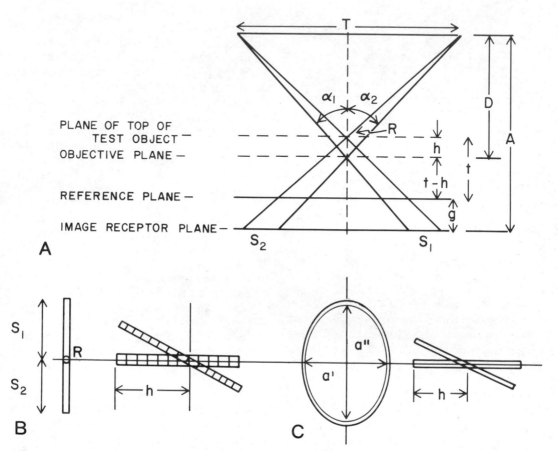

Figure 7.23. Geometry necessary to determine exposure angle (*A*) and reconstructed tomographic images for linear (*B*) and elliptical (*C*) motions. *A* is the source-image receptor distance; *D* is the source-objective plane distance; *h* is the distance to the objective plane from the top of the test object; *t* is the height of the test object; *g* is the image receptor reference plane distance; *T* is the distance moved by the source; and S_1 and S_2 are the excursions of the central ray.

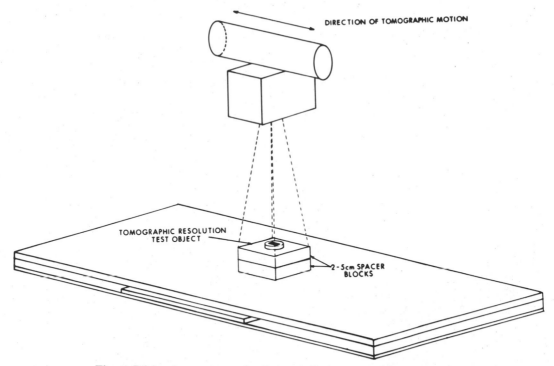

Figure 7.24. Arrangement for determining tomographic resolution.

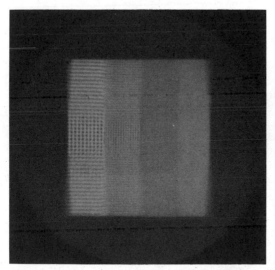

Figure 7.25. Tomographic image from which system resolution capability is determined.

Equipment for Acceptance Testing

To conduct a successful program of acceptance testing for radiological equipment, a few instruments are necessary. A general description of the required items of equipment, their normal use, and their approximate cost are provided in Table 7.6.

Summary

Table 7.7 presents a summary of equipment parameters to be tested, test methods, and levels of reasonably anticipated performance.

NUCLEAR MEDICINE

The most common piece of imaging equipment in nuclear medicine is the single crystal scintillation camera. This unit will be used to illustrate the details of acceptance testing procedures in nuclear medicine. Scintillation camera acceptance testing has been addressed by three major organizations: (1) the National Electrical Manufacturer's Association (NEMA) (51); (2) the Center for Devices and Radiological Health (CDRH) (52, 53); and (3) the American Association of Physicists in Medicine (AAPM) (54). Many of the techniques suggested in this section are taken directly or adapted from measurements suggested by one or more of these organizations.

Procedures for Scintillation Camera Acceptance Testing

Acceptance testing should be undertaken only after all components of the imaging

Table 7.6
Typical Instrumentation Required for Performance of Acceptance Testing

Item	Normal use	Approximate cost
High voltage dividers with jumper cables	kVp, timer evaluation	$2000.00
Dual trace storage oscilloscope with Polaroid camera	kVp, mA, timer evaluation, wave form recording and documentation	$7000.00
Digital multimeter (DMM)	mA evaluation, general voltage measurements	$350.00
mAs meter (may be part of DMM)	mA evaluation	$350.00
Dosimetry system (ion chambers, electrometer)	Exposure, exposure rate measurements	$3000.00
Densitometer	Film density measurements	$900.00
Sensitometer	Processor evaluation	$500.00
Resolution meshes, contrast penetrameters	Image intensifier evaluation	$500.00
Attenuation test object (variable thickness, acrylic)	AEC, ABC evaluation	$400.00
Tomographic test objects	Tomographic system evaluation	$600.00
Miscellaneous test objects, etc.		$500.00

Table 7.7
Summary of Parameters, Test Methods, and Levels of Acceptable Performance for Radiographic/Fluoroscopic Equipment

Parameter	Measurement method	Performance level
kVp	High voltage bleeder/ storage oscilloscope/ Polaroid recordings.	±4 kVp from indicated regardless of mA and ≤5 kVp overshoots.
mA (mAs)	Precision resistor in series with milliampere metering circuit/storage oscilloscope/Polaroid recordings. mAs meter. Dynalyzer II.	±5% of indicated, regardless of kVp.
Time	High voltage bleeder/ storage oscilloscope/ Polaroid recordings. kVp/mA sufficiently high to eliminate capacitive effects. Width of kVp pulse at vendor specified % of peak.	±5% of indicated. ±5% reproducible.
Tube protector	Comparison of system lock with vendor rating charts for tube.	+0% of allowed. −30% of allowed rating.
Focal spot size	Pinhole camera at NEMA technique. Star pattern at NEMA technique.	NEMA

Table 7.7—*continued*

Parameter	Measurement method	Performance level
Focal spot growth	Star pattern: $f(kVp, mA)$; (kVp^{min}, mA^{max}); (kVp^{min}, mA^{min}); (kVp^{max}, mA^{max}); (kVp^{max}, mA^{min}); consistent with tube ratings.	±40% with respect to NEMA technique.
Leakage radiation	Vendor supplied data.	≤100 mr in 1 hr at 1 m at leakage technique.
Exposure output	Exposure measurement with ion chamber.	20 mr/mAs ± 25% at 80 kVp at 24 inches from source.
Exposure reproducibility	Exposure measurement with ion chamber.	±5%, technique factors charged between each measurement ($\delta/\bar{x} \leq 0.05$).
Exposure linearity	Exposure measurement with ion chamber.	$$L = \frac{mR/mAs_{max} - mR/mAs_{min}}{mR/mAs_{max} + mR/mAs_{min}}$$ ≤0.10 over available mA range (mAs ≤ 200)
Beam quality	Exposure measurement with ion chamber using aluminum (1100) attenuators under conditions of good geometry.	HVL = BRH ≤ 1.40 BRH required minimum
SID indicator accuracy (rad)	Analysis of radiographic image of object of known dimensions and determination by triangulation.	±1% of indicated SID.
X-ray field to image receptor center (rad)	Analysis of radiographic image using specialized test cassette.	±1.5% of indicated SID on any edge, ±2% of indicated SID along length or width of film, ±3% of SID for sum of all edge misalignments.
Radiation field size/image receptor size congruence (rad)	Analysis of radiographic image using specialized test cassette.	±2% of indicated SID along length or width, ±3% for sum of length and width.
Radiation field size/numerically indicated field size congruence (rad)	Analysis of radiographic image using specialized test cassette.	±1% of indicated SID along length or width, ±2% of indicated SID for sum of length and width.
Intensity of light localizer (rad)	Photometric measurement.	160 lux at 100 cm or SID max, whichever is less.
Contrast ratio of light localizer (rad)	Photometric measurement.	4:1 at 100 cm or SID max, whichever is less.
Minimum source to skin distance (fluoro)	Analysis of radiographic image of object of known dimensions and determination by triangulation.	≥38 cm for stationary systems; ≥30 cm for mobile systems.
Radiation field center/image receptor center congruence (fluoro)	Analysis of radiographic image of specialized test device.	±1% of SID.

Table 7.7—*continued*

Parameter	Measurement method	Performance level
Radiation field/image receptor edge congruence (fluoro)	Analysis of radiographic image of specialized test device.	±1% of SID for any edge, ±2% of SID along diameter, ±3% of SID sum.
Radiation field size/image receptor size congruence (fluoro)	Analysis of radiographic image of specialized test device.	±2% of SID along length or width, ±4% of SID for sum of length and width.
Grid alignment	Mechanical verification of correspondence of grid center line to x-ray beam central ray. Application of lateral de-centering grid cut off with recording of optical density on film using specialized test device.	±½ inch
High contrast resolution of image intensifier	Wire mesh pattern or line pair plate placed directly (as close as possible) to input phosphor; grid removed, 60 kVp, ½ inch. Al attenuator at tabletop, small focal spot, IT 12 inches above tabletop; system nominal dose rate at IT input.	TV systems—10/9 inch—20; 7/6 inch—24; 5/4 inch—30 mesh. Film recording systems or direct view 10/9 inch—30; 7/6 inch—40; 5/4 inch—50 mesh.
Image intensifier low contrast resolution	2% thickness hole penetrameter (1/32-inch Al, in 1.5-inch Al) placed at tabletop, IT 12 inches above tabletop, grid in place; small focus, system operated at nominal dose rate, 80 kVp.	TV systems—10/9 inch—¼ inch, 7/6 inch—1/8 inch, 5/4 inch—1/16 inch. Film recording system All—1/16 inch.
Image intensifier input exposure rate/exposure	Measurement of exposure rate/exposure at input phosphor at 80 kVp with homogeneous phantom using suitable ion chamber/dosimetry system.	In agreement with manufacturer's specification (anticipate 3.6 mR/min for fluoro 9 inch)—100 μR/frame (fr) for photospot and 20 μR/fr 35 mm cine.
Image intensifier input exposure rate/exposure mode tracking	Measurement of exposure rate/exposure at input phosphor at 80 kVp with homogeneous phantom using suitable ion chamber/dosimetry system.	Input exposure rate/exposure to track with magnification rate of multimode image tube.
Consistency of image intensifier input exposure rate/exposure (ABC)	Measurement of exposure rate/exposure at input phosphor f(kVp, phantom thickness) using suitable ion chamber/dosimetry system.	Constant to within energy dependence of input phosphor.

Table 7.7—*continued*

Parameter	Measurement method	Performance level
Function of automatic brightness (dose) control	Measurement of exposure rate on entrance side of homogeneous phantom and exit side using suitable ion chambers/dosimetry systems $f(kVp$, phantom thickness).	Exit exposure rate to remain constant for given intensifier mode to within energy dependence of input phosphor. Entrance exposure rate evaluated dependent on type of ABC employed.
Maximum patient entrance exposure rate	Measurement of exposure rate at geometrical location corresponding to CDRH regulations for type of system using homogeneous phantom and suitable ion chamber and dosimetry system.	For systems with ABC ≤ 10 r/min max. Maximum exposure rate to be independent of kVp.
Magnification rate for multimode image tubes	Specialized test object consisting of wire circles at 1-cm radius increments placed at input phosphor. Ratio determined from image of circles on TV monitor or from film-recorded images.	Specification of manufacturer.
Distortion of image intensifier	Specialized test object consisting of wire mesh (square) on 1-cm spacings placed at input phosphor. Ratio determined from assessment of film-recorded images by comparing size of square (radial and tangential) at field center to field edge.	Specifications of manufacturer.
Image intensifier contrast ratio	Suitable method for field measurement unavailable.	
Automatic exposure control system (AEC) reproducibility	Measurement of exposure on beam entrance side of homogeneous phantom using suitable ion chamber/dosimetry system. Measurement of film optical density.	±5%, $\delta/\bar{x} \le 0.05$ for exposure times ≥5 msec. $\delta OD/OD \le 0.05$
AEC field matching	Measurement of exposure on beam entrance side of homogeneous phantom using suitable ion chamber/dosimetry system. Measurement of film optical density.	Individual fields and/or field combinations matched to within ±5% unless otherwise stated by manufacturer. OD matched to ±5%.

Table 7.7—*continued*

Parameter	Measurement method	Performance level
AEC field selection wiring	Individual fields blocked lead and selected. Exposure made with a backup time set.	Exposure time to run to backup.
AEC kVp compensation and thickness tracking	Measurement of film optical density as a function of kVp and phantom thickness. Additional parameters such as exposure time, actual kVp and mA, AEC reference and integrator voltages may also be measured.	±0.3 OD over working kVp range and phantom thickness range within system constraints as designed by the manufacturer.
AEC backup time	AEC pickup devices blocked with ¼-inch thick lead plate and exposure made.	Exposure to be determined by preselected backup time, automatically programmed backup time, or mAs limit.
Objective plane	45° inclined scale.	The measured objective plane shall coincide with the machine indicated objective plan within ±0.25 cm.
Exposure angle	45° inclined scale.	The measured exposure angle shall coincide with the machine indicated exposure angle (if any) within ±3°.
Flatness of plane	45° inclined scale.	The measured flatness of plane shall be in accordance with the manufacturer's specified tolerance for flatness of plane.
Tomographic resolution	Inclined mesh.	The measured tomographic resolution shall be in accordance with the manufacturer's specified tomographic resolution capabilities.
Section thickness	45° inclined scale.	The measured section thickness shall be within ±50% of the section thickness specified by the manufacturer.
Exposure uniformity	Aperture plate.	Uniform over entire geometrical motion.

system have been installed. The complete list of components, options, and accessories, along with the performance specifications for the system, should be reviewed, and a log book for acceptance testing should be initiated. The first entry in the log book should be the inventory list for the scintillation camera. Operator and service manuals should be checked for accuracy and completeness and should cover all accessories on the system. The manuals should be reviewed thoroughly before and during the acceptance testing procedure.

The mechanical function of all moving components should be inspected. Detector and yoke motion should be checked for travel to their specified limits. Limit switches should be checked, and braking mechanisms should be exercised to verify their proper operation. For whole body imaging systems, the camera or table travel should be checked for smoothness, speed, and total travel. For rotating camera tomographic systems, the detector rotation should be checked for smoothness, speed, and constancy of speed, both on the uphill and downhill sides of detector rotation. Alignment of the axis of a rotating detector with the patient imaging table should also be checked. Electrical cables should be inspected for mechanical protection during detector motion. For each component of the system, cable entry points should be checked for proper isolation with grommets.

All electrical switches and lights should be tested for proper operation according to the user's manual. Electrical circuit breakers and replaceable fuses should be identified to the purchaser. Power down and power up procedures for the high voltage supply should be noted.

Shielding of the detector head should be checked with a point isotopic source with emissions near the maximum rated energy for the detector head. With this source, the count rate is recorded at multiple points around the detector head (55), with special attention to rotation points and cable and bolt entry points. If areas of noticeably high count rate are detected, extra shielding should be applied. If extra shielding is impractical, the areas of decreased shielding should be noted, together with the appearance and reproducibility of higher count rates in an image. To identify detector shielding problems at the γ-ray energies routinely employed clinically, the measurements should be repeated with a high activity point source of the isotope in most common use.

Collimator acceptance should include inspections for collimator uniformity and mechanical defects. In some collimators, usually the molded type, the surface near the detector is uncovered and can be examined visually. On the other hand, foil collimators require removal of the covering for visual inspection; alternatively, an indirect inspection for localized defects can be made with roentgenography, fluoroscopy, or with a ^{99m}Tc flood tank exposing a large x-ray film or film screen combination (Fig. 7.26). The scintillation camera itself can be used to evaluate the integrity of the collimator, provided that methods are available for extracting the correlated nonuniformities of the detector.

Prior to NEMA specifications, measurements of detector response were not standardized and, for the most part, were qualitative only. NEMA intrinsic detector response measurements are now well accepted by camera manufacturers. The first NEMA measurement to be made is the energy resolution of the system. A multichannel analyzer (MCA) is used to record the analog Z (energy) pulses from the detector in response to interactions of monoenergetic radiation in the detector. The test should be performed at relatively low count rates (i.e., count rates which produce less than 10% deadtime in the MCA being used). The MCA must be calibrated in kiloelectron volts per channel by locating the centroids of two known energy photopeaks relatively close to the energy where the resolution is to be measured. ^{57}Co and ^{99m}Tc are convenient sources for calibration, since the 140 keV photopeak of ^{99m}Tc is the energy most commonly quoted for energy response. After the centroid of the two peaks and the channel width of the MCA have been determined, the full width at half maximum (FWHM) of the ^{99m}Tc photopeak can be determined. To permit an accurate determination of the peak center, there should be at least 50 channels above the FWHM. Channels in the photopeak should contain more than 10,000 counts/channel for good statistical definition of the peak. The detector energy resolution is reported in percentage terms as the (FWHM/photopeak energy) $\times$ 100. A value on the order of 10% is expected for NaI(Tl) crystals at 140 keV.

System deadtime should be measured next, so that count rate limits of the camera can be established for future measurements of uniformity, spatial resolution, and linearity at both "low" and "high" count rates. For all time-response measurements, the configuration of the source and the upper and lower limits of the energy window are critical. Source configurations should either involve no scatter medium (neither absorption nor backscatter material) or provide adequate filtration so that the photofraction of the energy spectrum is constant (56). In deadtime measurements it is important to remember that all interactions in the detector contribute to deadtime, whether they are interactions of primary or secondary photons and whether or not they are within the energy window. Maximum count rates will be observed for sources with no scatter and for energy windows encompassing the entire energy spectrum. Two time response meas-

Figure 7.26. Collimator quality assurance. Collimators with surfaces inaccessible for visual evaluation can be investigated by placing the collimator between a ^{99m}Tc-filled flood tank and a film-screen combination. This high-energy collimator was exposed to a 30-mCi flood source for 5 hr. Dupont Quanta III intensifying screens with Cronex 4 film was used as the image receptor.

urements should be made: (1) the count rate response curve and (2) the system deadtime. The count rate response curve can be generated with a point source and a collection of absorbers of equal thickness positioned in subsets in front of the uncollimated detector. (Any edge packing should be masked with lead.*) The sum of all the absorbers should provide a photon reduction of at least 100.

---

*Electronic masking is not sufficient since crystal deadtime and much of the deadtime of the electronic circuits is included before electronic masking occurs.

The count rate response curve should be recorded for all camera configurations, including low and high count rate modes, and with correction circuits engaged and disengaged. Camera deadtime can be determined by the dual source method without scatter material, as described by NEMA, or with scatter material as described by Adams (56). In either case, activities of the dual sources should provide a count loss of less than 20% for a single source, and a loss above 20% when the two sources are combined. From the count rates (R_1 and R_2) for each source singly and the combination count rate (R_{12}) expressed in counts per second, the camera deadtime (τ) can be computed:

$$\tau = \left[\frac{2 R_{12}}{(R_1 + R_2)^2} \ln \frac{(R_1 + R_2)}{R_{12}} \right] \times 10^6 \; \mu sec.$$

The count rate at which 20% of the counts are lost ($R_{-20\%}$) can be calculated from these data if the camera is considered as a paralyzable system (a good assumption for most cameras):

$$R_{-20\%} = \frac{1}{\tau} \ln \frac{10}{8} = \frac{0.2231}{\tau} \; cps.$$

This count rate can also be read directly from the count rate response curve.

Most of the remaining measurements are reported for the entire imaging area of the detector (the useful field of view or UFOV) and for the central 75% of the detector (central field of view or CFOV), as defined in Figure 7.27. Both fields of view are reported because camera performance usually is better in the center of the crystal, compared to the periphery.

The variation in intrinsic detector sensitivity over the detector is measured by placing a point source at a matrix of locations on the detector face (>100 points for a 15-inch field of view) and observing the count rate at each point. Counts must be measured for a time sufficient to provide statistically significant results (i.e., >100,000 counts per time period). These counts should be corrected for decay of the source, if significant, over the course of the measurements. The

variation in system sensitivity is reported as a percentage defined as:

Variation in system sensitivity

$$= \frac{\text{Maximum counts} - \text{Minimum counts}}{\text{Maximum counts} + \text{Minimum counts}} \times 100\%.$$

Values in the range of 3 to 5% can be expected.

Detector nonuniformity probably is the most frequently monitored parameter for quality assurance. As a benchmark for future quality assurance, acceptance testing measurements of detector nonuniformity are measured according to the NEMA protocol. The uncollimated detector (edge packing mask in place) is exposed to a point source of activity positioned far enough from the detector that the photon flux density is uniform at the detector. The recommended distance is greater than 5 UFOV diameters. The resulting data are digitized and stored in a 64 × 64 matrix at an average pixel depth in excess of 4,000 counts/pixel. This matrix of data is then smoothed using a standard 9 point 4:2:1 smoothing kernel and searched for the minimum and maximum value pixels. The integral nonuniformity is then reported in percentage terms as:

Integral nonuniformity

$$= \frac{\text{Maximum counts} - \text{Minimum counts}}{\text{Maximum counts} + \text{Minimum counts}} \times 100\%.$$

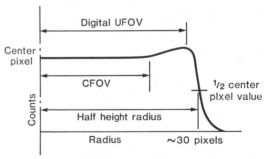

Figure 7.27. Definition of the field of view of a scintillation camera. From a 64 × 64 image of a uniform flood source, the average counts in the central portion of the crystal (central 10 × 10 pixel area) is determined. Following any radius, the half central pixel value is found, and 95% of this distance is defined as the UFOV (Useful Field of View) radius. The CFOV (Central Field of View) is 75% of the UFOV.

The maximum nonuniformity over a small area of the detector is reported as the differential nonuniformity. The computation is identical to that above, except that the maximum and minimum count pixels are derived from a 5-pixel horizontal or vertical strip (i.e., the strip of pixels with the largest difference in counts). Both of these nonuniformity indices are computed over the UFOV and the CFOV. They should be determined both with and without correction circuits engaged and should be reported for both low (<30,000 cps or < $R_{-20\%}/2$, whichever is smaller) and high (75,000 cps or $R_{-20\%}$ or both) count rates. Uncorrected, low count integral nonuniformity should fall in the range of 10 to 12%, and the differential nonuniformity may be near half of the integral nonuniformity. With correction circuits, the integral nonuniformity should be near 5%. Both nonuniformity indices will deteriorate with increasing count rate (57). Many other nonuniformity indices have been suggested (58–61), but only the measurements described above are currently reported by manufacturers.

Intrinsic spatial resolution usually receives the greatest attention in camera purchasing, even though the 3- to 4-mm intrinsic resolution is seldom approached in clinical situations. Three major measurements are made for spatial resolution: (1) the modulation transfer function; (2) the line pair or points per inch resolution; and (3) the line spread function. The MTF is the most complete characterization of camera response but is rarely provided as a performance specification by manufacturers. Resolution from line pair or hole phantoms (Fig. 7.28) is often used as a qualitative indication of spatial resolution. Line pair or hole phantoms usually are preferred for quality assurance measurements, and one usually is provided at the time of delivery of a new scintillation camera. The most commonly quoted specification of intrinsic resolution is the NEMA specification. This parameter averages measurements of the full width at half maximum (FWHM) of line spread functions in the image of 1-mm wide slits in a lead plate (Fig. 7.29). The slits are spaced at 3-cm centers, and images are collected with the slits oriented in both the X and Y directions. Analysis includes averaging the data over 3-cm line lengths and does not include any corrections for the 1-mm source width. Spatial resolution is reported in millimeters as the average of these measurements over the CFOV and the UFOV. Resolution should be determined at both low and high count rates, with the high count rates including both 75,000 cps, a NEMA standard, and the count rate for 20% data loss. The intrinsic spatial resolution of current cameras is in the range of 3 to 4 mm at low count rates, with some deterioration in this range at higher count rates.

Detector nonlinearity usually increases at the periphery of the field of view. Many newer cameras have incorporated computer correction schemes to place events where they should be registered to produce straight line patterns of straight line sources. To specify the nonlinearity in a quantitative fashion, images of the lead sheet with straight 1-mm slits on 3-cm centers can be utilized. These images can be fit with an "ideal grid" (62) of straight lines on 3-cm centers. The absolute nonlinearity is reported as the maximum deviation of any line in the image from the "ideal fitted grid." Differential nonlinearity is computed as the standard deviation of all 3-cm line segments from the same ideal grid. Typical values for absolute nonlinearity range from 0.5 to 4 mm for the UFOV on current cameras. Differential nonlinearity values might approach 0.1 mm. The CFOV value is usually far better than the UFOV. Nonlinearity values should also be reported for both high and low count rates in both the CFOV and the UFOV.

The final intrinsic parameter to determine is the multiple window spatial misregistration. This determination is accomplished visually by overlaying flood images with edge packing from each of the available energy windows (63). If these images do not overlap perfectly, then adjustments are required. To quantify the misregistration, two point sources on either side of the detector CFOV can be imaged in each of the energy windows. The maximum displacement of the centroids of each point source can then be calculated and reported in millimeters as the multiple window spatial misregistration.

Properties of the scintillation camera system that should be measured include the sensitivity and resolution. These properties

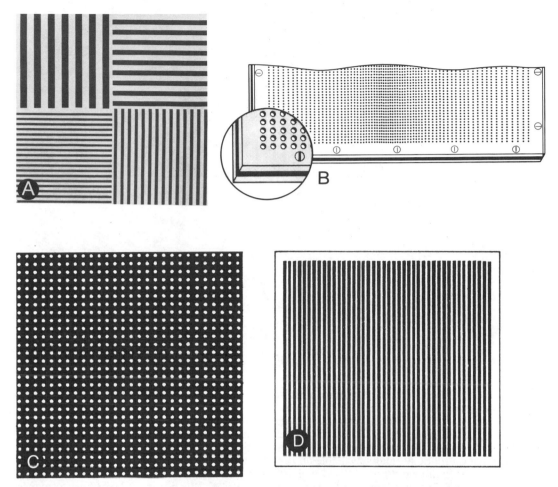

Figure 7.28. Spatial resolution phantoms. Resolution phantom images such as (*A*) the quadrant bar phantom and (*B*) the CDRH test phantom allow some quantitation of the intrinsic spatial resolution of a scintillation camera. A quadrant bar phantom is chosen so that the most closely spaced bars cannot be resolved by the camera. The CDRH test phantom is available in only one configuration, but has horizontal hole spacings ranging from 0.40 to 0.95 mm in 0.5-mm steps. The pattern contains 7200 holes, 2.5 mm in diameter on vertical 0.5-cm centers. The Orthogonal Hole Phantom (*C*) and the PLES (Parallel Line Equal Spacing) phantom (images in *C* and *D*, respectively) must be chosen at the resolution limits of the camera. They provide the additional advantage of a good qualitative demonstration of the detector's linearity. (Courtesy of Nuclear Associates, Inc.)

should be determined for each collimator. System sensitivity is determined by observing the camera's count rate when a small Petri dish with a calibrated amount of activity is placed on top of the collimator. For a pinhole collimator, the activity should be placed at a known distance similar to that to be used for imaging (e.g., 3 inches for thyroid imaging) and sufficient to include the entire source in the field of view. The system sensitivity is a single value for each

collimator and has units of counts per minute per millicurie.

System resolution is measured both with and without scatter. Two line sources of activity (1-mm ID capillary tubes) are suspended 10 cm above the collimator. Analysis of the FWHM of these two lines in the CFOV is performed in the same way that intrinsic resolution measurements were made. Measurements are repeated with an absorber thickness of 10 cm of plastic and 5

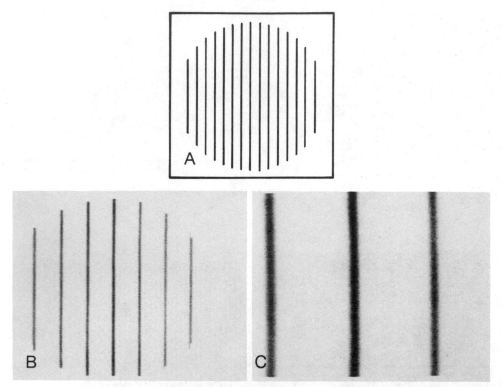

Figure 7.29. NEMA intrinsic resolution measurements. The NEMA phantom (*A*), when placed directly on the detector face and exposed to a point source of ^{99m}Tc at greater than 5 UFOVs, produces the image shown in (*B*). The image should be collected so that a 3-cm slice through the lines produces peaks with maxima greater than 10,000 counts per channel and with at least 10 channels above the FWHM of the peaks. One way to accomplish this (although the field of view is diminished) is with the magnification mode normally available on the camera and/or computer. The line images at (*C*) will meet the 10 channels above FWHM and 10,000 counts per channel criteria. (*A*, Courtesy of Nuclear Associates, Inc. *B*, From Raff U, Spitzer V, Hendee W: Practicality of NEMA performance specification measurements for user-based acceptance testing and routine quality assurance. *J Nucl Med* 25:679–687, 1984.)

cm of material for backscatter (Fig. 7.30). Values should be averaged over the X and Y directions and determined for both high and low count rates.

Whole body scanning devices should be checked for alignment if multiple passes are required for a complete scan. Systems that control their speed by monitoring the count density in a region can be tested by attaching a few different sources to the detector and monitoring the speed and speed constancy of the scanning motion. Two or three different count rate sources should be used. System spatial resolution tests should also be repeated with whole body scanning systems, but the X and Y directions should not be averaged. The greatest degradation in spatial resolution should occur in the direction of

motion; however, the perpendicular direction should also be measured to evaluate the smoothness of motion.

Computer-Assisted Imaging

Many of the tests (spatial resolution, nonlinearity, and nonuniformity) in the previous sections assume computer acquisition and analysis of scintillation camera data. For these measurements, the computer is part of the system to be evaluated. With the ever increasing utilization of computers in nuclear medicine, there is some benefit in including the computer as part of the imaging system during acceptance testing, since it will be part of the system during routine imaging (64). Resolution measurements can be made in magnification or zoom modes,

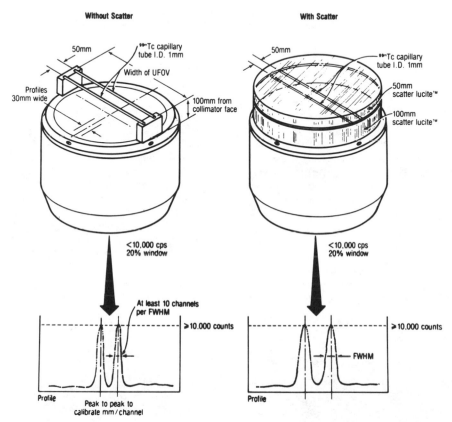

Figure 7.30. System resolution. NEMA measurements of system (extrinsic) resolution are made with two capillary tubes (1 mm ID) at 10 cm above the collimator. These measurements are repeated with scatter material between the sources and the collimator (10 cm) and above the line sources (5 cm). The line spread functions are analyzed as were the intrinsic measurements, and the FWHM is reported in mm.

so that the computer resolution or pixel size is small (<20%) compared to the resolution of the camera (<3 mm). Linearity and uniformity of the camera-computer system can be affected by nonlinearities in the analog-digital converters (ADCs) of the interface. Often these effects can be demonstrated in a very high count density flood image as straight line discontinuities at regular intervals. The discontinuities correspond to preferential states of particular bits in the analog to digital conversion process (Fig. 7.31). Deadtime measurements should also be made with the computer in the system. Multiple window spatial registration and energy resolution, on the other hand, should be unaffected by inclusion of the computer, since the Z signals are used only as gating signals. A summary report of representative acceptance testing measurements, their results, required sources and equipment, estimated times to perform the tests, and relevant comments are included in Table 7.8.

ULTRASOUND

The evolution of ultrasound equipment is still in its infancy. Still, many types of ultrasound equipment have been developed, and most ultrasound departments contain a variety of designs. The variations in equipment

design and the rapid advances in equipment development have presented obstacles to the development of standardized performance tests. To date, such tests have been widely accepted only for B-mode, single element static ultrasound scanners. Even for these scanners, the test procedures must be modified somewhat for each specific piece of equipment. With similar modifications, the test procedures are adaptable in many cases to real-time, echocardiographic, and doppler ultrasound systems.

The performance tests described below are more extensive than the routine quality assurance tests described in Chapter 8. To provide baseline values for routine preventive maintenance, the quality assurance tests should be performed along with the acceptance tests. Most of the acceptance tests are described in the following references:

1. Pulse Echo Ultrasound Imaging Systems: Performance Tests and Criteria. AAPM Report No. 8, available from the American Association of Physicists in Medicine, AIP, 335 East 45th Street, New York, NY, 10017.
2. Standard Methods for Testing Single-Element Pulse-Echo Ultrasonic Transducers—Interim Standard. Supplement to *J Ultrasound Med* 1(7) (Sept

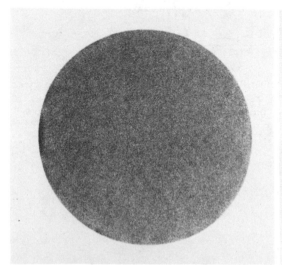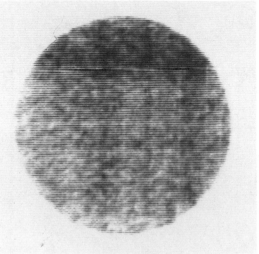

Figure 7.31. Analog to digital converter artifacts: The image on the *left* is a 5-million count ^{99m}Tc point source uniformity flood. The *right* image is a 120-million count flood collected in a 128 × 128 × 16 matrix. The flood is displayed with 86% background subtraction and clearly demonstrates striping in both the X and Y directions. (The X and Y signals are multiplexed to the same ADC in this system.)

Table 7.8
Scintillation Camera Acceptance Testing Example Report

Measurements	Results	Sources	Equipment	Time	Comments
Inventory	Complete			2 hr	See enclosed packing slips and purchase order (PO).
Detector motion	15–50 cm vertical yoke travel 360° yoke rotation			15 min	Unrestricted rotation applies stress to cabling.
Controls and lights	All properly functioning	^{99m}Tc (300 μCi)		2 hr	Repairs made to position indicating lights. Preset energy window set for indicated isotopes. High voltage (HV) power up requires 30-min stabilization.
Shielding	All measurements low and symmetrical	^{131}I (200 μCi) ^{99m}Tc (30 μCi)		30 min	See accompanying diagram.
Collimators	No obvious defects			15 min	Visual inspection.
Energy resolution	12.4% at 140 keV	^{57}Co and ^{99m}Tc	2048 ADC-MCA	2 hr	5,000 cps
Maximum Count Rate					
High count mode	166,000 cps	^{99m}Tc (500 μCi)		5 min	All correctors off.
Normal mode	115,000 cps	^{99m}Tc (500 μCi)		5 min	All correctors on.
Count rate response					
High count mode	See accompanying diagram	^{99m}Tc (500 μCi)	15–0.1 inch thick calibrated Cu absorbers.	30 min	
Normal mode				30 min	
Intrinsic deadtime					
High count mode	$\tau = 1.6$ μsec $R_{-20\%}=140$ kcps	^{99m}Tc (300 μCi)		20 min	All correctors off.
Normal mode	$\tau = 2.4$ μsec $R_{-20\%}=93$ kcps	^{99m}Tc (300 μCi)		20 min	All correctors on.
System deadtime					
High count mode	$\tau = 6.0$ μsec $R_{-20\%}=37$ kcps	^{99m}Tc (7 mCi)	Adams scatter phantom	20 min	High resolution collimator. All correctors off.

Table 7.8—continued

Measurements	Results	Sources	Equipment	Time	Comments
Normal mode	$\tau = 7.1$ μsec $R_{-20\%}=31$ kcps	^{99m}Tc (5 mCi)	Adams scatter phantom	20 min	High resolution collimator. All correctors on.
System deadtime with computer			Computer		
High count mode	$\tau = 4.6$ μsec $R_{-20\%}=48$ kcps	^{99m}Tc (7 mCi)	Adams scatter phantom	30 min	High resolution collimator. All correctors off.
Normal mode	$\tau = 7.5$ μsec $R_{-20\%}=30$ kcps	^{99m}Tc (5 mCi)	Adams scatter phantom	30 min	High resolution collimator. All correctors on.
Point source sensitivity	3.6%	^{99m}Tc (250 μCi)	3 cm² detector grid 3-mm hole Pb pig	30 min	All correctors off.
Detector uniformity			Computer		Correction floods were stored at low CR.

Detector uniformity results:

	CFOV Int	CFOV Diff	UFOV Int	UFOV Diff	Sources	Time
Correctors on						
$<R_{-20\%}/2$	5%	3%	5.6%	3%	^{99m}Tc (300 μCi)	30 min
75,000 cps	9%	6%	11%	6%	^{99m}Tc (750 μCi)	20 min
Correctors off						
$<R_{-20\%}/2$	11%	7.5%	13%	8%	^{99m}Tc (300 μCi)	30 min
75,000 cps	18%	10.5%	19%	11%	^{99m}Tc (750 μCi)	20 min

Intrinsic spatial resolution (Computer with zoom mode; Central 5-inch field of view only.):

Intrinsic spatial resolution	Results	Sources	Equipment	Time
Correctors on				
$<R_{-20\%}$	3.3 mm	^{99m}Tc (8 mCi)	NEMA phantom	3 hr
75,000 cps	3.9 mm	^{99m}Tc (30 mCi)	NEMA phantom	30 min
Correctors off				
$<R_{-20\%}/2$	3.4 mm	^{99m}Tc (8 mCi)	NEMA phantom	3 hr
75,000 cps	3.9 mm	^{99m}Tc (30 mCi)	NEMA phantom	30 min

Table 7.8—continued

Measurements	Results		Sources	Equipment	Time	Comments
				Computer		
Intrinsic linearity						
Correctors on						
$R_{-20\%}/2$	1.6 mm		^{99m}Tc (8 mCi)	NEMA phantom	30 min	Only 4 channels above
75,000 cps	3.7 mm		^{99m}Tc (30 mCi)	NEMA phantom	20 min	FWHM if peak.
Correctors off						
$R_{-20\%}/2$	3.5 mm		^{99m}Tc (8 mCi)	NEMA phantom	30 min	
75,000 cps	4.8 mm		^{99m}Tc (30 mCi)	NEMA phantom	20 min	
System resolution	Low energy collimators					
	Hi Res	GAP				
$<R_{-20\%}/2$	6.3 mm	8.4 mm	^{99m}Tc (10 mCi)	2 1-mm capillary tubes	40 min/collimator	
75,000 cps	7.1 mm	9.2 mm	^{99m}Tc (20 mCi)	2 1-mm capillary tubes	40 min/collimator	
Res. with scatter						
$<R_{-20\%}/2$	7.6 mm	9.8	^{99m}Tc (10 mCi)	2 1-mm capillary tubes	40 min/collimator	
75,000 cps	8.9 mm	12 mm	^{99m}Tc (80 mCi)	2 1-mm capillary tubes	40 min/collimator	
Multiple window spatial registration	Acceptable		Ga-67 (50 μCi)		15 min	By edge packing overlay.
System sensitivity						
High resolution collimator	240 cpm/μCi		^{99m}Tc (3 mCi)	3-inch Petri dish	10 min/collimator	
GAP collimator	373 cpm/μCi					
System sensitivity collimator	495 cpm/μCi					

1982), available from AIUM, 405 East-West Highway, Suite 504, Bethesda, MD 20814.

3. Safety Standard for Diagnostic Ultrasound Equipment. AIUM/NEMA Standards Publication No. UL 1-1981, Supplement to *J Ultrasound Med 2*(4) (April 1983), available as above.

Electrical and Mechanical Safety Tests

The requirements and test procedures for the electrical and mechanical safety of ultrasound equipment follow the guidelines of the American Association of Medical Instrumentation (AAMI)/American National Standards Institute (ANSI) document, "Safe Current Limits for Electromedical Apparatus" (65). Because the ultrasonic pulse is generated by applying a high voltage pulse to the transducer, the possibility always exists for electrical shock to the patient and technician. Transducer housings are electrically insulated to minimize this possibility; furthermore, the piezoelectric crystal itself is always operated at ground potential. Initial acceptance testing for electrical hazards should include inspection of the transducer housing and crystal for cracks or any other types of physical deformation. Additional electrical tests are designed to measure leakage current from the chassis, scanning arm, and transducer housing, as required by the Joint Commission on Accreditation of Hospitals (JCAH). Maximum limits in leakage current range from 10 to 100 μA, depending on the source of the current and the use of the instrument. Information on commercially available equipment to perform these tests is available in the literature (66). A thorough inspection of the equipment should be performed for mechanical defects, excessive vibration, noise, instability of the suspended scanning arm, and improper movement of parts (67–70).

Ultrasonic Emissions

Emission parameters described in Chapter 4 include the absolute maximum values of SPTA, SPPA, and SATA intensities, and output power (71). Typical values for these parameters are listed in Table 7.9. Because the values are relatively low, specialized equipment and techniques are required for their measurement. Ultrasonic power usually is measured with a radiation force balance; intensities are measured with a hydrophone scanning system (72). Intensity values should be reported by the manufacturer to an accuracy of ±20%. If available, the ultrasonic output power control should be calibrated by the manufacturer to an accuracy of ±25% of maximum power.

Because of the difficulty in measuring ultrasonic intensity and power, the manufac-

Table 7.9
Intensity Ranges Produced by Current Ultrasound Systems[a]

Type of equipment	Spatial average-temporal average intensity on the radiating surface (milliwatts/cm^2)	Spatial peak—temporal average intensity (milliwatts/cm^2)	Spatial peak—pulse average intensity (watts/cm^2)
Static pulse echo scanners and M-mode equipment	0.4–20	10–200	0.5–280
Automatic sector scanners (phased arrays and wobblers)	2.7–60	45–200[b]	25–100
Sequenced linear arrays	0.06–10	0.1–12	25–100
Pulsed Doppler, primarily for cardiac work	3–32	50–290	3–14
		Spatial peak intensity (milliwatts/cm^2)	
Doppler instruments, primarily for obstetric applications	3–25	9–75[c]	
Continuous wave doppler, primarily for peripheral vascular	38–840	100–2500[c]	

[a] From AIUM: Appendix B—survey of exposure levels from current diagnostic ultrasound systems. *J Ultrasound Med* 2(Suppl):S31–S32, 1983.
[b] This value was measured with the scanning mechanism arrested for M mode and at the maximum system *pulse repetition rate.*
[c] Estimate based on the *spatial average-temporal average.*

turer's reported values are seldom verified. It should be noted that data supplied by the manufacturer apply to the general line of equipment and not to the particular instrument purchased. In addition, the values vary with the transducer and scanning mode employed; hence, the reported values should be the absolute maximum for each technique. If an ultrasound unit is modified, emission parameters should be remeasured. If the modifications are provided by the manufacturer, they should be accompanied by new emission parameters. Often, new transducer assemblies are purchased from vendors other than the manufacturer. In this case the transducer manufacturer should provide the emission data.

Frequency and Bandwidth

The ultrasound system's sensitivity and resolution depend significantly on the frequency and bandwidth of the output ultrasonic pulse. Hence, both of these parameters should be verified. The measured center frequency of the output pulse should lie within ±10% of the vendor's stated value, and the bandwidth should be accurate to ±15%.

Although the frequency and bandwidth of the output pulse are affected by the pulser and receiver electronics, they are influenced primarily by the transducer assembly. Consequently, methods to measure these parameters should be independent of the ultrasound electronics. Appropriate tests should be performed on all transducers supplied with the system. For single element transducers, test procedures are described in the literature (73). To perform the tests, the echo from a flat reflective interface is analyzed to yield a plot of the frequency amplitude spectrum of the transducer (Fig. 7.32). From this plot, the peak frequency (f_p) and the upper (f_u) and lower (f_l) frequencies where the pulse echo response is half (−6 dB) the peak are determined. The center frequency is then calculated with the equation:

$$f_c = \frac{f_u + f_l}{2}.$$

The fractional bandwidth is calculated with the equation:

$$BW = \frac{f_u - f_l}{f_c} \times 100.$$

For instruments where the transducer

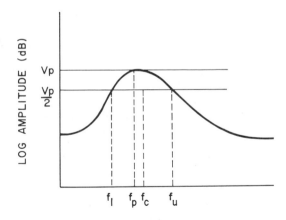

Figure 7.32. Pulse echo response profile. f_l = lower frequency, f_p = peak frequency, f_c = center frequency, f_u = upper frequency.

cannot be detached from the pulser, only system-dependent frequency and bandwidth measurements can be obtained. One method of measurement uses the system's broadband pulser to generate an ultrasonic pulse. The first echo returning from a planar interface is recorded on a spectrum analyzer. The peak, lower, and upper frequencies are identified, and the center-frequency and bandwidth are calculated as described above.

A coarse estimate of center frequency can be obtained with the zero crossing frequency method (74). In this method the first echo is viewed on an oscilloscope and the number, n, of half cycles above a set amplitude in the wave form is counted. The center frequency, f_c, is then calculated from the equation:

$$f_c = n/2t_n$$

where t_n is the time measured between the zero crossing points. The first point lies at the start of the first half-cycle and the second at the end of the nth half cycle. The accuracy of the center frequency obtained by this method may deviate by as much as ±10% from that determined by the former two methods.

The latter two methods require electrical access to the echo signal. For systems where the echo signal is inaccessible, a method such as spectral analysis of the transmitted ultrasonic pulse as detected by a hydrophone must be used (75). The use of ultrasonic frequency test objects (76) also has been suggested; however, appropriate test objects are not yet available commercially.

Calibration of System Sensitivity Controls

Diagnostic ultrasound scanners allow both range-independent and range-dependent control of signal amplification (gain). A range independent (i.e., overall system gain) control affects either the acoustic output or the receiver gain, or both. Calibration of this control is not essential for clinical use of the equipment but is required for many of the system performance checks. A measurement of the total gain available with the range-independent control is important, however, because it affects the instrument sensitivity. The range-dependent control (i.e., the swept gain or time-gain control (TGC), time varied gain (TVG), etc.) permits compensation for attenuation of the ultrasound beam by tissue. Calibration is necessary to determine if the change in gain is sufficient to compensate for tissue attenuation. The attenuation can be as great as 1 dB/cm at 1 MHz and, in most tissues, is directly proportional to frequency. Higher swept gain is required for "body wall" compensation and echocardiography. It is essential that the total swept gain be at least 60 dB. Detailed procedures for testing system sensitivity are given in the literature (75).

In general, the range-dependent control that is considered to be in calibration is the one that is tested. In some systems there is no calibrated control; in this case one chooses a control to calibrate by marking the calibration points with graph paper, using polar coordinate paper for rotating knobs. Calibration is performed easily with systems that provide electrical access to the pulser or to a linear portion of the received signal. The equipment required is a calibrated radiofrequency (rf) attenuator, water tank, planar reflecting interface (preferably stainless steel), and mounting system for the transducer. The transducer is aligned in the water tank to produce the maximum echo signal from the stainless steel plate as determined by the echo amplitude on the A-mode display. Attenuation is introduced into the system by the calibrated attenuator, and the system gain required to compensate for the added attenuation is recorded. Specific procedures should be followed to compensate for insertion loss and impedance mismatching of the calibrated attenuator (75).

The result of the calibration is a plot of the rf attenuator versus system gain settings, as shown in Figure 7.33. This procedure also provides an absolute calibration of system sensitivity versus that of a perfect planar reflector. If only a relative calibration is required, a simplified version of the test can be performed (75).

System gain controls should be accurate to within ±10% of the full range of the gain control. In Figure 7.33, for example, system controls should be accurate to ±3.3 dB. At the lower and upper range a change in system attenuator settings of 3 dB is an actual change of 1 dB in signal intensity. This change is within the expected accuracy. For every change of 10 dB the differential error should be less than 2 dB. In the above example this is only true in the central range of values. If there are other system-independent gain controls or a swept gain "initial" control, the calibration procedure described above should be obtained for a variety of control settings. An overall system gain of at least 80 dB should be calibrated.

When electrical access to the system is not available, more difficult calibration procedures can be performed using an acoustic gray wedge in place of the attenuator and planar interface (75).

Range-dependent (swept gain) controls can be calibrated with the AIUM 100-mm

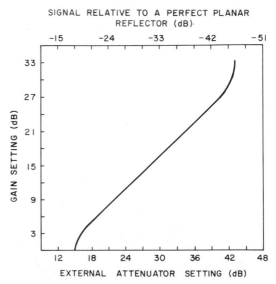

SIGNAL RELATIVE TO A PERFECT PLANAR REFLECTOR (dB)

Figure 7.33. Results from calibration of system gain control. At the lower range of system settings (0–6 dB) the actual measured attenuator change is 4 dB (15–19 dB).

test object described in Chapter 8, or with an electronic tone-burst generator (77). In the former method, the transducer is aligned over the vertical rod group spaced at 2-cm intervals in the AIUM phantom. With the swept gain off, the system gain required to produce echoes of a predetermined amplitude from each of the rods is recorded. A specific swept gain is set, and the measurement is repeated. The difference in range-dependent gains required at each depth yields a plot of the actual swept gain.

Use of the electronic burst generator is the simplest technique for calibration of a range-dependent control. However, it requires electrical connection of the burst generator to the system in place of the transducer. In most B-mode units this connection is possible. A burst generator can be obtained that provides a calibrated exponentially decaying signal in response to the transducer excitation pulse. Swept gain is then set to provide an A-mode signal of constant amplitude with depth. At this point the swept gain is equal to the signal decay rate of the burst generator. The swept gain should be 0 to 2 F dB/cm, where F is the center frequency of the highest frequency transducer in use.

System Sensitivity

The ability of an ultrasound system to detect low level echoes can be assessed by measuring the system sensitivity or signal to noise ratio. This measurement should be made at all display modes on the system, including the photographic display. It is particularly important to verify that the same range of echo amplitudes is visible on the photographic copy and on the image monitor. These tests are also used to evaluate the uniformity in sensitivity of a linear array transducer.

Equipment required for measurement of sensitivity includes a transducer mount and a planar reflecting surface. The system range-independent gain should have been calibrated as previously described. For cross correlation with other instruments, one should measure the absolute signal to noise ratio with respect to that of a perfect reflector. This measurement requires a knowledge of the ratio of the reflection coefficient of the planar reflector test object to that of a perfect reflector. Common test objects are a stainless steel plate in water, a water-CCl_4

interface (78), and an acrylic block (75). Choice of a test object depends on the sensitivity of the unit to be tested. Sometimes, for example, the stainless steel reflector provides an echo signal that is too large even at the lowest gain settings. Surfaces of lower reflectivity, such as an acrylic block, do not yield an absolute signal to noise ratio with the same level of accuracy. Their reflective characteristics are not as well understood as the stainless steel plate; furthermore, they depend on the transducer frequency and beam profile characteristics. Use of a small target such as a rod in the AIUM phantom is not recommended, because the echo strength is highly dependent on the transducer beam profile. Additional data using this or another routine preventive maintenance test object should be obtained at this time, however, so that baseline data are available for future quality assurance testing.

For the measurement of signal to noise ratio, the system gain required to obtain a preset A-mode echo signal and a barely discernible B-mode display from the reflecting surface are recorded. These two values should agree to within -1 to $+10$ dB. Subsequently, the system gain is increased until the noise level on A-mode echo and B-mode display are at the same levels as previously recorded. The difference in gain settings for the two measurements provides a measure of the signal to noise levels for both A- and B-mode displays. Absolute values for system sensitivity with respect to a standard perfect planar reflector in water, ideally, should be obtained. For transducers operating at a frequency of 1 to 4 MHz the sensitivity should be at least 105 dB greater than the noise. For measurements with weakly reflecting surfaces, similar units can be compared using relative values of signal to noise, provided that the measurements are obtained with transducers of similar frequency, diameter, and focal length. Stability of the measurements should be ± 3 dB with the stainless steel plate and ± 6 dB with the weaker reflecting test objects.

A simpler, but perhaps more subjective, test of system sensitivity utilizes a tissue-mimicking phantom such as the RMI 431 (79). These phantoms have attenuation and scattering properties qualitatively but not quantitatively similar to those of liver tissue. In such a phantom one can determine a penetration depth by adjusting the gain controls to yield echoes from the maximum possible depth in the phantom (Fig. 7.34). Although this measured depth may not be directly comparable to that expected in normal liver, it yields an adequate assessment of the effective system sensitivity in a clinical situation. Penetration depths of 120 to 130 mm are typically obtained with a phantom of this type.

System sensitivity tests can also be used to test the uniformity in sensitivity of the individual crystals in a linear array. This test usually is performed by coupling the linear array transducer to an acrylic block test object and viewing the linear echo from the far surface of the block. The threshold sensitivity required to display the strongest echoes from any portion of the array is recorded. The sensitivity is then increased to yield a display of the weakest echo section of the line. The difference in the two gain settings should be ≤6 dB to yield clinically acceptable images.

Dynamic Range

In addition to knowing the minimum echo strength discernible in an image, it is also important to know the range of echo

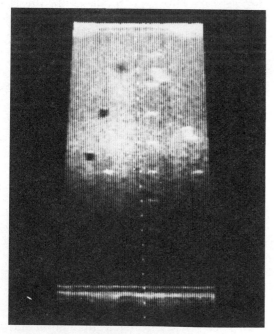

Figure 7.34. Penetration depth of B-mode scanner in tissue mimicking test phantom. Measured depth is 13 cm.

strengths visible. This range is known as the dynamic range; typically it is 40 db for A-mode, B-mode, and photographic displays employing standard (normally linear) signal processing. Measured values should agree with manufacturers specifications to within ±5 dB.

Dynamic range is measured by examining echoes from some stable echo source (75), such as an isolated target or a tone-burst generator. For A-mode dynamic range measurements, one determines the difference in system sensitivity required to produce a barely discernible A-mode echo from the target compared to that required to produce a maximum strength A-mode signal. For the B-mode test, two techniques are commonly employed. The first utilizes the M-mode display available on most B-mode units with the assumption that the M-mode and B-mode display characteristics are identical. The target echo is displayed in M-mode, and during an M-mode sweep the system sensitivity is changed. The sensitivities which produce a barely discernible echo and a saturated screen are recorded; their difference is the measured dynamic range.

The second method utilizes the tone-burst generator to provide a display of an exponentially decaying train of echoes. The echoes can be displayed in M-mode, or the transducer can be sectored through air to yield a B-mode image (Fig. 7.35). System gain is adjusted to yield a train of echoes varying in intensity from saturation to barely perceptible as a function of depth. The separation in depth of these two outlying signals is related to the gray scale dynamic range.

The dynamic range of the photographic hard copy device may be measured from an image of the gray bars or other test pattern normally supplied with the unit, provided that the pattern covers the full range of display levels available on the monitor. A second approach is to use a coin coupled to the transducer face. With the sensitivity high, the upper corner of the monitor is saturated by scanning the transducer over a small area of the scan plane. Then the gain is reduced, and the transducer is scanned to fill in the central portion of the image with barely discernible echoes. One section of the image is left blank for a background measurement.

The image is recorded on transmission film or on positive/negative Polaroid film. Optical density measurements are obtained with a portable densitometer, such as that commonly used for quality control in film processing. The optical density readings should be stable to ±0.15 OD.

Resolution

Both axial and lateral resolution should be measured as part of the acceptance testing procedure. Axial resolution (i.e., resolution parallel to the beam axis) is the finest resolution provided by the system. Values measured should not exceed those specified by the manufacturer. Either the AIUM 100 mm or the sensitivity, uniformity, and axial resolution (SUAR) test object can be used for axial resolution measurements. Use of the SUAR phantom is preferred because it provides a continuously varying range of reflector spacings (Fig. 7.36). Axial resolution normally is measured in the transducer far field for a number of different display modes, including zoom, as well as in the hard copy images (75). These measurements are repeated with the reflectors rotated 90° to obtain the resolution both parallel and perpendicular to the TV raster lines. Values of axial resolution might range from 2 mm for large FOV (40 cm) to less than 1 mm on zoom or for small FOV (10 cm). Measured values may also vary with different display criteria. The criterion of barely resolvable echoes is used most frequently. Less often, the clearly resolved criterion also is employed.

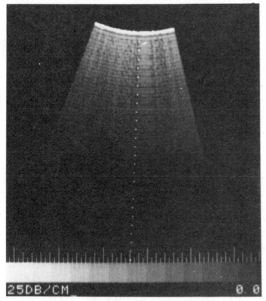

Figure 7.35. Gray scale dynamic range as measured on B-scanner using the pulse burst generator. The dynamic range is equal to the measured depth of visible echoes times the attenuator setting (dB/cm) on the pulse burst generator. In this example, dynamic range = (1.25 dB/cm) (15 cm) = 19 dB.

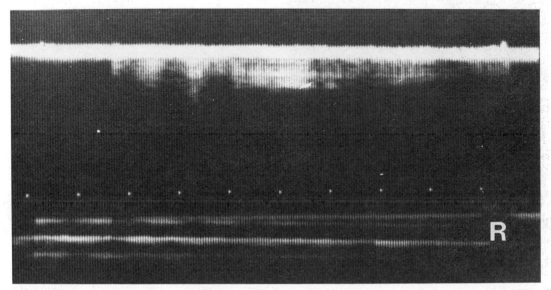

Figure 7.36. Axial resolution as measured with the SUAR phantom. Resolution is obtained by measuring with marker dots the distance from raised portion of wedge (R) to point at which the upper and lower surfaces of the wedge appear to converge. This distance multiplied by the known slope of the wedge (0.25 mm/cm) gives the axial resolution.

Lateral resolution (i.e., resolution perpendicular to the beam axis) should also not exceed the manufacturers specifications. A rigorous testing of this parameter requires mapping of the pulse echo response profile at several depths within the transducer field, as described in a recent AIUM document. In the field, lateral resolution is commonly described as the beam width, or, more accurately, the pulse echo response width. This width may be obtained by scanning a phantom containing rods lying perpendicular to the beam at several distances from the transducer face, including the focal length, twice the focal distance, and half the focal distance (Fig. 7.37). For asymmetrical transducers (e.g., linear arrays) measurement should be performed in at least two orthogonal directions. At each distance, the beam width is the length of the line in the B-mode image that corresponds to the appropriate rod. Readings should be taken at sensitivity settings of 6, 12, 20, and 40 dB. The tests should be performed for all transducers supplied with the system. Tissue mimicking test objects have also been used for measurements of lateral resolution (80).

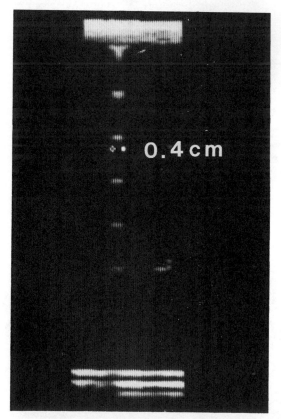

Figure 7.37. Lateral resolution as measured from reflections from rods in the AIUM 100-mm test object. Length of linear echo from rod is measured using system calipers.

Geometrical Accuracy

Ultrasound images are frequently used to determine object sizes (e.g., the biparietal diameter). For this application, images must not be spatially distorted, and accurate scales for measuring objects must be available. Acceptance tests for geometrical accuracy include assessment of the system's depth calibration (marker dots and arm registration), caliper accuracy, M-mode time markers, image distortion (video and photographic display), beam alignment, and scan plane accuracy.

Marker dots and calipers should be accurate to 1% or ±1 mm. At distances of at least 10 cm, arm registration should be ≤5 mm. M-mode time marker accuracy should be within 3%, and the seconds time markers on recordings should not vary more than 5% per 10 sec. Tests for these parameters are identical to those performed during routine preventive maintenance, as discussed in Chapter 8.

Image distortion can be evaluated by using the marker dots to generate an image of horizontal and vertical lines of centimeter-spaced dots. A ruler is used to determine if the monitor or photographic image is distorted by more than 2% (±1%) over a distance of half the image height in any part of the inner 80% of the image area, and more than 5% over the entire image. This specification is normally not met but is used as a guideline. However, measurement inaccuracies in distorted images can be corrected by using marker dots in the same scan plane and at the same scan angle as the object to be measured. More stringent conditions or measurement accuracy must be applied when ultrasound images are being used for radiation therapy treatment planning (75).

Alignment of the central axis of the ultrasound beam with the axis of the transducer assembly can be checked quickly with the AIUM 100-mm test object. The vertical rod group spaced at 2-cm intervals is imaged from the top. The transducer is then rotated from 90 to 180° in the transducer assembly, and the object is reimaged over the original image. Images from the targets should be superimposed with a maximum separation of 1 mm.

A common problem associated with B-mode scanners is play in the scanning arm, causing poor definition of the scan plane. The separation of scan planes is used clinically to estimate organ volumes. Hence, it is important to measure inaccuracies in transducer positioning devices and variations in the scan plane caused by force exerted on the scanning arm when it is moved across oblique surfaces. Positioning devices can be tested with a protractor fixed to a stand on the tabletop. After moving or angling the transducer assembly, one determines if the assembly still corresponds to within 0.5% or 2° of the reading indicated by the positioning device. Arm rigidity is determined by attaching a force gauge to the transducer and measuring movement of the arm when applying a known force perpendicular to the scan plane. For a force of 100 g wt, the angular deflection should be less than 1°; for a 300 g wt, the deflection should be less than 2°.

Scan plane shifts and variations in scan plane angulation with scan orientation may be caused by a bent scanning arm (81). This possibility can be investigated by scanning a solid rectangular block at all orientations and determining where the transducer face lies flush on all surfaces.

An example of a typical acceptance testing report utilizing these tests is presented in Table 7.10.

COMPUTED TOMOGRAPHY

Upon completion of installation and calibration by the manufacturer, the performance characteristics of a CT scanner should be verified. Outlined in Table 7.11 and Table 7.12 are a number of tests and performance criteria that should be addressed during the verification process. The manufacturer may take exception to any of these tests, provided justification is offered, together with an alternate test for the specific performance characteristic. The tests below are generally accepted by the medical physics community (see references 82, 83, 84, 85, 86, 87) and by most manufacturers; however, reasonable modification by either are acceptable.

In addition to serving as acceptance tests, the following measurements may be used as baseline data against which future performance of the CT scanner may be compared. For example, if suboptimal performance is suspected at a later date, the results of similar tests performed at the time may be compared with the original acceptance tests to identify any deterioration of performance. Acceptance tests may also be used as a gauge for periodic quality assurance tests.

The technique variables selected for a particular test can greatly influence the results of the test. Consequently, a "standard body" technique should be defined prior to any tests, and these techniques should be employed for all performance tests thereafter. The standard techniques may be chosen in consultation with the vendor and should be based on the techniques used most often in other installations possessing the same model CT scanner. In most cases, the "standard" techniques will be medium range techniques representing a compromise of the qualities of spatial resolution, contrast resolution, radiation dose, image noise, and others. In some cases, additional tests will be made to evaluate certain performance characteristics when the unit is operated under a particular set of conditions most favorable to reveal those characteristics.

Safety and Operational Tests

Several safety and miscellaneous operational checks should be performed initially. These are listed in Table 7.11. If all aspects of the system are operational and performing satisfactorily, then it is possible to proceed with more specific tests (Table 7.12).

Specific Tests

Table 7.12 outlines specific tests for selected performance characteristics of a CT scanner. Many tests rely on images of phantom test objects to evaluate the performance of some particular aspect of the scanner. A typical set of phantoms, containing a complete set of test objects, is described in Appendix 1. The table lists the test object and the performance level expected for each test. All of the tests (except 26) are noninvasive and require no dismantling of any part of the scanner. This feature should allay most fears of damaging the equipment or changing the calibration of the scanner during acceptance testing. It is prudent to invite the manufacturer to send a representative at the

Table 7.10
Example of Acceptance Testing Results from a Static B-Mode Ultrasound Unit

Measurement	Measured result	Phantom/equipment	Comments
1. Electrical	0.01 μA	DVM	No obvious defects. Current levels within guidelines.
2. Frequency/bandwidth (transducer 1)	fc = 3.5 MHz	Sine wave generator Stainless steel plate Water tank	Within specifications.
3. Gain calibration a. System gain	Maximum error = ±2 dB Differential error: Maximum = ±2 dB Range = 0 dB over 6–27 dB	RF attenuator Stainless steel reflector Water tank	See Figure 7.33. Within specifications.
b. TGC 1.25 dB/cm 2.5 dB/cm Maximum rate	Accuracy = ±1.5 dB/10 cm Accuracy = ±2 dB/10 cm 10 dB/cm	Electronic burst generator Electronic burst generator AIUM 100 mm	Within specifications.
4. Sensitivity (transducer 1)	S/N = 60 dB Sensitivity = 125 mm	SUAR RMI 413	Within specifications.
5. Dynamic range A-Mode B-Mode Photographic	40dB 40dB 30dB	Electronic burst generator Electronic burst generator Electronic burst generator	Within specifications. Within specifications. Within specifications.
6. Resolution Axial (transducer 1) Lateral (transducer 1) 6dB	1.8 mm 2 mm minimum 6 mm maximum	SUAR AIUM 100 mm	Within specifications. Within specifications.
7. Geometrical accuracy Marker dots Calipers Arm registration Image distortion Central axis Scan arm play Arm movement	 <1% <1% 7 mm <5% <1 mm 100 g: 2° 300 g: 3° ±0.5% horizontal ±2% rotation	 AIUM 100 mm AIUM 100 mm AIUM 100 mm AIUM 100 mm AIUM 100 mm Protractor Force balance Ruler, protractor Ruler, protractor	 Within specifications. Within specifications. Not within specifications (5 mm). Within specifications. Within specifications. Not within specifications. (1°, 2°) Within specifications. Within specifications.

Table 7.11
Safety and Operational CT Scanner Tests

Test	Performance
1. Radiation interlocks	Radiation exposure should be impossible until all interlocks (e.g., doors) are closed or in "safe" position.
2. Safety switches	All "Emergency Off" switches should be operational; i.e., they should stop the motion of the gantry and turn off the x-ray beam. Also, safety switches that forbid the accidental collision of the patient or patient couch with the gantry should be operational. Collisions are more likely to occur at the extreme tilt positions of the gantry.
3. Bed motion	Bed should be operational in both manual and computer-controlled modes.
4. Reconstruction time	The length of time for reconstructing an image should be ≤time quoted by the manufacturer. A stopwatch is convenient for this and measurement number 5.
5. Scan time	The actual scan time should match that selected on the control console. It is often difficult to determine exactly when data sampling begins and ends; however, there is usually a visual or audio indication of the presence of an x-ray beam. The presence of the beam may be somewhat longer (a second or two) than the actual data sampling period.
6. Other computer operations	Verify that data are being transferred to disk, stored, reconstructed, etc., correctly. Check that the data and images are present until they are no longer needed and that they may be then erased from the memory device (e.g., disk). Verify that images and data can be retrieved from archival storage devices, when necessary.

time of the tests so that the measurements and any performance questions may be discussed and resolved.

RADIATION THERAPY

The success or failure of curing cancer by radiation is often depicted by a sigmoid dose-response curve (see Fig. 7.38). In the low dose portion of the curve, the probability of local cancer control is unacceptably low. In the high dose portion of the curve, the probability of local control is high, but the likelihood of producing undesirable effects in normal tissues may be significant. In radiation therapy, the objective is to obtain an acceptable balance between the high probability of cure and a low rate of complications. To meet this balance, it is generally believed that an accuracy of ±5% in the delivery of absorbed dose is required (94).

Suboptimal performance of radiotherapy equipment leads directly to a compromise in patient benefit (95). After installation of radiotherapy equipment, and prior to clinical use, the equipment should be acceptance tested to verify that the equipment is operating according to the manufacturer's stated specifications. In addition, the testing process provides the physicist with additional knowledge and confidence in working with the equipment.

In radiation therapy centers of moderate size, the three types of equipment typically encountered are treatment planning computers, simulators, and megavoltage treatment units. In some centers, hyperthermia instrumentation and computed tomographic scanners to provide treatment planning information are becoming increasingly popular.

Treatment Planning Computer

Although computer-assisted radiation therapy treatment planning is an integral part of modern radiation therapy, there is still little guidance for the practicing clinical physicist to verify the accuracy of computerized treatment planning systems. System verification is a major undertaking that requires extensive comparisons of computed results with dose measurements. A recent protocol presented by McCullough and

Table 7.12
Specific CT Scanner Tests

Test no.	Test	Technique	Phantom or test tool	Parameters to be measured	Performance level
1	Low contrast resolution (normal head)	Head technique normally used	8-inch diameter phantom with low contrast hole pattern ($\Delta\mu \cong 0.5\%$)	Smallest hole visible	Smallest visible hole must be equal to or smaller than specified by manufacturer
2	Low contrast resolution (best head)	Best head technique (high dose) available	Same as 1	Same as 1	Same as 1
3	Low contrast resolution (normal body)	Body technique normally used	12-inch diameter phantom with low contrast hole pattern ($\Delta\mu \cong 0.5\%$). Alternatively, same phantom as in test 1	Same as 1	Same as 1
4	Low contrast resolution (best body)	Best body technique (high dose) available	Same as 3	Same as 1	Same as 1
5	High contrast resolution (normal head)	Head technique normally used	8-inch diameter phantom with high contrast hole pattern ($\Delta\mu > 10\%$). Alternatively, see note 1.[a]	Same as 1	Same as 1
6	High contrast resolution (best head)	Best head technique available	Same as 5	Same as 1	Same as 1
7	High contrast resolution (normal body)	Body technique normally used	Same as 5	Same as 1	Same as 1
8	High contrast resolution (best body)	Best body technique available	Same as 5	Same as 1	Same as 1
9	Patient dosimetry (head)	Normal and best head techniques	Phantom described in reference 88. 16-cm diameter × 14-cm long acrylic	Radiation exposure converted to dose at five locations within phantom.	Radiation dose should be less than or equal to that quoted by manufacturer at corresponding techniques.
10	Patient dosimetry (body)	Normal and best body techniques	Phantom described in reference 88. 32-cm diameter × 14-cm long acrylic	Same as 9	Same as 9
11	CT number flatness (head)	Normal head technique	8-inch diameter water phantom	CT numbers averaged over ~100 pixels at several locations in phantom	"Range" (defined in Chapter 4—"CT Technical Information" 22e) should be less than or equal to that quoted by manufacturer for this size phantom

12	CT number flatness (body)	Normal body technique	12-inch diameter water phantom	Same as 11	Same as 11
13	CT number calibration	Normal head technique	8-inch diameter water phantom	Average CT number in center of water phantom and outside of phantom in air	CT number (water) = 0.0 ± 1.5 CT number (air) = −1000. ± 3.0
14	Effective energy of x-ray beam	Normal head or body (depending on size of phantom)	Phantom with pins of several types of plastic	Find effective energy that gives the best CT number linearity (reference 89)	No specified energy. Usually in range 75–85 keV effective.
15	CT number dependence on beam width	Normal head technique at several different slice widths	8-inch diameter water phantom	Average CT number at center of phantom	Variation of average CT number from zero (water) should be less than a few (~3) numbers.
16	CT number dependence on algorithm	Normal head technique reconstructed with all practical algorithms	Same as 15	Same as 15	Same as 15
17	CT number dependence on phantom position	Normal head technique, move phantom up, down, right, left from center of gantry for different scans	Same as 15	Same as 15	Variation of average CT number from value at center of gantry should be less than a few (~5) CT numbers (see note 2)[b]
18	CT number dependence on phantom size	Normal technique for each phantom size	Several water phantoms with diameters from 2 to 12 inches	Same as 15	Variation of average CT number should be less than 20 CT numbers over range of phantom size
19	Light field/radiation field congruence	Normal head technique, narrowest width	Prepackaged film	Position of radiation beam relative to light field (see note 3)[c]	Center of radiation field should coincide with center of light field to within 1 mm or less
20	Bed indexing accuracy	Normal head technique, narrowest beam width bed loaded with approximately 150 lbs (70 kg)	Prepackaged film	Distance between successive scans as measured from film	Bed movement should agree with indicated movement very accurately. Disagreement should be less than 2 mm over 10 scans

Table 7.12 continued

Test no.	Test	Technique	Phantom or test tool	Parameters to be measured	Performance level
21	Backlash in bed movement	Same as 20	Prepackaged film	On same film as 20, move bed past desired position by a few cm, then return to desired position from opposite direction	Backlash should be less than 1 mm
22	Accuracy of anatomical localization system	Localization technique	Bead or small object in phantom, narrow beam width	Ability of scanner to scan at a location defined on the localization radiograph	Position of scan should be within 1 mm of the localization defined on the localization radiograph
23	Sensitivity profile	Scans at several beam widths	45° wire in phantom (see note 4)[d]	FWHM of profile obtained from image	Agreement to within 1 mm of nominal slice width
24	Artifact resistance	Normal head and normal body	One or more high density pins in phantom	Qualitatively assess the amount of streaking	No quantitative level specified; a "reasonable" amount or less. Substantial streaking may indicate mechanical misalignment
25	Noise characteristics	Various mA's	8-inch diameter water phantom	Standard deviation of CT numbers at center of phantom	Standard deviation (σ) should decrease approximately as $\sigma \sim (mAs)^{-1/2}$ except at very high mAs (See reference 90 and note 5)[e]
26	kVp and mA waveforms (optional)	Various kVp's and mA's	HV divider and storage oscilloscope	Wave shape, accuracy and stability	Measured kVp and mA should agree with nominal values to within ±5%. Wave forms should be reasonably free of ripple, spikes, and should be reasonably constant for the duration of the scan
27	Accuracy of distance measuring device	Images reconstructed at various magnifications	Phantom with a series of 1-cm spaced holes	Distance between arbitrary pair of holes	Actual distance and indicated distance should agree to within 1 mm

28	Distortion of video monitor image	Normal body technique	Same as 27	Measure distance between several pairs of holes at several locations on CRT image	Distance between pairs of holes on CRT image should be identical to within ±1% anywhere on the image (see note 6)[b]
29	Distortion of hard copy device (camera)	Same as 27	Same as 27	Same as 28, except that hard copy image is used instead of CRT	Same as 28
30	Radiation scatter and leakage, personnel monitoring	Normal head technique or most frequently used technique	8-inch diameter phantom for scatter. Use very large volume ionization chamber or survey meter	Measure radiation dose per scan at selected locations in the CT suite. Include: control console, diagnostic console, hallways, adjacent rooms, and locations where attending nurse may stand	Scattered and leakage dose per scan times number of scans per 8-hr shift should be less than maximum permissible dose (MPD) for radiation workers. For extra margin of safety, dose per 8-hr shift should be less than 0.5 (or very conservatively, 0.1) times MPD. Leakage radiation at 1 m from tube should comply with CDRH specifications (less than 100 mR/hr at 1 m operated at maximum technique)

[a] Note 1: Other modes of measuring high contrast resolution are frequently used. These include the estimation of modulation transfer function (MTF) from a star pattern, from an edge response function, or from a point response function. In these cases, performance levels at all spatial frequencies must be better than or equal to (higher or equal MTF) the manufacturer's MTF curves submitted with the bid.

[b] Note 2: Care must be taken not to move the phantom too far off center. Frequently, the edges of the x-ray fan beam are used for referencing the output of the x-ray tube. If the phantom eclipses these detectors, then severe artifacts and large CT number changes are possible.

[c] Note 3: Poke two pinholes in the daypack film, align the holes with the light field, expose the film by initiating a scan, and then process the film. The pinholes indicate the center of the light field relative to the center of the radiation field as indicated by the exposed section of the film.

[d] Note 4: Wires that are too large and some inclined plates may cause "flaring" in the image and subsequent inaccurate measurements, especially at low beam widths. A molybdenum wire of diameter 0.010 inch works well. Other satisfactory techniques are patterns of beads and holes placed diagonally across the beam. References 90, 91, 92, and 93 deal with beam width measurements.

[e] Note 5: Often, the standard deviation of CT numbers in the image will increase near the center of the phantom. The pixel to pixel variations (or "noise" in the image) are usually determined by statistical fluctuations in the finite number of photons passing through the phantom. Fewer photons are present in the center of the phantom, causing statistical fluctuations to be greater.

[f] Note 6: In general, it is difficult to magnify the CRT and film images to the same size as the phantom to facilitate direct comparisons of object and images. Using a ruler or the CRT or film images, it is possible to measure spacing between two holes at several locations within the image. The measured spacing should remain constant at all locations on the image. Do not use the "distance measuring device" checked in test 27 for this test, since distortions produced by the electronics of the CRT or optics of the hard copy camera system will not be demonstrated by test 27.

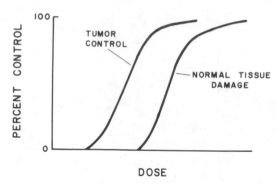

Figure 7.38. Schematic diagram of dose-response curves for tumor control and normal tissue damage.

Krueger documents system accuracy for plans commonly performed in the clinical setting for external photon beams (96). Another verification test package is being designed by the Computer Applications Task Group (TG-23) of the Radiation Therapy Committee of the American Association of Physicists in Medicine.

Simulator

An acceptance program for a radiation therapy simulator should initially test for compliance of all specifications applicable to a diagnostic unit of similar design. In addition, suitable tests should be performed to evaluate the extent of mechanical alignment errors in the simulator. Errors related to field size, treatment distance, table movement, gantry rotation, etc., must be documented and kept within appropriate specifications to provide accurate portal delineation and shielding of vital structures. A detailed protocol for testing a simulator for mechanical alignment errors is provided in a paper by McCullough and Earle (97).

Megavoltage Treatment Unit

The workhorse of most radiation therapy departments is the megavoltage treatment unit. As soon as a new megavoltage unit is able to produce radiation, a comprehensive protection survey should be performed. Electrical, mechanical, and radiation safety features peculiar to each make and model of equipment must be checked for proper operation. A radiation survey of all areas adjacent to the treatment room should be conducted, together with measurements of head leakage and an inspection of interlocks and other safety features.

After completion of the protection survey, a procedure for acceptance testing should be initiated. This procedure should be carefully prepared in advance and in proper sequence for the specific machine to be tested. The acceptance test procedure described below consists of a number of tests and performance criteria for the photon portion of a medical electron linear accelerator. The procedure evolved from the author's experience and by reviewing the performance test procedures of various manufacturers (i.e., Varian, Siemens, AECL) and other services (98, 99). It is written in a general fashion to be applicable to most accelerators. Manufacturer's specifications, and the corresponding tests designed to demonstrate compliance of a unit with the specifications, vary significantly from unit to unit. The procedures described here prepare a foundation upon which the physicist may build an acceptance testing procedure for evaluating the performance of any particular accelerator.

ACCEPTANCE TEST PROCEDURE
Collimator Jaws
SPECIFICATION

Misalignment between the collimator jaw closure position and collimator rotational axis shall not exceed 0.5 mm.

TEST PROCEDURE

Firmly close both pairs of jaws on the mechanical front pointer or on a straight, pointed rod of small diameter. With a sheet of millimeter-ruled graph paper taped to the treatment table surface and perpendicular to the mechanical pointer, raise the table to isocenter. Rotate the collimator through its complete arc, marking the paper about every 45° directly below the tip of the pointer. If the resultant pattern shows a misalignment exceeding 0.5 mm, the collimator jaws should be adjusted for proper alignment with the collimator axis before proceeding to the following tests.

Treatment Table
SPECIFICATION

The rotational axis of the treatment table and collimator shall coincide within ±1 mm.

TEST PROCEDURE

1. Attach to the collimator a mechanical front pointer that is accurately aligned with the collimator axis. Tape a piece of graph paper to the treatment table and raise the table to its highest elevation. Verify with a machinist's level that the table and pointer are orthogonal to one another. Rotate the table through 180° while observing that the tip of the mechanical pointer remains in a 1-mm radius circle.
2. Repeat test 1 with the table lowered to its lowest elevation.

Light Field Center and Crosshairs

SPECIFICATION

The position of the light field center, the cross hairs image, and the mechanical collimator rotational axis shall coincide within ±1 mm.

TEST PROCEDURE

1. With a sheet of graph paper taped to the treatment table surface, raise the table to its highest elevation. Verify with a machinist's level that the collimator face and tabletop are parallel. Rotate the collimator through its maximum arc, marking the points corresponding to the center of the light field. The light field center can be identified as the intersection of the diagonals of the light field. The light field center and cross hairs image should remain within a 2-mm diameter circle centered around the collimator axis.
2. Repeat test 1 with the table lowered to its lowest elevation. If adjustments are necessary, the position of the light field should be adjusted before modifying the cross hairs image, since repositioning the light field will displace the image of the cross hairs.

Light Field, Radiation Field, and Collimator Dial Settings

SPECIFICATION

1. The light field projected at a reference distance (e.g., the isocenter) shall be aligned with all collimator dial settings (mechanical and electronic) to within ±1.5 mm.
2. The light field edges shall be parallel and orthogonal to within 1°.

3. The light field shall coincide with the radiation field to within ±1.5 mm.

TEST PROCEDURE

1. Place a sheet of millimeter-ruled graph paper at the reference distance. The collimator face and graph paper must be parallel. Project a light field of moderate size (i.e., 10 × 10 cm) on the graph paper and observe that specifications 1 and 2 are satisfied. A precision ruler can verify the accuracy of the graph paper.
2. Place a sheet of x-ray film in a light-tight envelope at the reference distance and perpendicular to the central axis of the beam. Set a moderate field size and mark the light field edges by pressure from a ball point pen or 0.010-inch steel shim stock, leaving gaps for use of a densitometer. Pierce the corners of the light field with a needle. Cover the film with adequate buildup material to produce electron equilibrium and expose the film to yield an optical density in the useful optical density range (e.g., 1 to 2) of the film. Develop the film and confirm that the field size defined by the shim stock or other appropriate means coincides to within ±1.5 mm with the 50% isodensity lines of the radiation field. Also verify that the light and radiation field axes coincide to ±1.5 mm.
3. Rotate the collimator 90° and repeat tests 1 and 2.
4. Repeat tests 1 through 3 with 0, 90, 180, and 270° angulations of the gantry.
5. Repeat tests 1 through 4 for smaller and larger fields.

Mechanical Isocenter

SPECIFICATION

1. The position of the mechanical isocenter shall be contained within a 2 mm diameter sphere.
2. The target to isocenter distance shall equal the "expected value" to within ± 0.2 cm.

TEST PROCEDURE

1. Firmly attach a 2 mm diameter drill bit to the end of the treatment table or

other support and locate near the isocenter. Upon rotating the gantry, adjust the length of the mechanical front pointer and reposition the table as required. Rotate the gantry through 360° observing the mechanical pointer tip with respect to the drill bit. The pointer tip should not move outside a sphere of 2-mm diameter.

2. To verify that the location of the isocenter is in accordance with specification 2 (above), measure the distance from the collimator face to the mechanical front pointer tip. Once the isocenter has been established, calibrate (mark or adjust) the mechanical pointer so that the mechanical isocenter can be redetermined at any time.

Gantry Angle Indicators
SPECIFICATION

The true angular position of the gantry shall coincide with all gantry angle indicators (mechanical and electronic) to within ± 1.25°.

Test Procedure

1. Position the gantry to 0° (beam directed vertically downwards) with a machinist's level placed against the collimator assembly face. The true 0° position shall be read on the indicators in accordance with the specification above.
2. Repeat test 1 at 90, 180, and 270° angulations of the gantry.

Collimator Angle Indicator
SPECIFICATION

The true angular position of the collimator assembly shall coincide with all collimator angle indicators (mechanical and electronic) to within ±1.25°.

TEST PROCEDURE

1. With the gantry positioned at 90° (beam directed horizontally), rotate the collimator to a horizontal position using a small level placed on the lower jaw. Alternatively the level could be placed on a ledge formed by clamping a small thin piece of metal, such as a pocket ruler, between the jaws. Verify

that the collimator angle indicators coincide with the true angular collimator position in accordance with the above specification.

2. Repeat test 1 for other points along the collimator arc.

Optional Distance Indicator
SPECIFICATION

The optical distance indicator shall indicate the TSD in the range of ±30 cm from the isocenter to within ±2 mm.

TEST PROCEDURE

1. Place the gantry at 0° and position the treatment tabletop at the reference distance using the properly calibrated mechanical front pointer. Check that the optical distance indicator reading coincides with the isocenter value in accordance with the specification.
2. Repeat the test at ±30 cm from the isocenter by using a buildup surface and by lowering the treatment table.

Radiation Isocenter (Collimator, Treatment Table, Gantry)
SPECIFICATION

The rotational axis of the collimator, treatment table, and gantry shall coincide with the central axis of the radiation beam to within ±1 mm.

TEST PROCEDURE

1. Set gantry at 0°. Tape a sheet of x-ray film on the treatment table at isocenter and pinprick the point directly below the tip of the mechanical front pointer. Open the upper jaws wide and close the lower jaws of the collimator to yield a narrow slit of radiation 1 mm or less at the isocenter distance. Rotate the collimator and make several exposures (i.e., 7 or 8) on the same film at approximately equally spaced intervals. Each exposure should yield a film density of approximately unity and should not overlap the exposures from other orientations. On the processed film, construct lines parallel to and centered in each of the images. The intersection of these lines should be contained in a circle of radius 1 mm centered on the pinprick mark.

2. Close the upper jaws to a narrow slit; open the lower jaws and repeat test 1.

Beam Flatness and Symmetry
SPECIFICATION

1. The variation in intensity of the radiation beam over the central 80% of the longitudinal and transverse major axes of 10 × 10 cm fields and larger should not exceed ±3% of the arithmetic average of the maximum and minimum intensities in this region when measured at a depth of 10 cm in water and at the nominal TSD.
2. For fields of 10 × 10 cm and larger, measured along the major axes in water at a depth of 10 cm and at the nominal TSD, the intensity of the radiation beam shall not differ by more than ±2% when integrated over opposing halves of the field.

TEST PROCEDURE

1. Set gantry at 0° and field size to 10 × 10 cm. The scanning equipment must be level with respect to the gantry and shall include a reference probe. With the water surface at the nominal TSD, position the center of the small ionization chamber (e.g., 0.1 cc) at the depth of 10 cm below the water surface. With the radiation beam on, scan the ionization chamber in both the longitudinal and transverse planes through the radiation beam central axis. Verify that the resultant plots of the beam profile are in accordance with specification 1.
2. Repeat test 1 for a large field size (e.g., 35 × 35 cm).
3. Repeat tests 1 and 2 for 90, 180, and 270° angulations of the gantry.
4. Evaluate the beam profiles obtained in tests 1 through 3 for symmetry in accordance with specification 2. Areas may be measured by use of a planimeter or by counting squares on the graph paper.

Beam Energy
SPECIFICATION

1. The depth of maximum buildup for a 10 × 10 cm field at the nominal TSD

shall be the "expected value" ±0.2 cm.
2. The central beam axis intensity for a 10 × 10 cm field at the nominal TSD and 10 cm depth is the "expected value" of the intensity at the maximum buildup ±2%.

TEST PROCEDURE

Set gantry at 0° and field size at 10 × 10 cm. The scanning equipment must be level and shall include a reference probe. With the water surface at the nominal TSD, position the center of the ionization chamber at the water surface and at a depth of 10 cm, marking the corresponding location of the pen on the scan paper. Plot the central axis depth dose curve on the scan paper. Verify the depth of maximum buildup and the 10 cm depth dose value in accordance with specifications 1 and 2.

Dosimeter Linearity and Reproducibility
SPECIFICATION

1. Linearity of accumulated dose within a preset range of 10 to 999 monitor units shall be within ±2% or 1 monitor unit, whichever is greater.
2. Reproducibility of accumulated dose within any 5-day period shall be within ±2% or 1 monitor unit, whichever is greater.
3. In arc therapy, the reproducibility of accumulated dose shall be within ±3% or 1 monitor unit, whichever is greater, over arc angles greater than 45°.

TEST PROCEDURE

1. Set gantry angle at 0°, phantom surface at nominal TSD, and field size to 10 × 10 cm. With a suitable ionization chamber centrally positioned at the depth of maximum buildup in water or a suitable solid phantom, perform a series of irradiations at a fixed dose rate over the range of 10 to 999 monitor units. Linearity of the recorded accumulated dose readings for the various preset monitor unit settings shall be in accordance with specification 1.
2. Repeat test 1 with 90, 180, and 270° angulations of the gantry.
3. With the conditions in test 1, perform a series of 300 monitor unit irradiations over a 5-day period (AM and PM).

Reproducibility of the accumulated dose during this time period shall be in accordance with specification 2.

4. With the machine set so that the radiation will be terminated by the gantry stop angle, perform a series of arc irradiations with different starting gantry angles, dose rates, and gantry rotation speeds. Verify that the accuracy of the accumulated dose is within ±3% or 1 monitor unit, whichever is greater, of the console dose monitor reading.

References

1. Niemkiewicz, JM, Mulvaney JA, Rossi RP: Performance testing of diagnostic x-ray units. In: *Proceedings of the Society for Photooptical Instrumentation Engineers*. Bellingham, WA, 1980, vol 233, pp 112–121.

2. Stone T: Equipment performance analysis methods. In: *Proceedings of the Society for Photooptical Instrumentation Engineers*. Bellingham, WA, Sept 1976, vol 96, pp 26–30.

3. Federal Drug Administration: *Regulations for the Administration and Enforcement of the Radiation Control for Health and Safety Act of 1968*. HHS Publication (FDA) 80-8035. Washington, DC, US Government Printing Office, 1980.

4. Hendee WR, Rossi RP: *Quality Assurance for Radiographic X-ray Units and Associated Equipment*. HEW Publication (FDA) 79-8094, USDHEW. Washington, DC, US Government Printing Office, April 1979.

5. Hendee WR, Rossi RP: *Quality Assurance for Fluoroscopic X-ray Units and Associated Equipment*. HEW Publication (FDA) 80-8095, USDHEW. Washington, DC, US Government Printing Office, Oct 1979.

6. Hendee WR, Rossi RP: *Quality Assurance for Conventional Tomographic X-ray Units*. HEW Publication (FDA) 80-8096, USDHEW, Washington, DC, US Government Printing Office, Oct 1979.

7. Rossi RP: Acceptance testing of radiographic x-ray generators. In Lin PJ, Kriz RJ, Rauch PJ, Strauss KJ, Rossi RP (eds): *Acceptance Testing of Radiological Imaging Systems*. New York, American Association of Physicists in Medicine (AAPM), 1982, pp 110–125.

8. Rauch PL: Performance characteristics of diagnostic x-ray generators. In Lin PJ, Kriz RJ, Rauch PJ, Strauss KJ, Rossi RP (eds): *Acceptance Testing of Radiological Imaging Systems*. New York, AAPM, American Institute of Physics, 1982, pp 126–156.

9. Direction 13288E, Bleeder, High Voltage Dual Type, T8005G and C1515A, Connections . . . Applications, Medical Systems, General Electric Company 4-2977.

10. *Operating and Maintenance Instructions for Dynalyzer II High Voltage Unit*, (ST-2914-1). Stamford, CT, Machlett Laboratories, Inc., 1976.

11. Lin PJ, Kriz R: A four conductor to three conductor junction box. *Appl Radiol* Nov/Dec:61–62, 1978.

12. Kanamori H: Analysis of high-voltage waveforms in x-ray units: I. Single phase. *J Franklin Inst* 279:147–159, 1965.

13. Kanamori H: Analysis of high-voltage waveforms in x-ray units: II. Abnormal voltages. *J Franklin Inst* 279:246–253, 1965.

14. Kanamori H: Analysis of high voltage waveforms in x-ray units: III. Three Phase. *J Franklin Inst* 279:347–359, 1965.

15. Rauch PL, Block RW: Acceptance testing experience with fourteen new installations. In: *Proceedings of the Society for Photooptical Instrumentation Engineers*. Bellingham, WA, 1976, vol 96, pp 12–18.

16. Brezovich IA, Barnes GT: An investigation and explanation of the fall-off of x-ray tube current during an exposure. *Phys Med Biol* 25:241–249, 1980.

17. National Electrical Manufacturers Association: *Measurement of Dimensions of Focal Spots of Diagnostic X-ray Tubes*. NEMA Standards Publication No. XRS-1974. New York, NEMA, 1974.

18. Spiegler P, Breckinridge WC: Imaging of focal spots by means of the star test pattern. *Radiology* 102:679–684, 1972.

19. Robinson A, Grimshaw GM: Measurement of the focal spot size of diagnostic x-ray tubes—a comparison of pinhole and resolution methods. *Br J of Radiol* 48:572–580, 1975.

20. Bernstein F: Specification of focal spots and factors affecting their size. In: *Proceedings of the Society for Photooptical Instrumentation Engineers*. Bellingham, WA, Oct 1974, vol 56, pp 159–163.

21. Scheid C: Acceptance testing—is it worth the effort? In: *Proceedings of the Society for Photooptical Instrumentation Engineers*. Bellingham, WA, Sept 1976, vol 96, pp 392–396.

22. Strauss KJ: X-ray tube acceptance testing in the field. In Lin PJ, Kriz RJ, Rauch PJ, Strauss KJ, Rossi RP (eds): *Acceptance Testing of Radiological Imaging Systems*. New York, AAPM, 1982, pp 157–182.

23. Chaney EL, Hendee WR: Effects of x-ray tube current and voltage on effective focal spot size. *Med Phys* 1/3:141–147, 1974.

24. Federal Drug Administration: *Suggested Optimum Survey Procedures for Diagnostic X-ray Equipment*. USDHEW Publication (FDA) 76-8014. Washington, DC, US Government Printing Office, July 1975.

25. Federal Drug Administration: *BRH Routine Compliance Testing for Diagnostic X-ray Systems or Components of Diagnostic X-ray Systems to Which 21 CFR Sub-Chapter 3 Is Applicable*. USDHEW Publication (FDA) 77-8001. Washington, DC, US Government Printing Office, revised Oct 1976.

26. Van Roosenbeck E: A new method of aligning a light localizer x-ray beam. *AJR* 117:175–177, 1973.

27. National Electrical Manufacturers Association: *Test Methods for Diagnostic X-ray Machines for Use during Initial Installation*. NEMA Standards Publication No. XR8-1979. Washington, DC, 1979.

28. Federal Drug Administration: *Test Method for Fluoroscopic Beam Alignment*. USDHEW Publication (FDA) 72-8016. Washington, DC, US Government Printing Office, Nov 1971.

29. Relihan GF: Automatic brightness control of image intensifier systems. In Lin PJ, Kriz RJ, Rauch PJ, Strauss KJ, Rossi RP (eds): *Acceptance Testing of*

Radiological Imaging Systems. New York, AAPM, 1982, pp 61–73.

30. Siedband MP: How the user may specify and measure the performance of image intensifier systems. In: *Proceedings of the Society for Photooptical Instrumentation Engineers, Medical X-ray, Photo-Optical Systems.* Bellingham, WA, 1974, vol 56, pp 99–106.

31. Godbarsen R: Automatic brightness control of fluoroscopic image systems. In: *Proceedings of the Society for Photooptical Instrumentation Engineers, Application of Optical Instrumentation in Medicine,* III. Bellingham, WA, August 1–2, 1974, vol 47.

32. Siedband MP: Automatic brightness stabilizers. In: *Proceedings of the Society for Photooptical Instrumentation Engineers, Application of Optical Instrumentation in Medicine,* III. Bellingham, WA, August 1–2, 1974, vol 47.

33. Rich JE: *The Theory and Clinical Application of Television in the Radiology Department.* General Electric Company, 1969.

34. Rich JE: *The Theory and Clinical Application of Intensified Fluoroscopy in the Radiology Department.* General Electric Company, 1970.

35. Siedband MP: Choosing and setting up TV systems for fluoroscopy. In: *Proceedings of the Society for Photooptical Instrumentation Engineers, Application of Optical Instrumentation in Medicine.* Bellingham, WA, 1972, vol 35, pp 159–164.

36. Mulvaney JA, et al: System-level performance testing of image-intensified x-ray equipment. In: *Proceedings of the Society for Photooptical Instrumentation Engineers.* Bellingham, WA, 1981, vol 273, pp 153–159.

37. International Commission on Radiological Units and Measurement: *Cameras for Image Intensifier Fluorography.* Washington, DC, ICRU Report 15, 1969.

38. Casperson LW, Spiegler P, Grollman JH Jr: Characterization of aberrations in image-intensifier fluoroscopy. *Med Phys* 3:103–106, 1976.

39. National Electrical Manufacturers Association: *Test Methods for X-ray Equipment.* NEMA Standards Publication No. XR3-1970, New York, 1970.

40. International Commission on Radiological Units and Measurement: *Methods of Evaluating Radiological Equipment and Materials.* ICRU Report 10f (NBS Handbook 89), 1962.

41. Rossi RP, Bromberg N: Evaluation of the contrast ratio of intensified fluoroscopic imaging systems. In: *Proceedings of the Society for Photooptical Instrumentation Engineers.* Bellingham, WA, 1981, vol 347, pp 229–237.

42. Stanhope G: X-ray automatic exposure control. In: *Proceedings of the Society for Photooptical Instrumentation Engineers.* Bellingham, WA, 1975, vol 70, pp 171–175.

43. Mulvaney JA, Niemkiewicz JM, Rossi RP: Compatibility of rare earth screens with automatic exposure control systems. In: *Proceedings of the Society for Photooptical Instrumentation Engineers.* Bellingham, WA, 1980, vol 233, pp 170–175.

44. Rauch PL: Performance characteristics of diagnostic x-ray generators. In Lin PJ, Kriz RJ, Rauch PJ, Strauss KJ, Rossi RP (eds): *Acceptance Testing of Radiological Imaging Systems.* New York, AAPM,

1982, pp 126–156.

45. Craig JR: Characteristics and evaluation of automatic exposure controls. In: *Proceedings of the Society for Photooptical Instrumentation Engineers, Application of Optical Instrumentation in Medicine,* IV. Bellingham, WA, 1975, vol 70, pp 189–195.

46. Joseph ES, Schneble JE: X-ray automatic exposure timing and control circuitry. In: *Proceedings of the Society for Photooptical Instrumentation Engineers.* Bellingham, WA, 1975, vol 70, pp 166–170.

47. Rossi RP: Acceptance testing of geometrical tomographic equipment. In Lin PJ, Kriz RJ, Rauch PJ, Strauss KJ, Rossi RP (eds): *Acceptance Testing of Radiological Imaging Systems.* New York, AAPM, 1982, pp 275–289.

48. Littleton JT: A phantom method to evaluate the clinical effectiveness of a tomographic device. *AJR* 168:847–856, 1970.

49. Littleton JT, Winter FS: Linear laminagraphy, a simple geometric interpretation of its clinical limitations. *Am J Roentgenol Radium Ther Nucl Med* 95:981–991, 1965.

50. Kieffer J: Analysis of laminagraphic motions and their values. *Radiology* 33:560–585, 1939.

51. National Electrical Manufacturers Association: *Performance Measurements of Scintillation Cameras.* Standards Publication No. NU1-1980. Washington, DC, 1980.

52. Federal Drug Administration: *Measurements of the Performance Parameters of Gamma Cameras: Part I.* HEW Publication (FDA) 78-8049, US Department of Health, Education, and Welfare, PHS, Bureau of Radiological Health. Washington, DC, US Government Printing Office, Dec 1977.

53. Hine GJ, Paras P, Warr CP, et al: *Measurements of the Performance Parameters of Gamma Cameras: Part II.* HEW Publication (FDA) 79-8049, US Department of Health, Education, and Welfare, PHS, Bureau of Radiological Health. Washington, DC, US Government Printing Office, June 1979.

54. AAPM Report No. 6 Nuclear Medicine Committee: *Scintillation Camera Acceptance Testing and Performance Evaluation.* AAPM, Chicago, American Institute of Physics, 1980.

55. International Electrotechnical Commission (IEC): *Characteristics and Test Conditions of Radionuclide Imaging Devices,* 62C Revision March 1979 (Paris). Report of Technical Committee No. 62, Sub-Committee 62C, High-Energy Radiation Equipment and Equipment for Nuclear Medicine, International Electrotechnical Commission, 1 Rue de Verembe, Geneva, Switzerland.

56. Adams R, Hine GJ, Zimmerman CD: Deadtime measurements in scintillation cameras under scatter conditions simulating quantitative nuclear cardiography. *J Nucl Med* 19:538–543, 1978.

57. Strand SE, Larsson E: Image artifacts at high fluence rates in single-crystal NaI(T*l*) scintillation cameras. *J Nucl Med* 19:407–413, 1978.

58. Wooten WW, Graham LS: Analysis of anger camera flood field uniformity based on order statistics. *Med Phys* 9:41–51, 1982.

59. Keyes JW, Gazella GR, Strange DP: Image analysis by on-line minicomputer for improved camera quality control. *J Nucl Med* 13:525–527, 1972.

60. Nusynowitz ML, Benedetto AR: A mathematical

index of uniformity (IOU) for sensitivity and resolution. *Radiology* 131:235–241, 1979.

61. Cox NJ, Diffeg BL: A numerical index of gamma-camera uniformity. *Br J Radiol* 49:735–36, 1976.

62. Raff U, Spitzer VM, Hendee WR: Practicality of NEMA performance specification measurements for user-based acceptance testing and routine quality assurance. *J Nucl Med*, in press, 1985.

63. Chapman DR, Garcia EV, Waxman AD: Misalignment of multiple photopeak analyzer outputs: effects on imaging. *J Nucl Med* 21:872–874, 1980.

64. AAPM Report No. 9, Task Group of the Nuclear Medicine Committee: *Computer-Aided Scintillation Camera Acceptance Testing.* AAPM, Chicago, American Institute of Physics, 1982.

65. AAMI/ANSI: *Safe Current Limits for Electromedical Apparatus.* New York, American National Standards Institute, December, 1978.

66. *Quest Guide to Essential Test Instrumentation for Medical Equipment.* Diamond Bar, CA, Quest Publishing Company, 1978.

67. *Standard for Medical and Dental Equipment.* UL-544, Melville, Long Island, NY, Underwriters Laboratories, 1977.

68. National Fire Protection Association: *Safe Use of Electricity in Patient Care Areas of Hospitals,* NFP-76B. Quincy, MA, NFPA, 1980.

69. IEC: *Safety of Medical Electrical Equipment, Part I: General Requirements,* IEC 601-1. Geneva, Switzerland, IEC, 1977.

70. Canadian Standards Association (CSA): *Electro-Medical Equipment,* CSA C22.2, No. 125. Ontario, Canada, CSA, 1973.

71. AIUM: *AIUM Recommended Nomenclature, Physics and Engineering.* Bethesda, MD, AIUM, August 28, 1979.

72. AIUM/NEMA: *Safety Standard for Diagnostic Ultrasound Equipment.* AIUM/NEMA Standards Publication No. UL1-1981, Supplement to *J Ultra Med* 2(4), April, 1983.

73. *Standard Methods for Testing Single Element Pulse-Echo Ultrasonic Transducers—Interim Standard.* Supplement to *J Ultra Med* 1(7), September, 1982.

74. Brendel K, et al: *Ultra Med Biol* 2:343–350, 1976.

75. *Pulse Echo Ultrasound Imaging Systems: Performance Tests and Criteria.* AAPM Report No. 8. AIP, 335 E. 45th Street, New York, NY.

76. Goldstein A: B-scan transducer peak frequency measurement by diffraction grating spectroscopy. *J Ultra Med* 1:53–66, 1982.

77. Carson P: Rapid evaluation of many pulse echo system characteristics by use of a triggered pulse burst generator. *J Clin Ultrasound* 4:259–263, 1976.

78. AIUM: *AIUM Standard Specifications of Echoscope Sensitivity and Signal to Noise Level, Including Recommended Practice for Such Measurements.* New York, AIUM, 1980.

79. Burlew MM, Madsen E, et al: *Radiology* 134:517–20, 1981.

80. Banjavic RA, et al: Imaging characteristics of clinical ultrasonic transducers in tissue equivalent material. In Meterell A (ed): *Acoustical Imaging 8.* New York, Plenum, 1979.

81. Zagzebski JA: Ultrasound equipment acceptance tests. In Fullerton G, Zagzebski (eds): *AAPM Monograph Medical Physics of CT and Ultrasound:* *Tissue Imaging and Characterizations.* New York, AIP, 1980.

82. McCullough EC, Payne JT: X-ray transmission computed tomography. *Med Phys* 4:85–98, 1977.

83. Cacak RK, Hendee WR: Performance evaluation of a fourth generation computed tomography (CT) scanner. In: *Proceedings of the Society for Photooptical Instrumentation Engineers.* Bellingham, WA, 1979, vol 173, pp 194–207.

84. Weaver KE: Imaging factors and evaluation: computed tomography scanning. In Haus AG (ed): *The Physics of Medical Imaging Recording System Measurements and Techniques.* Proceedings of the AAPM Summer School. New York, American Institute of Physics, 1979.

85. McCullough EC: Specifying and evaluating the performance of computed tomography (CT) scanners. *Med Phys* 7:291–296, 1980.

86. Bellon EM, Mivaldi FD, Wiesen EJ: Performance evaluation of computed tomography scanners using a phantom model. *AJR* 132:345–352, 1979.

87. Kelsey CA, Berardo PA, Smith AR, et al: CT scanner selection and specifications for radiation therapy. *Med Phys* 7:555–558, 1980.

88. Shope TB, Gagne RJ, Johnson GC: A method for describing the doses delivered by transmission X-ray computed tomography. *Med Phys* 8:488–495, 1981.

89. Millner MR, Payne WH, Waggner RG, et al: Determination of effective energies in CT calibration. *Med Phys* 5:543–545, 1978.

90. Cohen G, DiBianca FA: Information content and dose efficiency of computed tomography scanners. In: Haus AG (ed): *The Physics of Medical Imaging.* New York, American Institute of Physics, 1979, pp 356–365.

91. Brooks RA, Di Chiro G: Slice geometry in computer assisted tomography. *J Comput Assist Tomogr* 1:191–199, 1977.

92. Sorenson JA: Technique for evaluating radiation beam and image slice parameters of CT scanners. *Med Phys* 6:68–69, 1979.

93. Schneiders NJ, Bushong SC: CT quality assurance: computer assisted slice thickness determination. *Med Phys* 7:61–63, 1980.

94. Fletcher GH: *Textbook of Radiotherapy,* ed 3. Philadelphia, Lea & Febiger, 1980.

95. International Commission on Radiation Units and Measurements: *Determination of Absorbed Dose in a Patient Irradiated by Beams of X or Gamma Rays in Radiotherapy Procedures.* Washington, DC, ICRU Report No. 24, 1976.

96. McCullough EC, Krueger AM: Performance evolution of computerized treatment planning systems for radiotherapy: external photon beams. *Int J Radiol Oncol Biol Phys* 6:1599–1605, 1980.

97. McCullough EC, Earle JR: The selection, acceptance, testing, and quality control of radiotherapy treatment simulators. *Radiology* 131:221–230, 1979.

98. Wooten P, Almond PR, Holt JG, et al: Code of practice for X-ray therapy linear accelerators. *Med Phys* 2:110–121, 1975.

99. Chester AE, Jones JC, Massey JB: *A Suggested Procedure for the Mechanical Alignment of Tele-gamma and Megavoltage X-ray Beam Units.* London, Hospital Physicists Association (UK), Report No. 3, 1972.

CHAPTER EIGHT

Design of a Quality Assurance Program

WILLIAM R. HENDEE, Ph.D., RAYMOND P. ROSSI, M.S.
VICTOR M. SPITZER, Ph.D., RICHARD L. BANJAVIC, Ph.D.,
ROBERT K. CACAK, Ph.D., and GEOFFREY S. IBBOTT, M.S.

INTRODUCTION

A carefully planned and executed program of quality assurance (1–10) is an essential ingredient of any radiologic process of high quality. Perhaps the most critical element of a quality assurance program is the commitment of personnel to a standard of excellence in their working environment (11). This commitment is nourished by the support and encouragement towards excellence offered by those persons in charge of a radiologic facility; alternatively, a lack of support and encouragement can easily stifle the most determined efforts to establish a quality assurance program. Support and encouragement should be directed towards the objective of instilling pride in each individual for the work he or she does. Through this sense of pride in the quality of work performed, a sense of determination can grow to do even better work, leading ultimately to achievement of a standard of excellence that is the true hallmark of an effective program of quality assurance.

As aids in the development of a quality assurance program, a number of suggestions can be offered. In radiologic imaging, for example, standards of quality should be established against which the products of any particular study can be judged. In an ultimate sense, appropriate standards of quality are difficult to identify for any particular study, as preferences vary among individuals responsible for interpreting the study. Still, certain standards can be identified. In roentgenography, for example, selected aspects of the image can be evaluated as criteria of quality. Among these criteria are:

1. Is the anatomy of interest displayed properly in the images?
2. Are image density and contrast adequate for visualization of the region of interest?
3. Was proper collimation employed as revealed by an unirradiated margin on all borders of the image?
4. Is image degradation caused by patient motion, scattered radiation, film fogging, etc., at an acceptably low level?

These criteria can or should be applied to all roentgenographic studies performed in the facility; similar criteria can be developed for other radiologic modalities. The application of these criteria to any particular study is the responsibility ultimately of the staff radiologist in charge of the study. For roentgenography, areas that are amenable to the development of criteria for quality assurance are shown in Table 8.1.

Of considerable assistance in the implementation of a quality assurance program is the establishment of standard protocols for the performance of different examinations in the facility. It should be understood by all personnel involved in a particular study that deviations from the standard protocols are desirable only under exceptional circumstances.

A standard protocol for a radiologic study should include a brief description of the study and its purpose, together with the techniques to be employed in conducting the study and the methods to be used to accumulate and record data resulting from the study. In roentgenography, for example, the protocol should describe the projections desired, the number and size of films to be used, the desired method for patient preparation, acceptable ranges of technique factors, the contrast media to be employed, and all other factors which may affect the quality of the study. All protocols should be reviewed periodically and approved by the physician-in-charge in consultation with the radiographers performing the studies.

Table 8.1
Areas in Which Specific Standards of Image Quality Might Be Developed

1. General radiographic studies
2. Orthopedics
3. Emergency studies and ER trauma
4. Gastrointestinal radiography
5. Tomography
6. Urography
7. Pediatrics
8. General special procedures
9. Angiographic special procedures
10. Chest
11. Portable studies

Successful implementation (12, 13) of a quality assurance program in a radiologic facility ensures that the product of the facility (i.e., diagnostic information) is of maximum usefulness in the care of patients. It also contributes to pride and a sense of accomplishment on the part of individuals working in the facility and leads to an enjoyable and supportive work environment. Under the right circumstances, it can also be cost-effective by reducing repeat examinations and equipment downtime. For all these reasons, a program of quality assurance can be recommended to all radiologic facilities, irrespective of size and complexity.

ROENTGENOGRAPHY

Standardization of Radiographic Techniques

The quality of a roentgenographic image is influenced by many factors such as kilovoltage peak, exposure time, imaging geometry, image receptor, patient size and physical condition, and processing and viewing conditions. For each image of a patient to be of optimal quality, and for sequential images to be helpful in detecting changes by comparative analysis, it is essential that imaging techniques be standardized and utilized uniformly by all personnel responsible for a given examination. To achieve these objectives, standardized technique charts should be posted in the control area for each examination room. Posted technique charts should provide the information required for each study performed in each room and should include at least the following data.

1. Exam name.
2. Projection(s) to be used.
3. Image receptor type and size.
4. Source to image receptor distance.
5. Grid to be used.
6. Kilovoltage peak and milliampere second exposure factors to be used as a function of anatomical part thickness or patient size.
7. Tube/image receptor holder to be used.
8. Sensitive fields for anatomically controlled exposure techniques.
9. Any special notes concerning the conduct of the examination.

The radiographer in charge of each room should be responsible for developing and updating the technique charts for the room. These charts should be consulted for each procedure done in that room.

In developing standardized technique charts, the following guidelines should be utilized.

1. To minimize patient exposure, the kilovoltage peak should be as high as possible consistent with adequate image contrast.
2. To minimize motion unsharpness, the speed of the image receptor should be as fast as possible consistent with adequate image clarity.
3. To minimize motion unsharpness, the milliamperage should be as high as possible consistent with tube loading restrictions.

For rooms equipped with automatic exposure control devices, manual exposure techniques should be posted in the event of failure of the automatic exposure control device.

To facilitate the implementation of remedial action, all problems encountered in using standardized techniques should be reported immediately to the appropriate individual.

Image Receptor Control, Evaluation, and Certification

In roentgenography, the image receptors represent an important element in the production of high quality images. To assure the proper utilization performance of image receptors, the following measures should be implemented.

INVENTORY CONTROL

All radiographic film should be ordered by one individual who is responsible for maintaining records of the quantity, size, type, and cost of film purchased. From these records an annual summary should be prepared in conjunction with other departmental statistics to estimate next year's budget and to identify important departmental characteristics, such as the average number of films used for each examination.

All radiographic film in the department should be retained in locked storage and should be inventoried and distributed by a designated individual. Stock film should be dispensed so that proper rotation is ensured to preclude outdated film and an excessive supply in a particular working area.

SENSITOMETRIC CONSISTENCY

To verify the consistency of radiographic film used in the department, the working stock of film should be evaluated sensitometrically at least quarterly. These evaluations should be the responsibility of a designated individual. They should be conducted by randomly selecting a sheet of each size and type of film from each imaging area's working stock and exposing each film with a standard light sensitometer. These films are then run in the same processor and the sensitometric curve plotted, with the current sensitometric monitoring values compared to previous results. Results of these evaluations should be reviewed to determine sensitometric consistency.

SCREEN MAINTENANCE AND EVALUATION

Screens should be cleaned at least semiannually in accordance with the manufacturer's recommendations, and each cleaning should be documented in writing. Cassette/screen combinations should be tested for contact annually and any time a contact problem is suspected. The results of contact

testing should be documented. All cassettes should be numbered to facilitate identification.

IMAGE RECEPTOR EVALUATION

Prior to routine use of a new image receptor, the receptor should be evaluated for its suitability for the intended imaging task. This evaluation should include assessment of appropriate imaging characteristics as determined from physical measurements and phantom images. Results of this evaluation should be documented.

Processor Monitoring and Maintenance

Control of the photographic process represents a key element in the production of roentgenographic images of consistent quality (14–16). To achieve proper photographic control, all processors should be monitored routinely by sensitometric methods. Results of this monitoring should be documented, and corrective action should be initiated whenever necessary. All processors should be cleaned routinely, and all corrective maintenance should be documented. One individual should be made responsible for the processor monitoring and maintenance program.

Procedures utilized in the monitoring and maintenance of processors are described in the literature and in the service manuals of the manufacturers. The following procedures for processor monitoring should be performed routinely.

ROUTINE SENSITOMETRIC MONITORING

1. Exposing, processing, and measuring of sensitometric test films daily, with documentation of the results on the processor control charts and the processor monitoring record.
2. Measuring of chemical replenishment rates at weekly intervals, with adjustment as indicated by the sensitometric monitoring data and with documentation on the processor control charts.
3. Measuring and documenting processor solution temperatures three times a week.

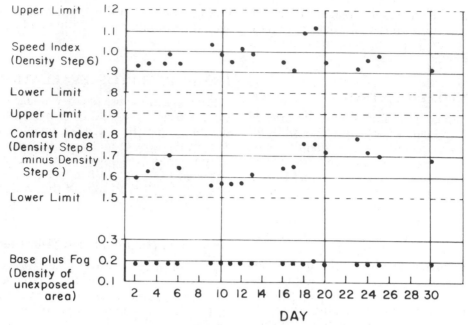

Figure 8.1. Example of a processor control chart.

An example of a processor control chart is shown in Figure 8.1.

ROUTINE PROCESSOR MAINTENANCE

1. Cleaning of crossover racks three times a week.
2. Cleaning of main racks once a week, with mechanical and electrical inspection of the processor for marginal parts and the replacement of these parts.
3. Changing processing chemistry whenever required as indicated by sensitometric control charts.
4. Establishing and posting a routine maintenance schedule for each processor.
5. Documenting all cleaning and corrective actions on the processor control charts.

CORRECTIVE PROCESSOR MAINTENANCE

1. Responding to and repairing processor malfunctions documented by a "Request for Service."
2. Documenting all action taken to repair processor problems.

RECORDS

1. Maintaining all processor control forms and monitoring summary forms in a current and complete manner.
2. Filing all processor control charts, monitoring summary forms, processor initialization records, emulsion comparison records, and film counter data.

Monitoring Equipment Performance

Monitoring the on-going performance of radiologic equipment may be centered at several levels (17–20). Primary monitoring should be the responsibility of a physicist or service engineer and should be correlated with a preventive maintenance program. Results of this monitoring should be documented, including a summary of the deficiencies identified and corrective actions taken. Performance verification of a radiologic system should be performed whenever a component that may affect system performance is repaired or replaced. In certain cases this verification may be limited to aspects of system performance that may be altered by the component.

Secondary performance monitoring may be conducted by staff radiographers on either a component basis utilizing procedures similar to those described in the literature (17–20) or on a systems basis utilizing a standard phantom imaged under reproducible conditions. With either approach, the results of secondary monitoring should be documented and reviewed periodically. A list of equipment performance parameters subject to primary and secondary performance monitoring is given in Table 8.2.

Radiation Safety of Personnel and Patients

The protection of personnel and patients from excessive radiation exposure is an important consideration in the performance of an overall quality assurance program. The following policies, procedures, and guidelines arc applicable to a radiation safety progam in a radiographic facility.

Table 8.2
Examples of Equipment Performance Parameters Suitable to Monitoring in a Quality Assurance Program

Radiographic beam restriction systems
Exposure timers
Tube protective circuitry
Exposure reproducibility
Exposure linearity
Beam Quality
Focal spot size and consistency
Kilovoltage peak accuracy
Grid alignment
Fluoroscopic beam restriction systems
Fluoroscopic exposure rate control
Fluoroscopic imaging system performance
  High contrast resolution
  Low contrast perceptibility
Automatic exposure rate control systems
  Reproducibility
  Field sensitivity
  Kilovoltage peak compensation
  Density control
  Response capability
  Milliampere second limit
  Backup timer
Tomographic equipment
  Level indicator
  Exposure uniformity
  Exposure angle
  Section thickness
  Resolution
Uniformity of screen speed
Film/screen contact
Uniformity of radiographic illuminators

FEDERAL AND STATE REGULATIONS

In any radiographic facility, compliance with all applicable federal and state regulations should be ensured. In particular, all equipment subject to the "Regulations for the Administration and Enforcement of the Radiation Control for the Health and Safety Act of 1968" (21) should be maintained in compliance with these regulations.

DEPARTMENTAL DESIGN CONSIDERATIONS

During the design of new facilities or renovation of existing facilities, the siting and layout of equipment should be structured to keep exposure of personnel and patients to levels well below maximum exposure limits. Shielding requirements for all facilities should be determined by a qualified expert in accordance with recommended methods.

PERSONNEL SAFETY

In any radiographic facility, safe working practices should be followed by all personnel so that exposures to radiation are kept at minimum levels. In particular, the practices outlined below should be observed.

Monitoring of Exposure

All personnel who are routinely exposed to radiation in the course of their employment should be equipped with one or more film badges or other dosimetry devices. This monitoring procedure should be supervised by the Radiation Safety Office, and summary reports of radiation exposure should be made available to the employee. The summary reports should be reviewed periodically to evaluate the average levels of personnel exposures and to identify methods for their reduction. Personnel monitoring devices used to assess whole body exposure should be worn on the front of the body between the waist and neck. When a protective apron is worn, the monitoring device should be worn at its normal location under the apron. Some individuals recommend that the monitoring device for whole body exposure should be worn at neck level outside of the protective device. Departmental and other hospital personnel who are not routinely exposed to ionizing radiation need not be monitored if their anticipated exposures do not exceed one-fourth of the maximum permissible dose for occupationally exposed individuals.

Pregnant Employee

The recommendations of NCRP 53 with regard to exposure of the pregnant employee should be followed. A formal policy for the pregnant employee should be available.

Protective Clothing

Radiation protective devices (aprons, gloves, mobile shields) with a lead equivalence of 0.25 to 0.75 mm should be conveniently available in sufficient numbers in each imaging area. Aprons and gloves should be worn by all personnel whenever appropriate. All aprons and gloves should be inspected fluoroscopically on an annual basis to verify their integrity. Any protective device found to be defective should be immediately removed from service. All protective clothing should be sequentially numbered and inventoried to assure the proper maintenance of records.

Holding of Patients

Except during emergencies, no individual occupationally exposed to radiation should be permitted to hold patients during examinations, and no one individual should be employed regularly for this service. Anyone holding a patient during an x-ray exposure should wear a protective apron and gloves of at least 0.25 mm lead equivalence and should be positioned so that no part of the body is exposed to the unattenuated x-ray beam. Holders for the image receptor and patient restraint devices should be routinely available and used to reduce the need for patient holding.

General Practices

Personnel should make use of permanent shielding (control booth and room walls), mobile shields, and distance to minimize their exposure to scatter radiation.

PATIENT SAFETY

Although it is desirable to reduce the exposure to patients undergoing radiological examinations, it must be borne in mind that the goal of any radiological imaging procedure is to acquire information about the medical condition of the patient as an aid in clinical management. Overly zealous attempts to reduce patient exposure may significantly compromise this information. Within the scope of this limitation, the following principles can be applied to reduce patient exposure to radiation (22, 23).

Exposure Factors

Technique factors for a given examination should be selected to minimize patient exposure. In general, higher kilovoltage peak techniques are preferred within the limit of obtaining adequate image contrast. The factors of milliamperage and time should be chosen to minimize the degrading effects of anatomical motion while keeping tube loading at a reasonable level.

Image Receptors

The speed of the image receptor should be chosen as high as possible, consistent with required levels of image detail and limits of image noise.

Grid Ratio

The lowest possible grid ratio should be utilized, consistent with effective removal of scattered radiation.

Collimation

Collimation of the x-ray beam should always be restricted to the area of clinical interest and should never exceed the size of the image receptor. Proper collimation can be verified by the presence of an unexposed border on all sides of the roentgenographic image.

Gonadal Shielding

Gonadal shielding of the contact or shadow shield type should be employed in all appropriate procedures. Detailed guidance for the use of gonadal shielding is available in the literature (24–26).

Repeat Radiographs

Working practices and techniques should minimize the need for repeat procedures. Roentgenograms should be repeated only when the quality of the image is insufficient to reveal needed diagnostic information (27–31).

Patient Exposure Estimates

Estimates of the exposure received by patients undergoing roentgenographic procedures should be available in the department. These estimates may be developed for the average patient from measurements of exposure characteristics of various radiological imaging systems. From these data, exposures for a given patient can be estimated (32, 33).

Pregnant/Potentially Pregnant Patients

To minimize the exposure to a fetus, special consideration should be given to potentially pregnant patients and to patients known to be pregnant. For female patients of childbearing age, all requests for radiological studies should describe the pregnancy status of the patient. All requests for radiological procedures on patients known to be pregnant should be approved by a staff radiologist. To minimize fetal exposure, consideration should be given to altering the conduct of the study through the use of selected views, high kilovoltage peak techniques, and high-speed image receptors.

Equipment

All radiological imaging equipment should be surveyed periodically by a qualified expert to determine the radiation safety characteristics. Usually these surveys should be conducted in conjunction with a scheduled preventive maintenance program on at least an annual basis. The results of radiation safety surveys should be documented, and any deficiencies should be corrected prior to returning the equipment to clinical service.

Retake Analysis Program

An analysis of the causes of suboptimal roentgenographic images can provide valuable information for quality assurance and in-service educational activities (27–31). An ongoing retake analysis program should be coordinated by a single individual in the department and should encompass the following activities.

1. Periodic (at least weekly) review of all repeat radiographs and film wastage, with categorization and documentation as to number and type.
2. From the data collected in the periodic review, calculation of the monthly retake rate based on the number of films processed (obtained from film count data) and estimation of the cost of retake and wasted film.
3. Preparation of a graphical presentation of the retake and wasted film data.
4. Analysis of the retake data to determine the problem areas and development of corrective action plans to minimize the retake rate in these areas.

A quarterly summary of retake analysis results and corrective action measures taken should be compiled. From this compilation, the effectiveness of corrective action plans may be assessed by the trends demonstrated in the data. An example of a retake analysis worksheet is shown in Figure 8.2.

Continuing Education and Training

The need for continuing education and training of departmental personnel is an important aspect of a quality assurance program. Efforts should be made to provide personnel with opportunities to participate in continuing educational programs. Specific areas of education should include those described below.

STAFF ORIENTATION

All newly employed personnel should receive an orientation in departmental policies and procedures.

RADIOGRAPHIC REJECT ANALYSIS

FROM: _____ TO: _____

		DARK	LIGHT	COLLIMATION & POSITIONING	MOTION	PROCESSING	UNNECESSARY TO EXAM	ALL OTHER	TOTAL
CHEST	Adult								
	Peds								
	Mobile								
EXTREMITIES									
Shoulder, Clavicle, Humerus									
Knee, Femur									
Distal									
SPINE-RIBS									
C-Spine									
T-Spine									
L-Spine									
Ribs									
SKULL									
Complete									
Facial Bones									
Sinuses, Mastoids, Mandible									
UPPER GI									
COLON(BE)									
KUB									
Abdomen									
Fetus									
IVP									
GALL BLADDER									
PELVIS-HIPS									
MISC. SPECIALS									
Tomograms									
Arthrograms, Venograms									
Myelograms									
ANGIOGRAPHY									
Neuro									
Abdomenial, Peripherial									
TOTAL REPEATS									
WASTE FILM		14 x 17	11 x 14	7 x 17	10 x 12	8 x 10	14 x 14	DUP	SUB
Black									
Green									
Clear									
Test									
TOTAL WASTE									

TOTAL REJECTS

Figure 8.2. Example of a retake analysis worksheet.

EQUIPMENT OPERATION

All staff radiographers should receive training in the proper operation of the department's radiological imaging equipment.

IN-SERVICE EDUCATIONAL PROGRAMS

Routinely scheduled in-service educational programs should be provided for all departmental personnel. These programs should be coordinated so that all personnel may attend. The content and attendance of in-service educational programs should be documented.

OUTSIDE EDUCATIONAL OPPORTUNITIES

Departmental personnel should be encouraged to take advantage of outside educational programs, and attendance at these programs should be supported by the department whenever possible.

Record Keeping, Review, and Evaluation

The review of records and documentation generated by a quality assurance program can provide valuable information on the effectiveness of the program. All records relevant to a quality assurance program should be readily available for review and evaluation by the individual responsible for a given quality assurance activity. These records should be reviewed periodically and no less than annually. The conclusions of these reviews should be documented in the form of a report.

Corrective Action Policies

Corrective action includes those activities taken to correct deficiencies identified by the quality assurance program. In general, any deficiency should be followed by an appropriate corrective action so that the quality of radiological images is maintained at the level of departmental standards.

Review Cycles for Appropriateness and Effectiveness

Periodic reviews should be conducted of the quality and appropriateness of radiological services and the effectiveness of the quality assurance program. These reviews should be conducted at least annually, and more frequently if warranted.

In evaluating the effectiveness of a quality control program, a review of all quality assurance records and actions should be made, and recommendations for improvement of the quality assurance program should also be considered in the review. In assessing the quality and appropriateness of radiological services, each staff radiologist responsible for a given imaging area should provide a written report addressing the quality and appropriateness of studies performed during the reporting period. In developing this report, the staff radiologist should obtain appropriate input from referring physicians utilizing the radiological service. One individual should be responsible for preparing a report covering the areas of patient scheduling, file room functioning, and the delivery of radiological reports to referring physicians. In particular, this report should address specific problems brought to the attention of the author during the reporting period.

An ongoing review of the quality and appropriateness of radiological services should be maintained on an informal basis by dialogue among staff radiologists and referring physicians.

The Cost of a Quality Assurance Program

Costs associated with a quality control program can be divided into three general areas: (1) personnel; (2) equipment; and (3) supplies. While costs will vary, depending on the size of the facility, it is essential to recognize that substantial costs of a quality assurance program do exist and must be identified to determine their impact on departmental resources (34–36).

PERSONNEL

The accomplishment of any quality assurance activity requires the expenditure of personnel time, including that required for planning, test performance, documentation, and analysis of results and corrective actions. In a medium sized facility it is not unreasonable to allocate between 0.5 and 1 FTE (full-time equivalent) to the quality control program.

EQUIPMENT

To conduct a comprehensive quality control program, a substantial investment in equipment is required. This equipment includes a sensitometer and densitometer for processor monitoring, a dosimetry system for exposure measurements, and a variety of specialized test tools for monitoring equipment performance. The capital outlay for this equipment may be in the range of $4,000 to $7,000. For acceptance testing, additional equipment costing $8,000 to $12,000 may be required. Even though these costs can be amortized over the life of the equipment, they are still substantial. A list of typical test equipment for quality assurance is given in Table 8.3.

SUPPLIES

The cost of supplies for a quality assurance program also is not insignificant. Many tests require the use of considerable film, and each film requires a certain amount of chemistry for processing. Data forms for documentation of test results must be printed. While these costs may seem trivial, they add up rapidly when the repetitive nature of testing is considered. For example, assume that three processors are to be monitored daily with 10- × 12-inch film. In 260 working days per year, 780 sheets of film will be required for daily monitoring. This number will increase to 900 sheets when normalization and crossover checks are included. At current prices, the expenditure for this much film and chemistry would be approximately $1,000 per year. Depreciation of the sensitometer and densitometer and the cost of forms might add another $300 per year. A similar analysis with respect to other quality control tests will identify the actual costs involved in a quality assurance program.

Benefits of a Quality Assurance Program

Quantification of the benefits of a quality assurance program is difficult. The most

Table 8.3
Listing of Test Equipment Required for a Quality Assurance Program

Number required	Description of item
1 each	Radiographic beam restriction system test cassette
4 each	Radioopaque markers strips, $3 \times \frac{1}{2} \times \frac{1}{16}$ inch
1 each	Set of lead numbers and markers
1 each	Centering and alignment test tool
1 each	6-inch ruler (graduated in $\frac{1}{16}$ inch)
1 each	6-inch ruler (graduated in $\frac{1}{32}$ inch)
1 each	12-inch ruler (graduated in $\frac{1}{16}$ inch)
1 each	24-inch ruler (graduated in $\frac{1}{16}$ inch)
1 each	Bubble level
1 each	Plywood board (24- $\times \frac{1}{2}$- $\times$ 20 inch)
1 each	Digital x-ray generator timer
1 each	Remote detector for digital x-ray generator timer
1 each	Digital x-ray generator timer-remote detector interconnecting
1 each	Cable (12-inch long BNC-BNC)
1 each	Keithley model 35050 dosimeter
1 each	Keithley model 96030 ionization chamber
1 each	Keithley model 86204 ionization chamber triax cable with 5-inch aluminum stem, cable length 4 ft
1 each	Ionization chamber test stand
1 each	LCD digital readout for Keithley dosimeter
1 each	Dosimeter-readout interconnecting cable (12-inch long banana plug each end)
1 each	Focal spot test tool
1 each	Wide range kilovoltage peak test cassette
1 each	Grid alignment test tool
1 each	Radiographic automatic exposure control system evaluation phantom (consists of 1- $\times$ 2-inch base section of plexiglass containing an orientation marker and reference area for density measurements and four 11- $\times$ 14- $\times$ 2-inch plexiglass blocks)
1 each	Ring stand with clamp
1 each	Lead beam stop (8- $\times$ 8- $\times \frac{1}{8}$-inch lead plate)
1 each	Film-scrreen contract test pattern
1 each	Simpson model 408 illumination level meter
1 each	Radiographic illuminator mask
1 each	Resolution test pattern
1 each	Low-contrast perceptibility test pattern
1 each	Fluoroscopic exposure rate control/film recording system evaluation phantom (consists of one 8- $\times$ 8- $\times \frac{1}{2}$-inch base section of 3-inch legs of 1100 aluminum containing an orientation marker and reference area and four 8- $\times$ 8- $\times \frac{1}{2}$-inch 1100 aluminum blocks)
1 each	1.6-mm aluminum (1100) attenuator, $3\frac{3}{4}$- $\times$ 6-inch
1 each	2.5 mm aluminum (1100) attenuator, $3\frac{3}{4}$- $\times$ 6-inch
1 each	45° tomographic test wedge
1 each	Tomographic aperture plate
2 each	5-cm plexiglass spacer blocks, 6- $\times$ 6-inch
2 each	$\frac{3}{4}$-inch plexiglass attenuators, 12- $\times$ 3-inch
1 each	Sensitometer
1 each	Densitometer

obvious index of benefit is the radiograph repeat rate. The departmental repeat rate should be estimated prior to implementation of the quality assurance program, and continually thereafter. The actual cost of a re-peat radiograph has been placed at between $15.00 and $30.00, so that even a small reduction in the repeat rate can provide substantial savings.

Quality control also should result in more

reliable performance of radiological imaging equipment. Small changes in equipment performance can be detected prior to their exerting an adverse influence on clinical studies and often can be corrected at lower expense.

Finally, and perhaps most importantly, quality assurance improves the overall morale of the department by encouraging the staff to take pride in the work of the department and in the efficiency by which it is achieved.

NUCLEAR MEDICINE

A complete quality assurance (QA) program in nuclear medicine includes not only the topics common to all quality assurance programs in medical imaging (e.g., film exposure and development, record keeping, and monitoring of instrumentation), but also an area unique to nuclear medicine: radiopharmaceuticals. This section considers a quality assurance program specific to the instrumentation unique to nuclear medicine (i.e., scintillation cameras, single probe units, isotope calibrators, xenon gas dispensing systems, and survey meters). Included are some of the hardware concerns that should be monitored for the quality assurance of computers in nuclear medicine. Quality assurance of computer software also is an important issue; however, it is beyond the scope of this text and is covered only in general terms.

Quality assurance procedures generate massive amounts of data. Much of these data are required by state and federal regulatory agencies and hospital accreditation agencies. Hence, extensive documentation of all quality assurance procedures is very helpful during reviews by these agencies. Quality assurance procedures should be designed with a high frequency of measurement compared to the rate or pattern of performance deterioration expected for a piece of equipment or process. On the other hand, the extent and frequency of quality assurance procedures must not be so burdensome that the tasks are not performed. Some measurement protocols may satisfy record-keeping requirements but do little to assure the quality of instrumentation. One major ingredient of a quality assurance program is the inclusion of "action levels" for each measurement so that the demonstration of suboptimal per-formance of an imaging system or process will elicit a response to correct the cause of poor performance.

Scintillation Cameras

Ideally, all quality assurance tests are performed initially during acceptance testing of a scintillation camera, and the data accumulated at this time are used as a benchmark for the camera's quality assurance procedures. It is on these data that acceptable performance values and action levels are based. Daily quality assurance should include a flood image to assure camera uniformity. Although NEMA (National Electrical Manufacturers Association) uniformity measurements for acceptance testing utilize a point source (Chapter 6), many institutions and manufacturers prefer a ^{57}Co flood phantom (a disk source of ^{57}Co) or a liquid-filled flood tank of ^{99m}Tc (Fig. 8.3). These extended, large area flood sources provide the advantage of measuring the extrinsic uniformity of the system (i.e., the uniformity with the collimator attached). They have the disadvantage, however, of increasing the exposure of technologists to radiation because they employ a 5- to 10-mCi extended source in place of a 200- to 300-μCi point source of radioactivity. Furthermore, they provide only a limited uniformity of activity across the field of view. The uniformity of the point source of radiation depends on the distance from the source to the crystal and the total counts comprising the image. Therefore, the photon flux from a point source can be made as uniform as desired by placing the source far from the crystal and counting for long times. Most commercial ^{57}Co flood sources, on the other hand, have guaranteed intrinsic uniformity of only 5%. Many commercially manufactured flood tanks demonstrate bulging at the center and consequent nonuniformities of 5 to 10% if filled without special precautions (see Fig. 8.3); that is, the point source uniformity flood has an advantage so long as the radiation source can be placed far enough from the crystal (>5 useful field of view (UFOV) diameters) and high count images can be obtained (>12 million counts for a 15-inch UFOV). If the point source uniformity flood method is used, then an independent method for frequent collimator inspection should be employed to ensure extrinsic uniformity. Collimator damage

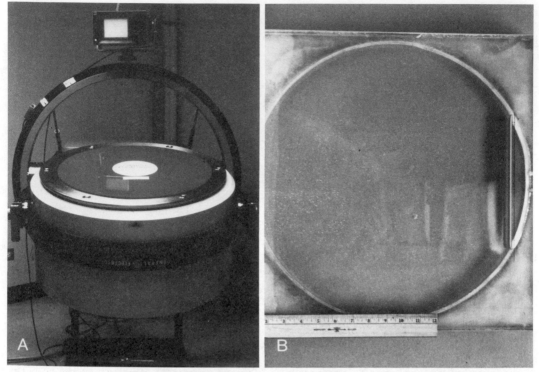

Figure 8.3. Uniform flood sources: The ^{57}Co, 10-mCi flood phantom (*A*) is on top of the collimator of the detector in position for uniformity flooding. (*B*) Demonstrates the volume of water or source nonuniformity due to bulging surfaces when a typical plastic tank is filled in a vertical orientation.

usually is caused by physical abuse, and the effects should be noticeable by visual inspection of both surfaces of the collimator. However, foil type collimators are subject to separation defects at the glue lines of adjacent foil strips without physical abuse. Some collimator defects are shown in Figure 8.4. Foil type collimators should demonstrate acceptable uniformity during acceptance testing and should be evaluated quarterly by quality assurance tests with a flood-type uniformity source.

In addition to uniformity images, data to be recorded during daily uniformity testing of a scintillation camera include the source activity, the counts in the image, the time required for image acquisition, and the high voltage and window width used to center the photopeak. Sensitivity data (observed counts/microcurie-minute) provide an indication of drift in the window level and width. A typical data sheet for daily quality assurance is shown in Table 8.4.

Resolution and spatial linearity of a scintillation camera should be checked at least weekly. Some phantoms, including the NEMA phantom, are designed to indicate both of these parameters simultaneously (Fig. 8.5). One particularly attractive phantom consists of an orthogonal array of uniform holes that allow the resolution and linearity to be checked simultaneously (measured, if a computer analysis of the point spread functions is done (37)) in both the x and y directions and even on the diagonals. If only a qualitative inspection of resolution and linearity is to be done, the phantom should have hole sizes that nearly match the resolution of the camera to be measured.

On most new cameras with an electronic mask or iris, the field of view is variable and should be checked periodically. Weekly measurements are suggested. Distance calibration on both the x and y axes can be accomplished quickly from images of any of the phantoms in Figure 8.5. The x and y calibration distances should be equal on the analog film and in the computer matrix, if utilized. The calibrated distances can be

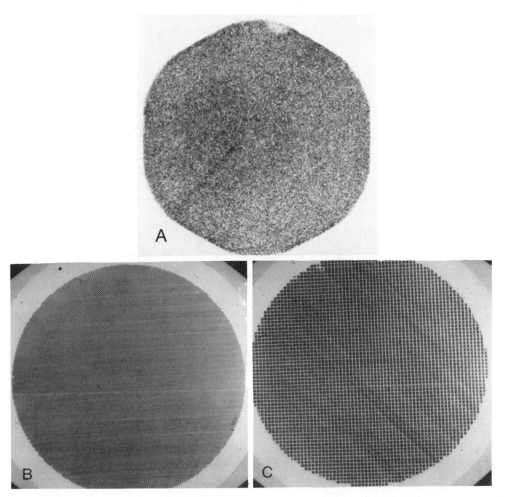

Figure 8.4. Collimator defects: The scintigraphic image in *A* demonstrates a collimator separation defect (7 inches long in the *lower left* quadrant) at the glue line of adjacent corrugated lead strips. The cold area at the top of the image is an air bubble in the liquid-filled flood tank. *B* is a radiograph of a normal foil-type, high resolution, low energy collimator. The collimator radiograph in *C* shows a large plug of lead in the *upper left* quadrant of a high sensitivity, low energy collimator. The corrugated lead strip nonuniformities typical of foil collimators are evident in both *B* and *C*.

used to measure the UFOV in the uniformity flood field image. Responses for these weekly measurements are included in Table 8.4.

More extensive quality assurance procedures to be performed quarterly include count rate response, uniformity at high count rates, more quantitative measurements of resolution such as those available with the Center for Devices and Radiological Health test pattern (38) or the NEMA resolution phantom (described in Chapter 6), and spatial linearity at low and high count rates, as provided by the NEMA method

described in Chapter 6. Energy resolution and point source sensitivity (both NEMA measurements) need be measured only annually. System resolution measurements with and without scatter should be obtained quarterly, together with some off-peak flood images to detect a hydrolyzing crystal (39).

Computer collection and analysis of the intrinsic tests described above (with the exception of energy resolution), have been developed at a number of institutions (40, 41). Computer-assisted quality assurance not only provides more quantification for routine measurements, but also often decreases

Table 8.4
General Electric 400: Weekly Quality Assurance

Technologist _____

Measurement	Monday	Tuesday	Wednesday	Thursday	Friday
Point source activity and time (~300 µCi)	**289** µCi @ **7:40** AM	**312** µCi @ **7:35** AM	___ µCi @ ___	___ µCi @ ___	___ µCi @ ___
Integral uniformity UFOV (correctors on)	@ **7.55** AM **5.2** %	@ **8:10** AM **5.6** %	@ ___ AM ___ %	@ ___ AM ___ %	@ ___ AM ___ %
Integral uniformity UFOV (correctors off)	@ **8:12** AM **13.6** %	@ **8:24** AM **12.9** %	@ ___ AM ___ %	@ ___ AM ___ %	@ ___ AM ___ %
Time required for 12 M (correctors on) flood	**740** sec	**690** sec	___ sec	___ sec	___ sec
Sensitivity (counts/µCi-sec)	**57.8**	**59.6**	___	___	___
High resolution collimator integrity	✓		___		
GAP collimator integrity	✓				
Medium energy collimator integrity	✓				
Resolution (CDRH test pattern)	**2.5**				
Linearity (CDRH test pattern)					
Field of view (analog) (digital)	X- **392** mm Y- **394** mm / X- **63** pixels Y- **64** pixels				

Comments

Please include service requested, including date and time, and the date and times of service.

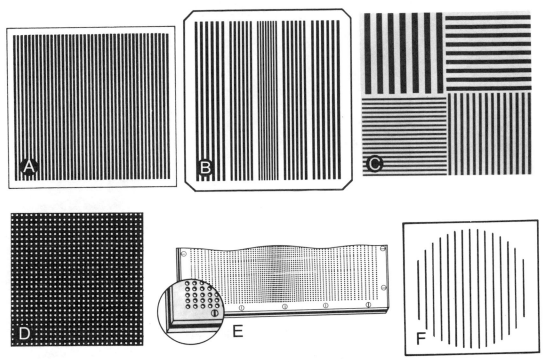

Figure 8.5. Linearity and resolution phantoms. The parallel line with equal spacing (PLES) phantom (*A*) demonstrates linearity and resolution. The line spacings should be matched to the camera resolution. The Hine Duly phantom (*B*) allows resolution to be determined. The quadrant bar phantom (*C*) also provides resolution measurement and demonstrates linearity, to a limited degree, in orthogonal directions. The orthogonal Hole Phantom (OHP) (*D*) must be selected to match hole sizes and spacings to camera resolution, but linearity is assessible on diagonals as well as along the orthogonal axes of the phantom. The CDRH test pattern (*E*) consists of equal size holes with center spacings which vary in 0.5-mm increments in the horizontal direction. The NEMA test pattern (*F*) is intended for quantitative assessment of both resolution and linearity and is widely accepted by camera manufacturers for determining performance specifications. (*A* to *F*, Courtesy of Nuclear Associates, Inc.)

the total quality assurance time by combining multiple measurements such as point source sensitivity, linearity, and resolution into a single image analysis. The major advantage of computer-assisted quality assurance is the immediate comparison of a set of quality assurance measurements to a data set completed over the last few months or any arbitrary time. When any measurement exceeds a preset limit of acceptability, the need for service may be indicated. A computer assisted quality assurance program is illustrated in Figure 8.6. The daily performance of a scintillation camera, along with acceptable limits, is demonstrated in the 120-day graph in Figure 8.7.

Single Probe Scintillation Devices

Single probe units include well counters, thyroid uptake units, and multiprobe units that have independent recording for each probe. Response variations in these systems usually are caused by instabilities in the high voltage source. Therefore, quality assurance for these systems should include monitoring of the high voltage by identifying window settings that bracket the photopeak of a standard long-lived isotope. A check of these units daily or before each use with a background count and a ^{57}Co or ^{137}Cs source in a constant geometry should yield reproducible count rates. If count rates deviate from those expected for constant window settings and a specific source, then the window level or width may have changed electronically and must be readjusted. Frequent or excessively large adjustments to the window indicate a need for service. The quality of the crystal should be checked on a monthly basis by plotting the energy spectrum of the pho-

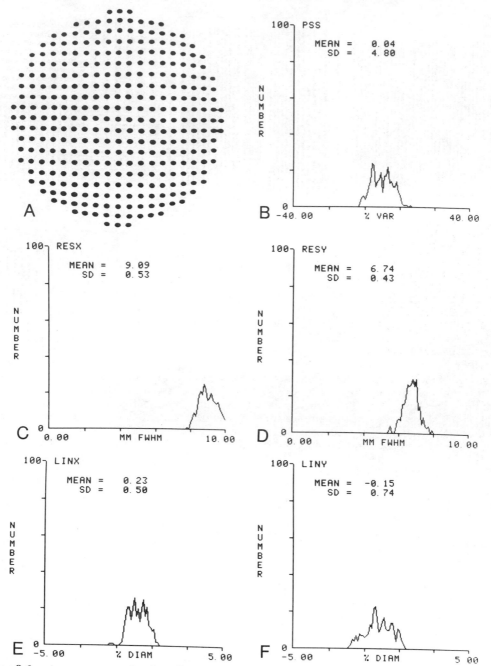

Figure 8.6. A computer-assisted quality assurance program. Five camera performance measurements are made from the single image of a precision machined orthogonal hole phantom (*A*). Point source sensitivity is derived from the total counts measured at each of the hole sites (*B*). Resolution in x and y directions (*C* and *D*) is determined from the point spread response of the camera to the activity flooding each hole. *E* and *F* show variations of the recorded hole patterns from the constructed hole distribution of the phantom. (From Hasegawa BH, Kirch DL, LeFree MT, et al: Quality control of scintillation cameras using a minicomputer. *J Nucl Med*, 22:1075–1080, 1981.)

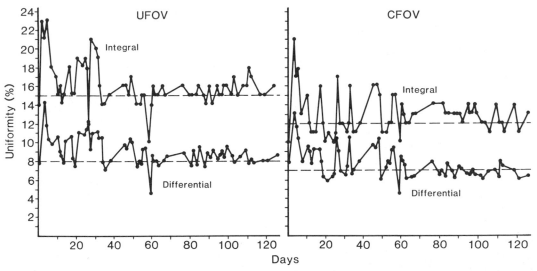

Figure 8.7. Uniformity variation over four months. Quantitative quality assurance measurements provide entries to a data base for automatic comparison of current measurements to the four previous months. Action thesholds (*dashed lines*) are set with consideration given to performance specifications, clinical image quality degradation, correctability without intervention, and the length of service required to bring the parameters back down to acceptable levels. The uniformity values shown in these graphs often exceed the action limits, and major overhaul of the detector system was required. (From Raff U, Spitzer M, Hendee WR: Practicality of NEMA performance specification measurements for user-based acceptance testing and routine quality assurance. *J Nucl Med* 25:679–687, 1984.)

topeak of standard radioactive sources. This is accomplished by moving a narrow window across the photopeak by varying the high voltage or amplifier outputs. A widening of the photopeak most often indicates a hydrolizing crystal.

Isotope Calibrators

The isotope calibrator (often referred to as a dose calibrator) is the single piece of instrumentation in a nuclear medicine department that commands the greatest attention from radiation protection agencies. Acceptable quality assurance methods are explicitly detailed in the Nuclear Regulatory Commission (NRC) Guide 10.8, Appendix C (41). The isotope calibrator should be checked daily for constancy of response to a long-lived isotope. A background count should be collected or background adjusted to 0 before measurement of the count rate from the long-lived source. Counts should be accumulated on all commonly used isotope settings and the background-corrected results compared to previous counts corrected for decay. Any measurement falling

above or below 2 SDs from the expected value should be remeasured. If the second measurement confirms the first, service should be requested on the calibrator.

In addition to daily checks of the constancy of response, quarterly determinations of linearity should be made. These determinations are accomplished by measuring the activity of multiple samples (or the same sample after decay or attenuation to different effective activities) over the range of activities encountered during use. The response of the isotope calibrator should reproduce the known activity to within 5%; otherwise, a correction factor or service is indicated.

The final quality assurance test for an isotope calibrator is performed on a semiannual or annual basis. This test measures the accuracy of response of the isotope calibrator to isotope sources emitting rays of different energies. The test requires sources of known activity traceable to sources certified by the National Bureau of Standards (NBS). Suggested sources include ^{137}Cs, ^{57}Co, and ^{133}Ba. The measured activity of these sources, corrected for background, should correspond to within 5% to the decay-corrected activity of the NBS-traceable sources. A correction factor may be applied to units that reproduce the correct activity to an accuracy between 5 and 10%. Any unit that exceeds that 10% error limit should be submitted for service.

Survey Meters

Survey meters should be calibrated at least annually and after any service or battery change. Procedures for survey meter calibration are also outlined in NRC Guide 10.8, Appendix D (42). An accepted method of calibration utilizes a high activity long-lived calibrated source (e.g., ^{137}Cs) traceable to NBS. Radiation fields of different exposure rates are obtained by placing the calibrated source at different distances from the survey meter. If necessary, calibrated attenuators can be used to extend the range of exposure rates. The survey meter is placed in appropriate locations to yield calibration points in each half of each scale on the instrument. The instrument should be adjusted to read the true exposure rate to within 10%; alternatively, calibration factors can be computed for the instrument so that the user can adjust each measurement to the correct exposure rate.

Computers

Quality assurance of computers involves both hardware and software considerations. Unlike most other instrumentation in this section, computer hardware operates in the digital or discrete domain. In this domain, problems usually do not arise slowly; instead, they occur in discrete and, therefore, much more noticeable steps. Two major causes of computer problems are humidity and heat; therefore, computer quality assurance should include close monitoring of the operative environment to ensure that it remains within the limits established by the manufacturer. In obtaining reliable digital results, the major concern usually rests with the input device where analog signals are converted to digital signals for processing. The analog to digital conversion (ADC) process should be monitored weekly with the uniformity flood of the scintillation camera. The ADC amplifier gains and offsets should be adjusted to provide a matrix-centered flood-field image that uses the maximum available matrix space and still includes the camera's UFOV (Fig. 8.8). The integrity of the ADC can be determined by acquiring a high count uniformity flood field image and comparing the uniformity of the field on the computer to the output of the photographic camera attached to the scintillation camera. As demonstrated in Figure 8.9, nonlinear ADCs will show striping artifacts in the image (striping artifacts are straight lines at bit borders; i.e., at power of 2 pixel locations).

An important consideration in the maintenance of computer hardware is cleanliness. Dust and smoke particles can damage hard platter disks and the read/write heads of the disk drive, as demonstrated in Figure 8.10.

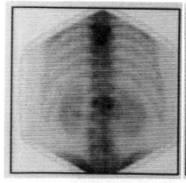 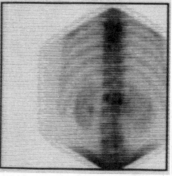 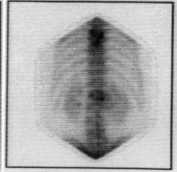

Figure 8.8. Misadjusted gain and offset. The left image shows a properly adjusted camera interface. Maximum computer resolution is achieved by filling the entire matrix with the camera's field of view (390 mm/128 pixels = 30.5 mm/pixel). Voltage offset may result in truncated images as in the center image. Improper gain adjustment (*right*) image degrades camera-computer system resolution with larger pixel sizes (390 mm/110 pixels = 3.54 mm/pixel).

Dirty environments also cause decreased lifetime and read/write errors on floppy disks and tape systems. Preventive maintenance for storage media includes semiannual cleaning of removable hard disk cartridges and monthly cleaning of hard disk drives and frequently used floppy disks.

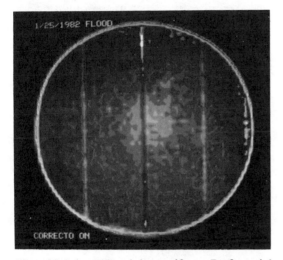

Figure 8.9. ADC striping artifacts. Preferential bit states in the X-ADC register are evident in the flood image. The center stripe is cold relative to its background, demonstrating a preferential off or zero state for the highest order bit of the conversion. The second highest bit is also malfunctioning. It is preferentially on or in the one state and consequently produces the hot stripes at one-fourth and three-fourths of the x-axis. Background subtraction has been applied to the image to visually emphasize the problem.

Tape system read/write heads require cleaning frequencies similar to those for floppy disk systems. Most types of disks can be used without verifying the integrity of each storage bit location. For nuclear medicine tests such as first pass and flow studies, each disk should be subjected to media verification at the time of first use and each time thereafter that the disk is totally erased for reuse. This process will identify bad sections of a disk as unreadable; many systems can still use a disk containing bad sections.

Dust also can cause overheating of electronic components in the computer and its peripherals. Overheating is caused by clogging of the Millipore filters on disk drives and the air filters on the cooling fans of electronic components. Routine filter cleaning and replacement should be established in every computer facility at least quarterly, and more frequently if the environment is particularly dirty. Hard disk drive filters should be inspected and possibly replaced at least semiannually.

Quality assurance of medical applications software should include the maintenance and documentation of data files for patients and phantom studies. Sometimes software replacements or revisions that analyze nuclear medicine studies yield results that can be compared to those of previous versions of acceptable software. However, new software often provides new or different data analyses that are accompanied by changes in the collection parameters of scintigraphic data. Consequently, benchmark data are not

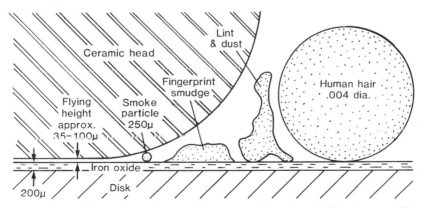

Figure 8.10. Debris on disk platters. One major cause of data loss is disk damage. The read/write head of hard disk systems flies approximately 100 μm above the magnetic oxide coating of the disk. Physical contact of the head with possible contaminants such as smoke particles, fingerprints, or dust can result in loss of data as well as damage to the disk and the read/write head.

available for newer software, and the evaluation is one of acceptance testing, rather than quality assurance.

ULTRASOUND

Once a piece(s) of new equipment has been delivered, installed, and shown by performance evaluation to be acceptable, the burden of maintaining image quality transfers to the user. By the use of periodic quality assurance tests (QA), the integrity of the images can be monitored, and the unit can be adjusted to maintain images of acceptable quality. In this manner, film usage, scan time, and repair costs can be reduced, as well as patient exposure to high frequency insonification. This chapter covers the design and execution of a quality assurance program for dedicated A-mode and M-mode units, compound articulated arm B-mode scanners, "real-time" mechanical autosectoring scanners, "real-time" sequential linear arrays, and electronically phased linear arrays. There are other dedicated scanners on the market, such as water-standoff sector systems and both singular and duplex Doppler units. Although some of the techniques discussed here may not be directly applicable to these units, similar methods can be identified to check selected performance parameters. Preceding the references is a list of quality assurance manuals from which many of the procedures discussed here have been taken.

Definition of Quality Assurance

A working definition for quality assurance is:

The periodic monitoring of a given performance parameter for a diagnostic instrument under constant conditions using known standards to assure that the parameter has not degraded (43).

The key phrases of this defintion are "periodic monitoring," "constant conditions," and "using known standards."

Quality assurance tests are designed to be performed by sonographers, and the results must be easy to interpret.

The most important part of any quality assurance program is its periodic application to all units in the clinical service. In any protocol, some tests should be scheduled for

performance more often than others; however, all tests should be performed at least bimonthly. Shown in Table 8.5 is an excerpt from a typical quality assurance schedule, delineating which tests to do and how frequently to do them. Included in Table 8.5 are the performance parameters considered to be most important because they yield the best overall estimate of image quality scan after scan, year in and year out.

The tolerance allowed for each result should not be neglected. Examples of tolerance levels for the maintenance checks in Table 8.5 are:

Maintenance function or test	Tolerance
Distance (or time) calibration check	2%
Caliper (marker dot) calibration check	2%
Sensitivity variation check	3 dB (i.e., 6 dB) variance (same as no change in depth of penetration in tissue-mimicking test phantom of more than ±5 mm out of 12 cm (±4%).
Misregistration check	5–7% (i.e., 5–7 mm over 10-cm path length).
Sector scan misregistration	2–3% (i.e., 2–3 mm over 10-cm path length).
Resolution checks (For largest field of view)	
Axial	±0.5 mm
Lateral	±1 mm
Uniformity of scan registration check	±3 dB
Accuracy of time markers in M-mode check	60 ± 2 cycles coincide with 1-sec time markers.

To remove as many variables as possible, quality assurance measurements should always be performed using the same transducer assembly and instrument settings. In

Table 8.5
Ultrasound Quality Control Schedule[a]

Maintenance function or test	Static-scanners (used frequently)	Static-scanners (used intermittently)	Real-time sequential linear arrays	Real-time mechanical electronic sector	M-mode units (used frequently)	Older A-mode and M-mode equipment
Distance (or time) calibration check	T	SM	W	W	SM	A
Caliper (marker dot) calibration check	T	SM	W	W	SM	A
Sensitivity check	T	SM	W	W	SM	A
Misregistration checks						
B-mode arm misregistration check	T	SM	T	T		
Sector scan misregistration check			SM	W		
Axial resolution checks—3 FOVs	W	SM	W	T	SM	A
Lateral resolution check—1 FOV	W	SM	W	T	A	A
Real-time scan uniformity check			T	T		A
Hard copy and gray scale photography checks	D	W	T	D	SM	A
Film processor quality control check (once a week for department)						
Filter checks (where present)	SM	SM	SM	SM	SM	A
Electrical and mechanical checks	M	SA	M	M	M	A

[a] Abbreviations used are: D, daily; T, twice weekly; W, weekly; SM, semimonthly; M, monthly; Q, quarterly; SA, semiannually; A, annually; FOV, field of view.

this manner, abnormal results are detectable, and the causes of these results are more easily identifiable.

The third part of the working definition of quality assurance refers to the use of "known standards." The techniques discussed here all use two types of test objects and one type of commercially available tissue-mimicking test phantom. (The suppliers of these and other test objects and test phantoms are given in Appendix II.)

The first test object is the American Institute of Ultrasound in Medicine (AIUM) Standard 100-mm test object. A sketch of the test object appears in Figure 8.11. Only a summary of its use is provided here; considerable additional information is available in the literature (44).

The second test object is the Sensitivity, Uniformity, and Axial Resolution (SUAR) Test Object. This device consists of an acrylic block 16 ± 0.1 cm $\times$ 14 ± 0.1 cm $\times$ 6.35 ± 0.1 cm, with a bottom wedge-shaped piece of dimensions 10.0 ± 0.01 cm $\times$ 4.0 ± 0.1 cm and a height that varies from 2.5 mm ± 0.05 mm to 0 mm along the 10-cm distance. The bottom of the block is then covered with a ¼-inch plexiglass plate. The wedge compartment normally is filled with a solution with a speed of sound of 1540 ± 3 m/sec.

The SUAR block is used for measurements of axial resolution and for sensitivity checks on dedicated A-mode and M-mode units, static articulated arm B-scanners, and real-time scanners with both mechanical and electrical drives. With the test object on its 6.35-cm side, it can be used for basic sensitivity tests in A-mode, M-mode, and B-mode static systems, and for system uniformity studies with linear sequential arrays or mechanical and phased array sector scanners (45). (If exact estimates are not required for axial resolution, uniformity checks can be made with a solid acrylic block of the same approximate dimensions as those for the SUAR phantom.)

The third test object is a tissue-mimicking Model 412 or 413 Resolution Registration Profile and Sensitivity Phantom, marketed by Radiation Measurements, Inc. (RMI), of Middleton, Wisconsin. A sketch of this phantom appears in Figure 8.12. The phantom consists of three 7.5-mm diameter clear cylindrical tubes in water-based gelatin and graphite substrate. The tubes are arranged normal to and at an angle to the scanning window at depths of 3, 5, and 9 cm. Nylon fibers of 0.3-mm diameter serve as line reflectors and are positioned vertically at depth spacings of 2 cm down the center line of the phantom, normal to the scanning window

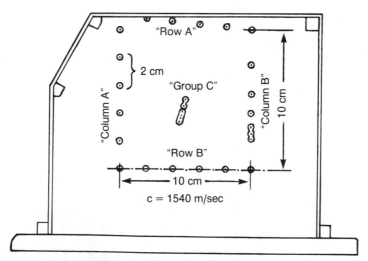

Figure 8.11.   AIUM standard 100-mm test object. The following are identified: The set of wires used for vertical calibration and precise beam width checks (*Column A*); the set of wires used for horizontal calibration and B-scan misregistration checks (*Row B*); the sets of wires used for gross axial (*Group C*) and lateral (*Group B*) resolution checks. The wires are 0.75-mm diameter stainless steel, and the fluid in the test object has a speed of sound 1540 ± 3 m/sec.

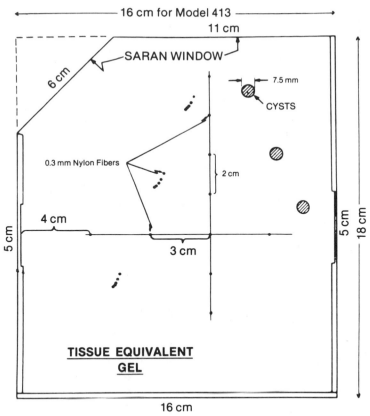

Figure 8.12. RMI model 412 or 413 tissue-mimicking phantom. Shown is the internal geometry of the nylon fibers and "cystic" structures in the test phantoms. The nylon fibers are all 0.3 mm in diameter. The tissue-mimicking gel has a speed of sound of 1540 ± 3 m/sec and an attenuation coefficient of 0.6 dB cm^{-1} MHz^{-1}.

and horizontally at intervals of 3 cm at a depth of 10 cm. The nylon fibers also are used to make three sets of groups of 5 lines, offset by 1 mm at vertical separations of 3, 2, 1, and 0.5 mm. The offset groups are positioned at depths of 3, 7, and 12 cm. The entire test phantom has an attenuation of 0.6 dB cm^{-1} MHz^{-1} (46).

The RMI phantom is one of many available tissue-mimicking phantoms on the market. Almost any value can be obtained for the attenuation coefficient and the backscatter coefficient (47). The RMI phantom was chosen for presentation here because it is one of the more popular and provides results which are easy to interpret.

Alignment of the Test Devices

In performing any of the tests with the AIUM 100-mm test object, the SUAR test object, or the RMI test phantom, the test devices must be properly aligned and remain *absolutely* stationary. Patient couches with cushioned pads and nonlockable wheels often create problems with alignment, since it may be impossible to determine a scan plane which is in contact at all times with the test device. For the case of a compound scanner, the tilt of the scan plane is first adjusted so that the transducer face can be placed flush on both the scanning window and the table surface. This adjustment assures adequate transducer-surface contact using test devices with solid surfaces. When a soft-surfaced scanning window phantom like the RMI models 412 or 413 is used, the procedure recommended above is the most practical way of assuring that the sound beam is directed perpendicularly on the targets in the test phantom.

The second stage in the alignment process is the positioning of the test device so that all windows are accessible for scanning. With the transducer aimed horizontally, the device is placed with the vertical window nearest the probe flush with the face of the transducer. Then the scanning arm is moved until the transducer is flush with the opposite vertical window. Occasionally, manual scanning arms are found where this motion is not possible because of slight mechanical flaws in the arm. If contact cannot be made, it should be brought to the attention of the instrument manufacturer's service representative.

Transducer Selection

A standard transducer should be employed for routine performance tests. For the RMI model 412 phantom, a 3.5-MHz, 19-mm diameter, long-focused probe is recommended, and this transducer should be kept out of routine use. If a lower frequency transducer is employed, the depth of penetration of the ultrasound beam may exceed the phantom's distal margin, and sensitivity measurements may be impossible. The selected transducer should be the only one used in all future quality assurance testing of all the available ultrasound units. Different connectors for different types of equipment may require more than one "standard" transducer.

Routine Performance Tests

Routine performance tests for dedicated A-mode and M-mode units, for articulated arm B-mode scanners, for "real-time" electronic linear sequential or phased arrays, and for mechanical autosector scanners should be conducted routinely. Quality assurance notebooks should be kept and inspected monthly to identify trends in equipment performance. The QA program consists of assessment of the following.

1. Distance (or time) calibration checks, including horizontal and vertical display size comparisons.
2. Assessment of accuracy of digital calipers.
3. Systems sensitivity checks.
4. Articulated arm B-scan misregistration checks.
5. Sector scan misregistration checks.
6. Axial resolution checks (three fields of view).
7. Lateral resolution checks (one field of view).
8. Real-time uniformity checks.
9. Gray scale and hard copy photography checks.
10. Film processor checks.
11. Electrical and mechanical checks. Each time the tests are conducted, the sonographer should follow a standardized worksheet developed for each type of ultrasound unit. The worksheet helps assure consistency in the test procedure and in the analysis of the results. It is completed and included in the quality assurance notebook kept with the scanner.

DISTANCE (OR TIME) CALIBRATION CHECKS
Scan Procedure

Distance calibrations can be conducted using any column of targets of physically known separation and spacing (e.g., column A and row B in the AIUM 100-mm test object shown in Fig. 8.11). The AIUM test object should be filled with a solution whose speed of sound is within 3 m/sec of 1540 m/sec. If a tissue-mimicking test phantom is used for any of the geometry-related tests, it should also contain material whose speed of sound is 1540 ± 3 m/sec. The scanner's field of view is set at 20 cm, and a smooth scan across the top of the test object is performed. The sensitivity settings of the instrument are recorded so that the test can be reproduced. Usually, all sensitivity controls (e.g., near gain, far gain, initial, delay, slope or time gain compensation (TGC)) are set near zero, and the overall gain control is set about 6 dB above threshold display.

The depth markers (centimeter marker dots) are positioned on the image vertically and horizontally. In addition, the cursors of the digital caliper are positioned to measure the distance between images of targets in the phantom that are separated by a known distance (e.g., 10 cm). A second image, or the image of the bottom row of targets in the phantom as described above, is used to check the accuracy of the calipers in the horizontal direction. A second hard copy can be recorded, if desired.

The time calibration for M-mode systems is checked by turning on the 0.5-sec time markers and the internal EKG. One of the metal contacts of one EKG lead is held motionless in one hand, while the EKG gain and position are adjusted until a 60-Hz oscillation is displayed on the EKG trace. A strip chart recording of the trace is obtained so that the number of 60-Hz oscillations in 1 sec of time markers can be counted (48).

Analysis

A set of dividers (hand-held calipers) is used to compare the distance on the film between the images of targets spaced over a 10-cm distance in the test object to the distance measured with the 1-cm depth markers. A disagreement of greater than 2 to 3 mm could mean that:

1. The depth marker circuitry is faulty.
2. The test object is faulty (this can be easily checked).

After the vertical 10-cm distance is recorded on the worksheet, the horizontal target spacing (row B in Fig. 8.11) is compared to the horizontal depth or the horizontal calipers. Imprecisions of more than 2 to 3 mm should be noted. They are often caused by distortion in the TV monitor but can originate from other sources as well. Discrepancies of 5 mm or more suggest a correction whenever distances are measured on an echogram. To avoid errors arising from TV distortion, distance measurements should be made by generating markers along the line of sight for the usual clinical measurements.

For M-mode systems, the strip chart recording should be checked to verify that 60 ± 2 cycles of 60-Hz oscillations coincide with 1 sec of time markers and that the 0.5-sec time markers are evenly spaced on the recording.

DIGITAL CALIPER CHECKS

Scan Procedure and Analysis

For ultrasound systems equipped with calipers and digital readout, the numerical indication of the caliper in the first two images should be compared with the actual spacing between the most distal reflectors. Imprecisions of 2 to 3 mm should be noted. All results should be recorded.

SYSTEM SENSITIVITY CHECKS

Scan Procedure

The system sensitivity characterizes the ability of the system to detect weak echoes, such as those from inhomogeneities embedded in an attenuating medium at some distance from the transducer. Abrupt changes in sensitivity usually are easily detected. Slow deterioration in sensitivity and in signal to noise ratio are much more difficult to assess without objective measurements. Two ways are suggested for verifying the consistency of system sensitivity.

One approach is to verify that the instrument gain settings required for a "threshold" display or for fixed display level for the echo from a fixed reflector are consistent from one trial to another. Suggested standard echo sources include the lowest rod in column A of the AIUM 100-mm test object, the distal echo obtained from transmitting the signal through a 14-cm × 16-cm × 5-cm block of acrylic as in the SUAR test object or the flat gel-perspex wall interface at the distal end of the RMI phantom. For example, a sensitivity check can be performed by obtaining a 3-division deflection on a dedicated A-mode unit or the A-mode scope of a B-mode system, using the most distal wire in column·A of the AIUM standard 100-mm test object. The overall gain value needed to achieve this value is recorded, as well as the other instrument settings. This check can then be repeated with only the overall gain as the variable.

Another approach is to observe if there are changes in the maximum depth of visualization of scattered echoes within a tissue-mimicking phantom (49). With the RMI model 412 or 413 phantom, the overall gain controls must be raised so that the maximum TGC (swept gain) is realized at a depth that is less than the maximum depth of visualization in the phantom. If this condition exists, a true indication of maximum penetration will be assured. A smooth, uniform scan is performed and the image photographed at a 20-cm field of view. This type of scan is shown in Figure 8.13.

Analysis

In the phantom image, the maximum depth that parenchymal scatterers can be

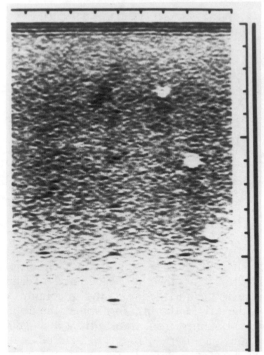

Figure 8.13. Depth of penetration in RMI test phantom. The measured depth of penetration for the ultrasound beam used here can be seen to be 10.5 cm. Small losses in equipment or transducer assembly sensitivity can be detected by decreases of more than 4% in this depth value.

visualized over the entire phantom is estimated. To add consistency to this estimate, the maximum penetration depth chosen should be that at which a 7.5-mm diameter cyst can barely be identified. Readings of a number of scans by 126 independent individuals using this criterion yielded a variation in depth of about ±5 mm or ±1 dB (50). This test is repeated twice a week to identify changes greater than ±5 mm out of 12 cm (4%).

B-MODE COMPOUND POSITION MISREGISTRATION

Scan Procedure

To produce an image for assessing compound B-mode position misregistration, generous amounts of coupling gel are applied to all windows of the AIUM 100-mm test object. With respect to the scanning arm, the test object should be positioned in about the same place as that for a patient being scanned. The test object is scanned using

each of the windows. Disengaging the Write switch between repositionings of the scanning arm facilitates the procedure. Depth markers are placed in vertical and horizontal directions on the image before photographing. When producing the image, the test object must remain perfectly stationary between each of the scan positions, so that the position of a line reflector that is stationary in space is being tested. If any slight movement of the test object occurs as a result, for example, of pressure against the sides of the object, the procedure must be repeated. Depending on the instrument being evaluated, a Zoom image of one or more wires with echoes from three or more distinct directions should also be obtained.

Analysis

Data to be analyzed include the maximum separation of the *centers* of individual echo images of the same line target, generated from different orientations of the scanning arm. If perfect registration is present, the image of a single wire will form an asterisk with the centers of individual echoes crossing at a single point. On a good machine, a 6% or greater error normally is not tolerated.

SECTOR SCAN MISREGISTRATION CHECKS

Scan Procedure

For "real-time" units, especially mechanical sector systems and electronic phased arrays, a test that is analogous to the misregistration check on an articulated arm system is a scan misregistration test, using row B in the AIUM 100-mm test object. For this test, the transducer assembly is coupled to the top window of the test object, using copious amounts of scanning gel (Fig. 8.14). The 20-cm field of view setting should be employed. The other gain controls should be those employed for the previous distance calibration checks. The transducer assembly is positioned to yield an image with row B of the test object parallel to the bottom edge of the display screen, and wire group C centered in the echogram. At this time, either the Write control for the instrument should be disengaged or the Freeze image control should be employed on those units equipped with this switch. If available, elec-

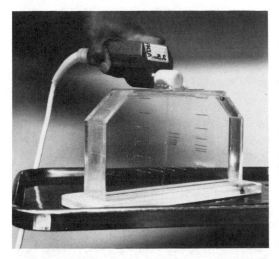

Figure 8.14. Sector scanner coupled to AIUM 100-mm test object. When an image of the entire wire array is centered within sector window on video display, the most distal wires in row B should show a separation (S) of 100 mm to within ± 3% (i.e., 97 mm $< S <$ 103 mm).

tronic calipers should be positioned horizontally alongside the most distal target echoes from row B. A hard copy recording of the scan can then be taken.

Analysis

With either a set of dividers or the reading from the previously calibrated digital calipers, the distance from echo center to echo center between the most laterally displayed echoes from the wire targets in row B should be within 3 mm out of 100 mm. If the digital readout indicates otherwise, it is imprecise and should be adjusted. When determining the vertical distances between echo images of small line or point targets, a rule to use in all quality control measurements is to measure from center to center at the top of the echoes when the beam direction is within 45° of normal incidence (90° to target) and 45° of reverse normal incidence (180° to target), and center of echo to center of echo elsewhere. This rule is especially important when checking digital gray scale systems for the B-scan articulated arm misregistration check and vertical and horizontal distance calibration. For medium and long focused transducers, the increased sensitivity near the focal plane of the transducer can yield up to a 6-mm discrepancy in measured distance (Fig. 8.15). Since tolerances of 2 to 3%

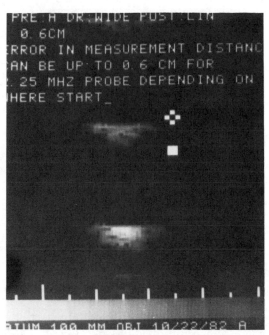

Figure 8.15. Thickness of echo images as function of depth. For focused transducers, the wire images within the focal region appear "thicker" than those close to, or farther from the transducer's face due to the effect of increased axial intensity in the focal region of the transducer assembly. This effect could cause a variation of up to 6 mm in vertical measurement.

are the maximum allowed, a consistent and reproducible method of determining distance is a necessity.

AXIAL RESOLUTION CHECKS

Scan Procedure

Measurements of longitudinal (axial) resolution along the central axis of the transducer indicate the consistency of signal processing; they also can sometimes provide information on the integrity of the transducer crystal, housing, and frequency-dependent matching layers. Assessment of the spatial resolution characteristics of an instrument (lateral or axial) should include consideration that this parameter is dependent on the echo signal level and the amplification of the receiver. A useful concept is that of "best achievable resolution." For this approach, the operator adjusts the sensitivity settings so that the desired target or sets of targets can be detected; he also adjusts these settings so that target size and, thus, spatial resolution, are as small as possible in the image.

Another approach is to create an image using sensitivity settings placed at predetermined values greater than the "threshold" level for detection of echoes from the reflector or sets of reflectors. The disadvantage of this approach is that the most meaningful measurements require a calibrated sensitivity control; this control is not present on every instrument. If such a control is present, it offers the most meaningful approach to resolution measurements. Axial resolution can be measured at a predetermined value above the threshold level by employing the sets of closely spaced nylon fibers in the RMI model 412 or 413 test phantom or the central wire rods in the AIUM 100-mm test object. Alternately, the wedge of water in the acrylic block (SUAR) test object can be used. The advantage of the latter test object is that a continuous range of target spacings is available.

When using the AIUM 100-mm test object and a 20-cm field of view (FOV), scans should be taken across the top of the phantom while the overall gain/sensitivity is increased slowly until the echoes from rods in group C are just barely visible on the display. The sensitivity control should be increased by a fixed amount, say 3 or 6 dB. For units with a calibrated sensitivity control, this increase is straightforward. For other units, the position of the gain control should be increased a fixed amount, and the position should be recorded for reproducibility. Then a new image can be obtained by rescanning the test object, followed by a second scan with a 30- or 40-cm FOV. Finally, a third scan can be made of rod group C with the instrument set for a 20-cm FOV and in the Write Zoom mode.

With the RMI model 412 or 413 phantom and a 20-cm FOV, the sensitivity is decreased to a point where only echoes from the three sets of nylon fibers are obtained. The image is then recorded. The phantom can be used for both static and "real-time" units to yield a qualitative estimate of the variation in the axial resolution as a function of depth in a tissue-mimicking attenuating medium.

When using the SUAR test object, the same general scanning procedures apply. On the rescan at increased sensitivity, the transducer assembly must be positioned as flat as possible with respect to the Teflon® strip

across the top. An image of the position of the two end points of the physical wedge is given by the "ribs" at the 2.5-mm wedge height thickness and 100-mm lateral where the physical thickness of the wedge is zero. The images will show an apparent point of convergence at some lateral distance less than 100 mm from the 2.5-mm high side. In the upper image of Figure 8.16, this distance is 42 mm.

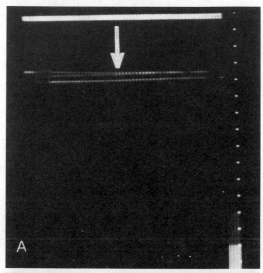

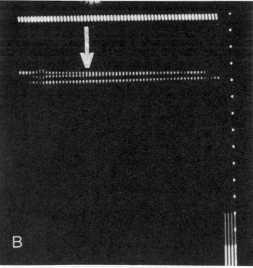

Figure 8.16. Echograms of SUAR test object with wedge. The images were made with the same sequential linear array with 120 scan lines per frame and 60 scan lines per frame (with twice as many scan lines per frame). The apparent change in axial resolution is a factor of about 2. The points at which the wedge apparently converges are indicated by *arrows.*

Analysis

When the AIUM 100-mm test object is employed, the smallest resolvable vertical separation between the echoes from the rods in group C is recorded for each of the three fields of view. The actual vertical separation between the array of six rods is 5, 4, 3, 2, and 1 mm. The observation of a gap in the echoes indicates that the axial resolution is between that distance and the following unresolvable gap. The rods are positioned at an angle to minimize shadowing and resonance effects of the wire. It is likely that the results from the three FOVs will be different, since a different region of the storage target area of the scan converter is being tested in each case.

For the RMI model 412 or 413 test phantom, evaluation of the axial resolution is incorporated into a general assessment of axial and lateral resolution (i.e., spatial resolution). A written record of the resolvable vertical separations between nylon fibers at each of the three depths (3, 7, and 12) helps determine a qualitative assessment of axial resolution under equipment control settings analogous to those employed for clinical scanning of soft tissue.

For more exact measurements of axial resolution, the images obtained from the top and bottom surfaces of the SUAR test object's wedge can be used. As shown in Figure 8.16, the objective is to determine the apparent point of convergence for the echo images away from the thick side of the wedge. By the use of similar triangles, the axial resolution (A) is then:

$$A \text{ (mm)} = \frac{100 - d \text{ (mm)}}{40}.$$

This test can resolve discrepancies to within 0.3 mm when done carefully (51). It is especially useful for testing real-time sequential linear arrays for all available FOVs. The largest FOV will appear to yield the poorest axial resolution, while the smallest FOV will appear to have the best axial resolution, since, in the latter case, more pixels can be used to display individual echo lines. Also, the number of scan lines per frame will influence the axial resolution. With a larger number of scan lines per frame, the axial resolution appears to improve.

With use of any of the test objects with vertical columns of stainless steel rods or nylon lines (as are present in the RMI models 412 or 413 phantoms) to evaluate axial resolution, it is important not to misinterpret an apparently better axial resolution because of the lateral displacement of echo images of the targets caused by the finite beam width of the transducer and the slight angulation of the targets in the axial resolution group. In Figure 8.17, two scans of the rods in group C are shown. In case A, the smallest resolvable axial distance is 2 mm and not 1 mm, as the displacement might lead one to believe. In case B, the smallest resolvable axial distance is indeed 1 mm. To be more exact, the axial resolution is less than or equal to 2 mm, but greater than 1 mm in case A, and less than or equal to 1 mm in case B. The degree of improvement in case B cannot be determined by the test object. The SUAR test object, however, can resolve the axial resolution more precisely (e.g., 1.20 mm for case A, 0.75 mm for case B, in Fig. 8.17).

LATERAL RESOLUTION CHECKS

Scan Procedure

To obtain lateral resolution checks, three different procedures can be performed. First the RMI model 412 or 413 tissue-mimicking test phantom can be used to determine the depth at which anechoic cylindrical tubes of specific diameter can be clearly defined when the object is scanned under fixed, clinical-type control settings. Second, the AIUM 100-mm test object can be scanned along the top window, and the lateral echo widths, as well as the echogram, can be recorded. In addition, the lateral pulse-echo beam width at 5 cm or at 15 cm can be determined by scanning vertically and recording the echograms produced when using column B of the AIUM test object. Third, a complete pulse-echo beam profile or lateral profile can be determined at various axial distances from the face of the transducer assembly. Manufacturers usually provide a set of lateral beam profiles with each transducer assembly. These plots should be checked at the time of purchase and whenever necessary thereafter.

Analysis

The recorded echograms from the RMI Model 412 or 413 test phantom may often

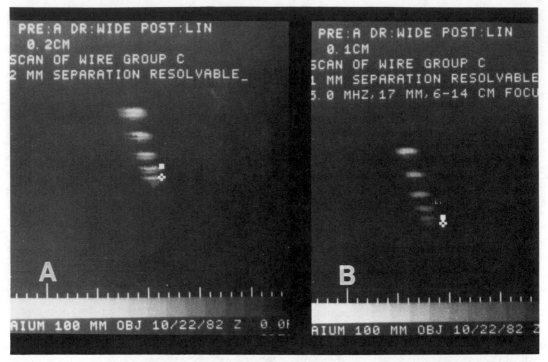

Figure 8.17. Echograms of group C of AIUM 100-mm test object. In both cases, the Read Zoom × 2 mode is used to display the images. In case *A*, the smallest resolvable separation is 2 mm, even though the beam displacement may imply it is 1 mm. In case *B*, 1 mm is resolved.

be difficult to interpret for these studies. The ATS Laboratories model 503 tissue-mimicking spatial resolution test phantom actually provides a three-dimensional check of spatial resolution. This phantom is excellent for intratransducer comparisons on one machine and for intercomparison of the same transducer or transducer assembly on different systems. With the ATS phantom, the depth range can be eliminated. Only the 6-mm diameter, echo-free cylindrical tubes are seen; furthermore, the depths and diameters at which smaller, clear cylindrical tubes are visible can be ascertained.

With the vertical rods of column A in the standard AIUM 100-mm test object, the unattenuated lateral resolution can be determined from the hard copy recording. For this test, an external measuring device, such as a pair of calipers, is used to determine the minimum and maximum lateral echo widths and the depths at which they occur. These values, and the echograms from which they were determined, provide a permanent record of the lateral resolution of the system.

The rods in column B can also be scanned

vertically along the scanning windows closest to and farthest from the face of the transducer assembly. If the transducer assembly is focused either proximal to 5 cm or between 5 and 15 cm, however, this measurement may yield a result that is not necessarily the optimum value. Use of the Write Zoom mode may make any of these lateral resolution measurements easier.

SCAN UNIFORMITY CHECKS

Scan Procedure

An important test of "real-time" units, particularly sequential linear arrays, is to determine if the transducer assembly's sensitivity is uniform for all apertures and array elements. This test is conducted by employing either the SUAR test object or a piece of acrylic or polyethylene of approximately the same external dimensions with the two opposing longest sides milled smooth and as parallel as possible (at least to within ±0.0005 inch). With the phantom resting on one of its long sides, the transducer assembly is coupled to the opposite long side with

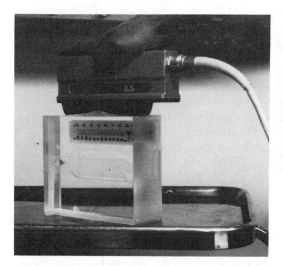

Figure 8.18. Sequential linear array coupled to SUAR test object. If precise axial resolution measurements are not required, a solid acrylic block of the same dimensions as the SUAR can also be used. Good coupling is a prerequisite to meaningful results.

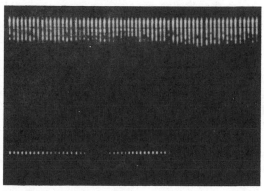

Figure 8.19. Echogram of SUAR test object using nonuniform linear array. The gaps in the echo produced from the distal acrylic-air interface indicate a nonuniform sensitivity across the elements and/or apertures of the array. The possible causes of nonuniformity encompass a spectrum of conditions from dead elements to broken electrical leads.

copious amounts of coupling gel (see Fig. 8.18). With the far and near gain controls set at maximum, the overall gain control or TGC is increased until the echo from the far wall of the test object appears on the monitor. Then, the gain is increased until the echo amplitude saturates the receiver.

Analysis

The "real-time" transducer assembly exhibits uniform sensitivity if the echo image appears simultaneously at the same brightness level for all scan lines across the entire linear array. For checking "real-time" mechanical sector systems, the transducer assembly may have to be rotated through the sector angle to ensure that all acoustic scan lines encounter the distal test object-air interface at normal incidence. There should be no visible gaps in the image, such as those in Figure 8.19. The gain setting at which the spontaneous image display first occurs should be marked so that the unit can be checked for changes in sensitivity by noting changes in the gain setting.

In performing this test, care must be taken to align the transducer assembly so that all scan lines intersect the distal test object-air interface at normal incidence. (For many of the sector scanning heads, this criterion may

require that a slight backward tilt to the scanning assembly, or a rocking motion to the linear array head, be employed.) The test requires good coupling between the transducer assembly and the test object.

HARD COPY RECORDING CHECKS (GRAY SCALE PHOTOGRAPHY)

Scan Procedure

Assessment of gray scale photography can be performed using clinical images of the liver or images generated with a tissue-mimicking phantom or with the gray bar pattern of the instrument, if one exists. The images contain gray patterns representative of those produced by large amplitude echoes, as well as by weak texture echoes produced by scatterers in the phantom. If the system photography is adjusted properly, the weak texture echo signals will be recorded on the hard copy images, and the contrast between high amplitude echo signals will also be visible.

If the ultrasound unit is not equipped with a gray bar pattern, it is useful to provide an additional high level echo pattern in the image. A convenient way to obtain this pattern is to arc the transducer slowly at a position close to the corner of the image, while a coin is coupled to the transducer face. During the rotation, the sensitivity is varied by about 10 dB in a single abrupt step. The resultant image is recorded and left on the display monitor to compare with the hard copy image.

Analysis

The hard copy images are compared with the images on the video monitor to determine if low-level texture echoes originating from small scatterers or from scatterers at the maximum depth of penetration are visible in the image. Also to be noted are whether variations in brightness for high-level echo signals are discernible in the image.

The gray scale appearance of the hard copy images may change as a function of time, since the source of the image is a CRT. If improvements in the hard copy process are desirable, camera settings should be adjusted by an experienced sonographer, sonologist, or physicist. In any adjustment, the preferred brightness level of background should be selected before changing the image contrast level. This procedure ensures that optimum viewing levels are maintained for the echograms. After the contrast is reset to yield an agreeable image, the brightness should be rechecked. For these procedures, variations in camera settings of not more than 5 to 10% are usually sufficient. Also, the glass face of the CRT and the lens surfaces of multiformat cameras should be kept free of dust and debris. For institutions using video recorders to photograph real-time images, the heads of the recorders must also be cleaned periodically. For institutions using Polaroid® film, the hard copy recording device should be checked at least twice weekly, since different batches of the film may have different speeds or latitudes and thus require adjustments in exposure parameters.

FILM PROCESSOR QUALITY CONTROL CHECKS

Scan Procedure and Analysis

Often a degradation in image quality or the appearance of artifacts on multiformat film is falsely blamed on problems with the ultrasonic unit or camera system, whereas the x-ray film processor is actually the true culprit. Chemical solutions in a film processor have a finite lifetime, and silver removed in the development process can accumulate to create problems. Usually, the processor is monitored daily, and an individual is assigned to its maintenance, cleaning, and replenishment of solutions when needed. For small institutions, where the budget precludes a separate maintenance individual, a few checks can still be made to determine if the film processor is functioning properly. These checks on performance include the identification of high or low density images, high or low contrast images, fog, the presence of stains, deposits, marks, or scratches on images, and streaks and fuzziness on the final films. These problems usually can be related to the film processor, and most processor service manuals contain suggestions for their solutions (52). For low volume film processors (less than about 100 films per day), chemical solutions should be changed with a frequency of once every month or two. For high volume systems (greater than about 200 films daily), the chemicals need only be changed approximately semiannually (53).

FILTER CHECKS (WHEN PRESENT)

Scan Procedure and Analysis

In order to draw outside air into an ultrasonic unit to dissipate the heat generated in the high voltage circuits, small circulating fans are placed in strategic locations in the side and back panels of the unit. In most cases, these fans are accompanied by either reticulated foam or wire mesh filters to trap dust and keep it from settling on the electrical components of the unit. Within a short time period, these filters can become clogged with dirt and dust. They should therefore be checked and cleaned periodically (at least twice a month). Sponge or foam filters should be easily removable from the unit and can be washed with mild soap, rinsed clean, and patted dry between two paper towels. The wire mesh filters have to be either vacuumed or rinsed with clear water. Dust and dirt may adhere more tenaciously to a wire mesh filter, and it may need to be replaced after several months. Replacement filters can be obtained from the service representative. If considerable effort is required to remove a filter, it should be left in place, since the manufacturer probably designed the system to prevent access to this part of the circuitry.

ELECTRICAL AND MECHANICAL CHECKS

Scan Procedure and Analysis

The ultrasound unit should also be checked periodically to verify the electrical safety of the patient and sonographer and the mechanical stability of any articulated arm which defines the scan plane. Electrical requirements are established by law in the American National Standards "Safe Current Limits for Electromedical Apparatus," ANSI/AAME SCL 12/78, as summarized in Table 8.6 (54). Also, no externally grounded components on the transducer assembly should come into contact with either the patient or the sonographer during a scan.

The mechanical stability of an articulated arm scanner depends on both the rigidity of the arm itself and the precision of alignment of the central beam in the plane determined by moving the arm. The mechanical rigidity of any articulated arm system should be sufficient to support a force of 100-g equivalent normal to the scan plane applied at the transducer position with an angular deflection of the scan plane no greater than 0.02 radians (1°). For a force of 300-g equivalents, the deflection should be no greater than 0.04 radians (2°), respectively. At all

Table 8.6
Electrical Measurments (All Measurements to DC to 1 Hz Current Limits)[a]

These tests should be performed with all permutations of the following test conditions:
1. Power line polarity normal and reversed.
2. Power on and off.
3. Ground contact open and closed.
   Allowed leakage currents
   Patient connections[b] to chassis, metal scanning arm, or transducer housing, and power ground 50 μA.[c]
   Chassis and metal scanning arm or transducer housing 100 μA.

[a] The ultrasound units are assumed to be portable for electrical safety considerations. The ANSI-AAME Standard should be consulted for units which are grounded permanently.
[b] Patient connections include the transducer face and EKG connections.
[c] Transducers and other connections which are to be placed in direct electrical contact with the heart or great vessels (e.g., in surgery or catheterization) must meet a 10-A current limitation.

times, the transducer face should remain normal to the scan plane to within 0.01 radians (½°) throughout the arm's motion (55). This requirement allows the transducer assembly's line of sight to be in the plane of the scan for all orientations. For "real-time" systems with the mechanical or electrical sectoring transducer assembly mounted in an articulated arm, the same requirements on mechanical stability apply.

A quality assurance program is only as thorough as it's performance and documentation. Copies of all films should be dated and kept, along with the results and general comments that constitute a complete record of the performance and stability of an ultrasound unit. A dated list of service calls also aids in assessing the overall imaging performance of a given item of equipment and the responsibility and quality of service on the unit. This information is often useful in planning the purchase of a new piece of equipment.

Not every quality assurance test for ultrasound instrumentation has been discussed in this section. The reader is encouraged to use other test objectives and techniques, and to develop methods designed for the instrumentation at hand. The purpose of this chapter is to help the reader understand the need for quality assurance and to encourage a program of system checks to detect changes in equipment performance.

COMPUTED TOMOGRAPHY SCANNER

Quality assurance (QA) tests for CT scanners are essentially abbreviated forms of the acceptance tests outlined in Chapter 7. Many of these tests examine characteristics of the scanner that are addressed by daily or weekly calibrations prescribed by the manufacturer. In these cases, the QA tests may be used primarily to verify the calibrations. If the manufacturer's periodic calibration protocols include tests similar to the specific tests listed below, then the manufacturer's tests may suffice. Many of these tests utilize CT scanner phantoms similar to those described in the appendix.

In Table 8.7, quantitative QA tests are listed in order of decreasing frequency of the test. The tests should all be performed at a prescribed "QA technique"; usually, the

Table 8.7
Quality Assurance Tests for CT Scanners

Frequency of tests	Test[a]	Test instrument(s)	Permissible deviation
Daily	CT Number Calibration*	20-cm diameter phantom	Air: −1000 ± 3 CT numbers Water: 0 ± 3 CT numbers
	Standard Deviation of CT Numbers*	20-cm diameter phantom	Norm +2 CT numbers
	Hard Copy Output	"Standard" image or gray scale and densitometer	Densitometric brightness and contrast not significantly different from baseline gray scale image, standard image not visually different from baseline image.
Biweekly	Effective Energy of X-ray Beam*	Phantom with plastic pins	±2 keV
	Low Contrast Resolution*	Low contrast phantom	+0.5-mm holes
	High Contrast Resolution*	High contrast phantom	+0.1-mm holes
	CT Number Flatness*	20-cm diameter water phantom	"Range" (defined in Chapter 4) ≤5 CT numbers
	Distortion of Video Monitor	1-cm spaced holes	±1.5 mm anywhere on image projected to actual size
	Distortion of Hard Copy	1-cm spaced holes	±1.5 mm anywhere on image projected to actual size
Semiannually	Patient Dosimetry*	Dosimetry phantom	±20% from norm
	Artifact Resistance*	Artifact phantom	Small qualitative changes
	Bed Indexing	Prepackaged film	≤2 mm in 10 scans
	Bed Backlash	Prepackaged film	≤1 mm
	Light Field/Radiation Field Coincidence*	Prepackaged film	≤2 mm
	Sensitivity Profile	45° wire in phantom	FWHM within 1 mm of nominal
	Noise Characteristics	20-cm water phantom	Verify: (Standard deviation of CT numbers) α (mAs)$^{-1/2}$
	Dependence of CT Number on Phantom Size	5- to 30-cm diameter water phantoms	≤20 CT numbers

Annually			
	Dependence of CT Number on Phantom Position	20-cm diameter water phantom	≤5 CT numbers
	Dependence of CT Number on Algorithm	20-cm diameter water phantom	≤3 CT numbers
	Dependence of CT Number on Beam Width	20-cm diameter water phantom	≤3 CT numbers
	Accuracy of Radiographic Localization	Small object in phantom	≤1 mm
	Kilovoltage Peak and Miliamperage Wave Forms	HV divider + oscilloscope	±5% of nominal
	Accuracy of Distance Measuring Device	1-cm spaced holes	±1 mm across image
	Radiation Scatter and Leakage*	Ion chamber or survey meter	Scattered radiation within permissible levels for controlled and uncontrolled areas.

ᵃ Tests marked with an asterisk should be performed each time an x-ray tube is replaced.

most commonly used clinical technique is a prudent choice. The column on the right, labeled "Permissible deviation," is intended for use only as a guideline for day-to-day (or month-to-month, etc.) deviation of a variable from the norm. Maximum permissible deviations may be tightened or relaxed, depending on the model of CT scanner. As experience with a particular scanner is gained, the normal range of values for each test will become familiar, and abnormal variations (including possible malfunctions) can be recognized as deviations outside of the normal range of values.

Tests marked with an asterisk (*) should be performed each time an x-ray tube is replaced.

RADIATION THERAPY

Of great importance in radiation therapy is the accurate delivery of the prescribed dose to the proper location within the patient. Thus, the therapist's dose prescription requires not only accurate calibration of treatment units and correct procedures for fulfilling treatment protocols but also exact functioning and use of devices used to position the patient and the treatment unit. A quality assurance program in radiation therapy must address all of these requirements. In addition, the safety of both the patient and operator must be maintained.

A comprehensive quality assurance program can be divided into several levels for optimum monitoring of various aspects of equipment and procedure performance. For example, an important component of all treatment units is the device or circuit that terminates the treatment. Most treatment units have a backup device or circuit that limits the delivered dose in the event of failure of the primary mechanism for termination of treatment. Backup devices rarely are needed; however, their operation must be dependable when they are needed. Therefore, frequent monitoring of backup devices is necessary. Some treatment units provide a means for checking these devices immediately before each treatment. For other units, daily testing is recommended.

At the other extreme, the degree of shielding provided by the treatment room is not likely to vary; hence, unless major changes occur in the equipment or room construction, annual or even less frequent checks are sufficient to verify the integrity of the shielding.

Because of the nature of different test procedures, it is often appropriate that they be conducted by various individuals. For example, daily checks of treatment unit operation can be conducted by the technologist who delivers the treatments. In most cases, parameters requiring less frequent checks should be performed by a physicist or service engineer as part of a more exhaustive evaluation of the treatment unit. This evaluation may include a test of many of the parameters checked frequently by the technologist; however, the procedure and test equipment used for the physicist's or engineer's evaluation would be more complex and thorough in most cases. Such a testing program provides redundancy and helps to ensure that aspects of performance are not overlooked by the test procedure.

The schedule of quality assurance procedures should be related to the normal operating schedule for the unit and the schedule for routine preventive maintenance. Daily procedures should be incorporated into a warmup sequence to be conducted each day immediately before the start of patient treatment. Such scheduling has two purposes: first, it ensures that events associated with turning the unit off and on, as well as disturbances experienced overnight, are detected before the first patient is treated; secondly, it reduces the likelihood that the procedure is overlooked or postponed because of a heavy work load.

Treatment Unit

Of great importance is assurance that the treatment unit is delivering the intended dose. Proper dose delivery is dependent upon several parameters, including the accuracy of the timer or dose monitor, beam flatness and symmetry, and beam energy. Variations may occur in any of these parameters as a result of mechanical or electronic changes. For example, both the dose rate and the uniformity of a radioisotope beam depend on accurate positioning of the source in the treatment location. Any change in position may produce partial shielding of the source and misalignment with the collimator central axis. A change in speed of the

source mechanism may alter the "shutter error" and influence the effective dose rate. Variations in timer accuracy will obviously affect the total delivered dose (56).

Compared to radioisotope units, linear accelerators are subject to many more possible alterations in equipment performance. Photon beam uniformity is dependent upon proper positioning of a flattening filter. In some accelerators the flattening filter is fixed, but in others the filter must be retracted when the beam energy or radiation mode is changed. In some accelerators, movement of a mechanical stop resulting in inaccurate repositioning of the filter has been reported (J. Barnes, personal communication, 1980). This incorrect positioning has produced both beam asymmetry and erroneous dose delivery.

Accelerators rely on intrinsic ion chambers and electronic dose integration circuits to monitor the delivered dose. Variations may occur in the sensitivity of the circuitry. In addition, the sensitivity of the ion chambers may vary, especially when unsealed chambers are used. Variations in chamber sensitivity with time of day and climatic conditions have been reported (57). In addition, variations in beam energy may occur; however, in accelerators with bending magnets, these variations should be limited to the energy bandwidth of the bending magnet, provided that the electrical current supplied to the bending magnet remains constant.

Monitoring of the quality assurance parameters associated with a treatment unit is best accomplished by a multilevel approach. On the first level, daily checks of the parameters should be conducted by the treatment technologists. A program should be designed that permits a rapid spot check of the central axis dose rate. This measurement should be made with sufficient accuracy that a variation of more than a few percent from prior measurements is detectable. This procedure is not an accurate calibration, but merely a constancy check. The measurement should be repeated for each beam energy and modality, and the results should be recorded. In addition to the dose rate check, the quality assurance program should include all of the readings, measurements, and test procedures recommended by the manufacturer.

Additional daily checks are warranted until the treatment unit demonstrates stable and reliable operation. Several devices are available commercially that permit a rapid measurement of beam symmetry and energy, as well as central axis dose rate. Sophisticated and expensive tools are not required for these tests. An adequate test of output constancy may be made with a Victoreen condenser chamber or similar instrument placed in a small plastic phantom. It is even possible to use the same instrument to verify beam symmetry by positioning the chamber at a suitable distance in each direction from the central axis. However, this practice is time-consuming and may be unlikely to be performed routinely. To ensure performance of the test, a more sophisticated instrument is desirable.

It should be emphasized that daily checks made by the technologist should not be substituted for more thorough checks made by the physicist. Recommendations for the frequency of these checks are shown in Table 8.8 and may be found in various references (58, 59). The actual frequency employed should be determined from the record of performance of the treatment unit. In addition, the frequency should be adequate to prevent the administration of an incorrect dose to a patient over a period too long for correction. Since the daily checks are designed to recognize only variations greater than 5%, misadministrations could conceivably reach or exceed 5% without detection. To prevent this potential problem, accurate dose rate measurements should be made at intervals considerably shorter than the length of a typical treatment. A frequency of 1 to 2 weeks meets this goal; a frequency of 1 month may be acceptable in some circumstances.

Measurements of dose delivery should be made in a suitable tissue-equivalent (water or plastic) material, according to published protocols (60). At a considerably lower frequency, a thorough evaluation of the entire dosimetry system should be conducted by the physicist. This analysis should evaluate and correct, if required, the timer or integrator accuracy, the symmetry and flatness of the beam, and the beam energy.

Table 8.8
Recommended Frequencies for Constancy Checks

Procedure	Treatment unit type	Frequency
Protection survey	All	At installation and after modifications
Isocenter stability	Cobalt units	Monthly
	Accelerators	6 months
Collimator rotational stability	All	6 months
Couch positions and isocenter stability	All	6 months
Accuracy of digital position indicators	All	Monthly
Accuracy of mechanical position indicators	All	6 months
Radiation/light field congruence	All	Weekly
Optical distance indicator	All	Daily
Other patient positioning devices	All	Weekly
Dose rate spot check	Cobalt units	Weekly
Dose rate (calibration)	Cobalt units	Annually
	Accelerators	Monthly
Beam energy	Cobalt Units	Annually
	Accelerators (photon beams)	Weekly
	Accelerators (electron beams)	Weekly
Flatness and symmetry	All	Monthly

Measurement of timer error should be made for cobalt units (61). Verification of the accuracy of the dose integrator or measurement of the dose rate should include evaluation of the effects of field size, source-to-skin distance, and dose rate in the case of the dose integrator. These data should be compared with previous measurements for consistency. Beam symmetry and flatness probably are best measured in a water phantom, although other acceptable methods such as film dosimetry sometimes are employed. Symmetry refers to the equivalence of dose rate at points equidistant from the central axis, while flatness describes the variation of dose rate with distance from the central axis. Specifications for both are exhibited by manufacturers, by the Center for Devices and Radiological Health and by the International Electro-Technical Commission. For linear accelerators, an indication of beam energy can be obtained from measurements of ionization vs depth in a water or plastic phantom. For photon beams, the nomimal accelerating potential may be estimated by comparing the ratio of ionization measured at depths of 10 and 20 cm to published data. Electron beam energy generally is determined from measurements of the range of ionization in water or plastic. These measurements may be used to determine the mean incident energy and the most probable energy of the electron beam.

While accurate delivery of the prescribed dose is of paramount importance, it is also important to ensure that the dose is delivered to the intended volume of tissue. This objective is accomplished by relating the internal anatomy and target volume to external landmarks. These landmarks then are used to align the patient and treatment beam so that the target volume is encompassed by the radiation beam, while healthy tissues are spared to the maximum degree possible. Once the external landmarks are identified on the patient, correct treatment depends on the accurate alignment of a variety of positioning devices. These devices include a field-defining light, positioning lasers, and a number of mechanical scales or digital position indicators. As before, a multilevel quality assurance program is most suitable to verify the integrity of these devices.

A rigorous test of the mechanical stability of the treatment unit should be performed by a physicist no less frequently than annually. It is prudent to conduct these tests at the time of a major calibration of the unit. The mechanical tests should include evaluation of the stability of the gantry, collimator, and treatment couch, assessment of the alignment of the field-defining light with the radiation beam, and alignment of positioning lights and lasers. The accuracy of all position indicators should be adjusted if necessary.

Daily spot checks of the indicators and devices most likely to vary may be made by the technologists. Straightforward and rapid tests can be devised that permit several parameters to be evaluated (e.g., light field, field size indicators, and lasers) (62). These tests will reveal if any of the devices are in error.

Finally, the safety of the patient, operator, and public must be assured. A quality assurance program should include procedures to evaluate the continued effectiveness of radiation shielding around the treatment unit. Protective devices for electrical and thermal hazards also should be checked. Most linear accelerators contain mechanisms to evaluate a variety of protective devices, such as the location of a retractable beam stopper, as well as various dosimetry-related items, such as the location of the x-ray target and the attachment of additional collimators or beam-shaping devices.

It is customary for a physicist to perform a thorough protection survey at the time of installation of a treatment unit. Unless major changes occur in the unit or in construction that affects a treatment room or use of the surrounding space, it should not be necessary to repeat the survey. However, replacement of major components in the unit or evidence of structural changes in the facility are indicators that another survey should be performed.

Evaluation of devices that protect against thermal or electrical hazard generally is the responsibility of a service engineer working under the supervision of a physicist. During service it is not unusual to bypass protective devices for brief periods. When protective devices are bypassed, alternative procedures or devices that afford equivalent protection should be in place. Personnel responsible for the safe operation of the treatment unit should guard against the bypassing of safety devices for longer than brief periods.

Simulator

A simulator is a hybrid device: it has characteristics of both a diagnostic and a treatment unit. Hence, it requires suitable quality assurance procedures for both types of equipment. The imaging capabilities should be evaluated with procedures and schedules determined from information in other sections of this chapter. Procedures for testing the mechanical alignment of accelerators can be followed for simulators.

Treatment Planning Computer

There is a strong tendency, especially among infrequent users of computers, to accept without question data generated by computers. This level of confidence has, on occasion, led to undesired consequences. These consequences are unfortunate, since it is relatively simple to conduct a program of quality assurance to verify the proper operation of each component of a computer system.

At the level of lowest frequency is the verification by a physicist of new software packages and data. New programs need to be evaluated only once when they are received by a facility. On the other hand, the maintenance of reliable duplicate copies of programs and data is a continuing operation. As in the cases of treatment units and simulators, a quality assurance program for a treatment planning computer is best conducted at several levels.

In the design of a quality assurance program, it is helpful to consider a computer system as five basic subsystems. The first subsystem includes the fundamental hardware, including the CPU, memory, storage devices, keyboard, and printer. These devices are unlikely to change in characteristics or to function improperly; if they do malfunction, the consequences will be obvious to all. Hence, they may be considered very reliable.

The second subsystem includes input devices employing analog-to-digital interfaces. Examples are graphics digitizers and isodose plotter interfaces. Analog devices may change in subtle ways with severe results. A good quality assurance program will rapidly reveal these subtle changes.

Output devices such as plotters and photographic hard copy imagers form the third subsystem. These devices are often analog and are therefore susceptible to electronic drift.

The fourth subsystem includes all the software for the system. Software may be purchased from a manufacturer, obtained from a colleague, or developed in the institution. It is very important that each new release of software and each new program introduced into clinical use is checked carefully for subtle changes that may have been introduced since the previous version of the same program. It is sometimes difficult, especially with complex programs, to ensure that the introduction of a software change does not produce undetected errors.

The data provided by the user to specify characteristics unique to the institution's treatment devices and procedures comprise the fifth subsystem. Once the data are stored it is unlikely that any undetected changes will occur. However, it is the user's responsibility to ensure that the data provided for clinical use continue to be appropriate.

It is prudent to maintain duplicate copies of all programs and data, since even the most reliable storage media fail occasionally. Many treatment planning computers utilize floppy disk drives that are relatively unreliable. Errors that occur with these devices are generally obvious and automatically detectable by the hardware. They may easily be corrected, provided up-to-date copies have been maintained.

Tests of accuracy of input and output devices should be made frequently. The frequency chosen depends upon the reliability of each component; a frequency of once or twice each month might be suitable in most cases. A series of simple tests could be designed for rapid evaluation of the accuracy of input and output devices, as well as computational reproducibility. The procedures should be capable of evaluating the full range of analog devices rather than simply the ranges most commonly used. The tests also should reveal if obsolete or incorrect treatment beam data have been used.

The accuracy of the entire treatment planning system should be checked on a daily basis by verifying that the output representations of patient contours conform to the input data and that computed dose distributions appear reasonable.

References

1. Berkhart Roger L: A proposed recommendation for quality assurance programs in diagnostic radiology facilities. In: *Proceedings of the Society for Photooptical Instrumentation Engineers*. Bellingham, WA, 1977, vol 127, pp 266–270.
2. Reagan TA: Dupont quality assurance program for the radiology department. In *Proceedings of the Society for Photooptic Instrumentation Engineers, Application of Optical Instrumentation in Medicine*, V. Bellingham, WA, 1976, vol 96.
3. Irvine WG: Management of the radiographic environment. In: *Proceedings of Society for Photooptical Instrumentation Engineers, Application of Optical Instrumentation in Medicine*, V. Bellingham, WA, 1976, vol 96.
4. Vucich JJ: Quality assurance: a fundamental whose time has come. In: *Proceedings of Society for Photooptical Instrumentation Engineers, Application of Optical Instrumentation in Medicine*, IV. Bellingham, WA, 1975, vol 70, pp 138–144.
5. Walker WJ Jr: A program for diagnostic x-ray quality assurance in the hospital radiology department. In: *Proceedings of Society for Photooptical Instrumentation Engineers, Application of Optical Instrumentation in Medicine*, IV. Bellingham, WA, 1975, vol 70, pp 151–153.
6. Winkler NT: Quality control in diagnostic radiology. In *Proceedings of Society for Photooptical Instrumentation Engineers, Application of Optical Instrumentation in Medicine*, VI. Bellingham, WA, 1975, vol 70, pp 125–131.
7. Taylor KW: Quality control in a large teaching hospital. In: *Proceedings of Society for Photooptical Instrumentation Engineers, Application of Optical Instrumentation in Medicine*, IV. Bellingham, WA, 1975, vol 70, pp 146–150.
8. Gray JE: Why quality control? In: *Proceedings of Society for Photooptical Instrumentation Engineers, Application of Optical Instrumentation in Medicine*, IV. Bellingham, WA, 1975, vol 70.
9. Federal Drug Administration: *Quality Assurance Programs for Diagnostic Radiology Facilities: Final Recommendation*. 21 CFR Part 1.000 (1.000.55) FR Docket 76N-0145, USDHEW (FDA), Washington, D.C., US Government Printing Office, Dec 1979.
10. Tuddenham WJ: Quality assurance in diagnostic radiology: an irreverent view of a sacred cow. *Radiology* 131:579–588, 1979.
11. Edgerton RE: Management by commitment: theoretical personnel management. *Radiol Technol* 47:382–384, 1976.
12. Cedars MM, Addison SJ, Henry CR, et al: Quality assurance in diagnostic radiology—an implementation program. *Appl Radiol* 4:77–78, 1975.
13. Koenig GF: Management of a quality assurance program for a diagnostic x-ray department. Proceedings of the Fourth International Conference on Medical Physics, Ottawa, Canada, July 25–30, 1976.
14. Gray JE: *Photographic Quality Assurance in Diagnostic Radiology, Nuclear Medicine, and Radiation Therapy: Volume I, The Basic Principles of Daily Photographic Quality Assurance*. HEW Publication FDA 76-8043; and *Volume II, Photographic Processing, Quality Assurance and the Evaluation of Photographic Materials*. HEW Publication FDA 77-8018. Washington, DC, US Government Printing Office, 1977.
15. Poznanski AK, Smith LA: Practical problems in processing control. *Radiology* 90:135–138, 1968.
16. Gray JE: Light fog on radiographic films: how to measure it properly. *Radiology* 115:225–227, 1975.
17. American Association of Physicists in Medicine (AAPM): *Basic Quality Control in Diagnostic Radiology*. AAPM Report No. 4. New York, American Institute of Physics, 1977.
18. Hendee WR, Rossi RP: *Quality Assurance for Radiographic X-Ray Units and Associated Equipment*. HEW Publication (FDA) 79-8094, USDHEW. Washington, DC, US Government Printing Office, 1979.
19. Hendee WR, Rossi RP: *Quality Assurance for Fluoroscopic X-Ray Units and Associated Equipment*. HEW Publication (FDA) 80-8095, USDHEW. Washington, D.C., U.S. Government Printing Office, 1979.
20. Hendee WR, Rossi RP: *Quality Assurance for Conventional Tomographic X-Ray Units*. HEW Publication (FDA) 80-8096, USDHEW. Washington, DC, US Government Printing Office, 1979.
21. *Regulations for the Administration and Enforcement of the Radiation Control for Health and Safety Act of 1968*. HHS Publication (FDA) 80-8035. Washington, DC, US Government Printing Office, 1980.
22. Report of the Subcommittee on Technic of Exposure Prevention: Background Report: *Recommendations on Guidance for Technic to Reduce Unnecessary Exposure from X-Ray Studies in Federal Health Care Facilities*. US Environmental Agency, Interagency Working Group on Medical Radiation. Washington, DC, US Government Printing Office, 1976.
23. US Environmental Protection Agency: *Radiation Protection Guidance for Diagnostic X-Rays*. Federal Guidance Report No. 9, EPA 520/4-76-019. Washington, DC, US Government Printing Office, 1976.
24. FDA: *Gonad Shielding in Diagnostic Radiology*. U.S. Department of Health, Education and Welfare, HEW Publication (FDA) 76-8024. Washington, DC, US Government Printing Office, revised 1975.
25. FDA Office, *Specific Area Gonad Shielding, Recommendation for Use on Patients During Medical Diagnostic X-Ray Procedures*. U.S. Department of Health, Education and Welfare, HEW Publication (FDA) 76-8054. Washington, DC, US Government Printing Office, 1976.
26. Church WW, Burnett BM: *The Clinical Testing of Male Gonad Shields*. HEW Publication (FDA) 76-8025, 1975. Washington, DC, US Government Printing Office, 1976.

27. Bourne D: Repeats—an aspect of department management. *Radiography* 35:257–261, 1969.

28. Burnett BM, Mazzaferro RJ, Church WW: *A Study of Retakes in Radiology Departments of Two Large Hospitals.* HEW Publication (FDA) 76-8016. Washington, DC, US Government Printing Office, 1975.

29. Mazzaferro RJ, Balter S, Janower MJ: The incidence and causes of repeated radiographic examinations in a community hospital. *Radiology* 112:71–72, 1974.

30. Mazzaferro RJ, Church WW, Burnett BM: Retakes in diagnostic radiography. *Proceedings of the Health Physics Society Seventh Midyear Topical Symposium, Health Physics in the Healing Arts.* Washington, DC, Health Physics Society, 1972, p 142.

31. Trout ED, Jacobsen G, Moore RT et al: Analysis of the rejection rate of chest radiographs obtained during the coal mine "Black Lung" program. *Radiology* 109:25–27, 1973.

32. Rosenstein M: *Organ Doses in Diagnostic Radiology.* HEW Publication (FDA) 76-8030. Washington, DC, US Government Printing Office, 1976.

33. Wochos JF, Cameron JR: *Patient Exposure from Diagnostic X-Rays, an Analysis of 1972–1974 Next Data.* HEW Publication (FDA) 77-8020. Washington, DC, US Government Printing Office, 1977.

34. Barnes GT, Nelson RE, Witten MW: Comprehensive quality assurance program—report of a four years' experience at University of Alabama. In: *Proceedings of Society for Photooptical Instrumentation Engineers.* Bellingham, WA, 1970, vol 96, pp 19–25.

35. Hall CL: Economic analysis of a quality control program. In: *Proceedings of Society for Photooptical Instrumentation Engineers.* Bellingham, WA, 1977, vol 127, pp 271–276.

36. Nelson RE, Barnes GT, Witten DM: Economic analysis of a comprehensive quality assurance program. *Radiol Technol* 49:129–134, 1977.

37. Hasegawa BH, Kirch DL, LeFree MT, et al: Quality control of scintillation cameras using a minicomputer. *J Nucl Med* 22:1075–1080, 1981.

38. Paras P, Hine GJ, Adams R: BRH test pattern for the evaluation of gamma-camera performance. *J Nucl Med* 22:468–470, 1981.

39. Lukes SJ, Grossman LW, Nishiyama H: Thallium-201 imaging artifacts not detected by technetium-99m or cobalt-57 quality control testing. *Radiology* 146:237–239, 1983.

40. Raff U, Spitzer VM, Hendee WR: Practicality of NEMA performance specification measurements for user-based acceptance testing and routine quality assurance. *J Nucl Med* 25:679–687, 1984.

41. Keyes JW, Gazella GR, Strange DP: Image analysis by on-line minicomputer for improved camera quality control. *J Nucl Med* 13:525–527, 1972.

42. U.S. Nuclear Regulatory Commission: Regulatory Guide, Office of Standards Development, Regulatory Guide 10.8, Revision 1. Washington, DC, US Government Printing Office, 1980.

43. National Electrical Manufacturers Association (NEMA): *Safety Standard for Diagnostic Ultrasound Equipment.* American Institute of Ultrasound in Medicine (AIUM)/NEMA Standards Publication No. UL 1-1981:33, Washington, DC, US Government Printing Office, 1981.

44. American Institute of Ultrasound in Medicine: Standard 100-mm test object, including recommended procedures for its use. American Institute of Ultrasound in Medicine, Oklahoma City, OK. *Reflections* 1:74–91, 1975.

45. The sensitivity, uniformity and axial resolution (SUAR) test object. In Carson PL, Dubuque GL, (eds): *Ultrasound Quality Control Procedure*, Report III:16–26. Chevy Chase, MD, Center for Radiological Physics, 1979.

46. Carson PL, Shabason, L, Dick DE, et al. tissue equivalent test objects for comparison of ultrasound transmission tomography by reconstruction and pulse-echo ultrasound imaging. In Linser ML (ed): *Ultrasonic Tissue Characterization II.* NBS Special Publication 525:337–342. Washington, DC, US Government Printing Office, 1979.

47. Madsen EL, Zagzebski JA, Frank GR: Oil-in-gelatin dispersions for use as ultrasonically tissue-mimicking materials. *Ultrasound Med Biol* 8:277–287, 1982.

48. M-mode quality control tests—instructions and data sheets. In Carson PL, Dubuque GL (eds): *Ultrasound Quality Control Procedure.* Report III:10–13, Chevy Chase, MD, Center for Radiological Physics, 1979.

49. Burlew MM, Madsen EL, Zagzebski JA, et al: A new ultrasound tissue equivalent material. *Radiology* 134:515–520, 1980.

50. Madsen EL, Zagzebski JA, Banjavic RA, et al: *Further Developments in Soft-Tissue Equivalent, Gelatin-Based Materials.* Presented at the 24th Annual Meeting of the American Institute of Ultrasound in Medicine, San Diego, CA, 1978. Bethesda, MD, AIUM.

51. Abstracts of bandwidth axial resolution. In Goldstein A (ed): *Quality Assurance in Diagnostic Ultrasound.* American Institute of Ultrasound in Medicine. Bethesda, MD, 1980, p 49.

52. McKinney WEJ: *Common Causes of Unsatisfactory Radiographs with Automatic Processors.* Imaging Services Processing Seminar, Denver, 1980, pp 19–23. Minneapolis, PAKO Corporation.

53. *PAKO 240 HC Processor Service Manual.* Minneapolis, PAKO Corporation, 1980.

54. *American National Standard: Safe Current Limits for Electromedical Apparatus.* Arlington, VA, American National Standards Institution/Association for the Advancement of Medical Instrumentation (ANSI/AAMI), 1978.

55. AAPM: Delineation of scan plane (Section 7.7). In Carson PL, Zagzebski JA (eds): *Pulse Echo Ultrasound Imaging Systems: Performance Tests and Criteria*, American Association of Physicists in Medicine, Report 8:65–67. New York, American Institute of Physics, 1981.

56. Lanzl LH, Grant WH III, Davis MJ: ^{60}Co therapy equipment malfunctions. *Radiology* 109:193–194, 1973.

57. Sharma SC, Wilson DL, Jose B: Variation of output with atmospheric pressure and ambient temperature for therac-20 linear accelerator. *Med Phys* 10:712, 1983.

58. Code of practice for x-ray therapy linear accelerators. *Med Phys*, vol 2, no 3, May/June 1975.

59. Mozer RF, King GA, Jones GL: *Practical Quality*

Assurance in Radiation Therapy. Exhibit presented at the Radiological Society of North America (RSNA), 1977.

60. AAPM: *A Protocol for the Determination of Absorbed Dose from High-Energy Photon and Electron Beams.* Report of Task Group 21, Radiation Therapy Committee, AAPM. *Med Phys* 10(6), 1983.

61. Orton CR, Siebert J: The measurement of telethapy unit timer errors. *Phys Med Biol* 17:198, 1982.

62. Ibbott GS, Bothe KA, Thyfault PJ, et al: Quality-assurance workshops for radiation therapy technologists. *Appl Radiol* Mar/Apr 1977.

APPENDIX I:
MANUALS ON PERFORMANCE
EVALUATION AND/OR QUALITY
CONTROL

Ultrasound Instrument Quality Control Procedure. CRP Report Series, Report 3; Paul L. Carson, Ph.D., and Gregory L. Dubuque, Ph.D. (eds)
   Available from:
      AAPM-CRP Coordination Office
      6900 Wisconsin Avenue—Suite 307
      Chevy Chase, MD 20015

Methods of Monitoring Ultrasonic Scanning Equipment. The Hospital Physicists' Association Topic Group 23; R. C. Chivers (ed).
   Available from:
      The Hospital Physicists' Association
      47 Belgrave Square
      London, SWIX, England

Quality Assurance in Diagnostic Ultrasound. American Institute of Ultrasound in Medicine (AIUM); Albert Goldstein (ed).

   Available from:
      AIUM Central Office
      4405 East-West Highway—Suite 504
      Bethesda, MD 20814

Pulse Echo Ultrasound Imaging System: Performance Tests and Criteria. American Association of Physicists in Medicine (AAPM), Report 8; Paul L. Carson, Ph.D., and James A. Zagzebski, Ph.D. (eds).
   Available from:
      Executive Director, AAPM
      American Institute of Physics
      335 East 45th Street
      New York, NY 10017

Implementation for a Quality Assurance Program for Ultrasound B-Scanners. HEW Publication (FDA) 800-8100; Hector Lopez, Ph.D., and Steve Smith, Ph.D. (eds).
   Available from:
      Superintendent of Documents
      U.S. Government Printing Office
      Washington, D.C. 20402

APPENDIX II:
SOURCES OF PERFORMANCE EVALUATION TEST TOOLS FOR ULTRASOUND: SOME SUPPLIERS OF THE AIUM STANDARD 100-MM TEST OBJECT

Joe Anderson 3360 Stuart Street Denver, CO 80212 (303) 458-5872	Enclosed test object with guide for precision A-mode and M-mode measurements.
ATS Laboratories P.O. Box 792 South Norwalk, CT 06856	Enclosed test object.
Dunning Plastics Company 2910 Frankling Boulevard Sacramento, CA 95818	Enclosed test object with guide.
Modern Electronic Diagnostic Corp. 820 W. Hyde Park Boulevard Inglewood, CA 80302 (213) 673-2201	Open test object; optional enclosing container.
Nuclear Associates, Inc. 100 Voice Road Carle Place, NY 11514 (516) 741-7614	Enclosed test object—model 84-301; Enclosed test object with thermometer model 84-316.
Ultra-Cal, Inc. 3014 Laurashawn Lane Escondido, CA 92026 (619) 741-7207	Enclosed test object; shipped filled, sealed with thermometer.

APPENDIX III
QUALITY ASSURANCE TEST OBJECTS

ATA Corporation
967 Welch Court
Golden, CO
(303) 233-9035

Model UC-2 Electronic Ultrasound Phantom.

Nuclear Associates
100 Voice Road
Carle Place, NY
11514
(516) 741-7207

SUAR Test Object (without thermometer)

Echo-Check Low-Cost Resolution Test Fixture:
84-310 (lines only)
84-311 (lines only)
Ophthalmic Ultrasound System Q.A. Kit 84-309
Ultrasound Electronic Test Pattern Generator 84-406 or 84-407

Radiation Measurements, Inc. (RMI)
P.O. Box 44
Middleton, WI
53562
(608) 831-1188

SUAR Test Object Model 420

APPENDIX IV:
TISSUE-MIMICKING PHANTOMS

Acoustic Standards Corporation   Model Echobloc
Distributed by Echosonics
Division of Cone Instrumentation
5380 Naiman Parkway
Solon, OH 44139
(800) 321-6964

ATS Laboratories	Model 503	Model 509
P.O. Box 792	Model 504	Model 510
South Norwalk, CT 06856	Model 505	Model 511
(203) 847-3510	Model 506	Model 512
	Model 507	Model 513
	Model 508	Model 514

Nuclear Associates   Model 84-308
100 Voice Road   Model 84-317
Carle Place, NY 11514
(516) 741-7614

Radiation Measurements, Inc. (RMI)	Model 410	Model 412
P.O. Box 44	Model 411	Model 413
Middleton, WI 53562		
(608) 831-1188		

CHAPTER NINE

Preventive and Corrective Maintenance of Radiological Equipment

RAYMOND P. ROSSI, M.S., and DAVID A. OWEN, B.S.E.E.

INTRODUCTION

The proper maintenance of radiological equipment is important to the consistent production of high quality radiologic images. Increasing sophistication of imaging technologies, stringent requirements for ongoing performance, high acquisition and upgrade costs, and the expense of repair costs demand the effective management of radiological imaging systems by use of a sound maintenance program. The purpose of this chapter is to outline the goals of a maintenance program, identify important requirements, and discuss possible approaches to implementing a satisfactory program.

Goals of a Maintenance Program

The goal of a maintenance program for radiological equipment is to assure that radiological images are of high quality on a consistent basis. This goal should be sought at reasonable cost and with minimum interruption to the normal use of the equipment (minimum "downtime"). All types of radiological equipment are subject to changes in calibration, mechanical and electrical wear due to age and use, and occasional unintentional abuse. These tendencies necessitate the implementation of a sound maintenance program to maintain the equipment in a satisfactory state of performance (1).

Categorization of Classes of Maintenance

An effective maintenance program should address both preventive and corrective maintenance. Corrective maintenance (repair) is any maintenance action that responds directly to a specific equipment malfunction that compromises the clinical use of the equipment. Corrective maintenance must be conducted on an unscheduled or "as needed" basis, with rapid response and resolution of the problem as its objectives.

In contrast to corrective maintenance, preventive maintenance includes all maintenance activities conducted on equipment to minimize the need for corrective maintenance. Preventive maintenance involves the periodic evaluation of the equipment, with identification and correction of potential problems before they impact adversely on the clinical utilization of the equipment. Preventive maintenance occurs on a scheduled basis and can be accommodated in the operational schedule of the department without undue disruption. When properly implemented and managed, an effective preventive maintenance program substantially reduces the amount of corrective maintenance required.

Management of A Maintenance Program

The management of a maintenance program should provide efficient performance of service, adequate documentation of maintenance to permit identification of specific problems, and delineation of the costs of the maintenance program. Whenever corrective or preventive maintenance is provided, a number of issues should be documented, including: the equipment involved; who initiated the service request and when; to whom was the request made; the reason for requested service; the service agency contacted and the response time; the service performed; when the service was completed; labor and travel hours and their associated costs; the parts required and their cost; and the total equipment downtime. By recording this information, it is possible to evaluate specific problem areas that may exist within a department so that appropriate corrective action can be taken. Furthermore, maintenance costs can be estimated on an equipment- and department-wide basis.

The approach taken to administration of a maintenance program should be tailored to the needs of the institution. The overall responsibility for coordinating the program should be placed with one individual who handles all maintenance scheduling and record keeping. This individual is responsible for making decisions regarding service and for knowing the status of all equipment within the department.

An approach to a maintenance program that has been used successfully for the past 6 yr is illustrated in Figure 9.1. An individual, designated as the service coordinator, is on call 24 hr/day. On a day-by-day basis, responsibility as service coordinator is shared among individuals in the department. Any equipment problem requiring corrective maintenance is reported to this individual, and he or she selects the appropriate action to be taken. To ensure that problems are not "lost in the shuffle" and to maintain adequate documentation, a written request form, such as that illustrated in

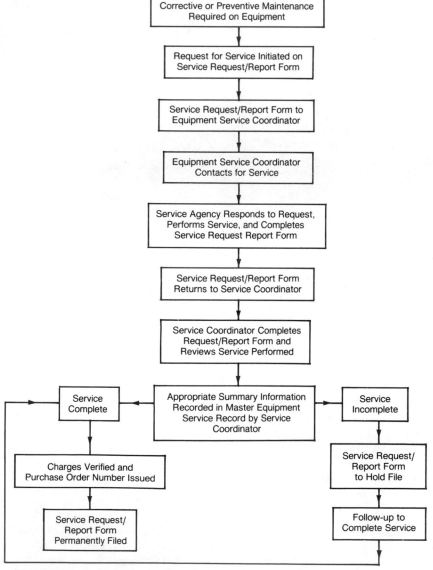

Figure 9.1.   Logistical operation for a service and maintenance program.

Figure 9.2, is utilized. This form consists of three parts. Part I is completed by the individual requesting the service and describes the date and time of problem occurrence, equipment identification, and nature of the problem. Part II is completed by the individual providing the service and describes the response time, service time and charges,

PART I: To be completed by individual initiating service request							
Date:	Time:	Requested by:				Reported to:	
Equipment Description Identification:						Room #/ Location:	
DESCRIPTION OF PROBLEM/REQUESTED SERVICE:							

PART II: To be completed by individual performing service							
SERVICE AGENCY		Date	Time	Date	Time		
	Arrival						
	Departure						

DESCRIPTION OF PROBLEM AS DIAGNOSED/CORRECTIVE ACTION TAKEN/SERVICE PERFORMED:

Date	Labor Hours		Travel Hours		Parts/Materials				
	RT	OT	RT	OT	Quantity	Part #	Description	Unit Cost	Total

Other Charges		
Description	Amount	

Billing Terms: ( ) Warranty ( ) Service Contract ( ) Billed Service ( ) Other

Service Representative Signature:	Status: ( ) Complete ( ) Incomplete

PART III: For internal use only– to be completed by service coordinator			
Problem Occurrence/Service Requested	Date:	Time:	Explanatory Remarks:
Service Agency Notified	Date:	Time:	
Service Agency Responded	Date:	Time:	
Problem Corrected/Service Completed	Date:	Time:	
Total Equipment Down Time:			

Equipment Manufacture:	Equipment Type:
Service Agency:	Service Agency Repsonse Time:

Problem Location	Primary	
	Secondary	
Component Failure	Primary	
	Secondary	
Failure Mode	Primary	
	Secondary	
Corrective Action		
Safety Hazard		

ADDITIONAL COMMENTS:	Charge Summary	
	Labor	
	Parts	
	Other	
	Total	

REFERENCE SERVICE REPORT #:	REFERENCE PURCHASE ORDER #:

Figure 9.2. Example of a "Request for Service" form used in an equipment service and maintenance program.

parts used and cost, billing terms, and status of the service. Part III is completed by the service coordinator and summarizes the services performed. In addition to handling all requests for corrective maintenance, the service coordinator is responsible for scheduling the preventive maintenance of the equipment and for keeping departmental staff informed about equipment status.

Preventive and Corrective Maintenance Costs

The execution of a maintenance program may be achieved through the use of vendor service, an in-house service group, or a combination of both (1–3). The suitability of these options for a particular institution reflects primarily their relative costs and the size of the institution. If maintenance is provided by a vendor, then the institution bears the cost of service performed by the vendor (labor, travel, parts) for a specific maintenance task. Items such as salary and

benefits, continuing education, test equipment costs, and parts inventory are assured by the vendor and are part of the vendor's charges.

When an in-house approach is used, the institution assumes the responsibility for hiring qualified individuals to perform the service and for budgeting for salary and benefits, test equipment, continuing education, parts inventory, etc. The institution must also allocate space for the maintenance program.

To compare the cost effectiveness of these alternatives, three types of service agreements offered by most vendors for corrective and preventive maintenance are examined. These agreements are:

1. Labor only.
2. Labor and parts, excluding glassware.
3. Labor and parts, including all glassware.

Charges for these different programs vary with the vendor, the age of the equipment, and the number of systems to be covered. Typical average charges are 4 to 5% (for 1), 6 to 7% (for 2), and 9 to 10% (for 3) of the replacement value of the imaging equipment.

Representative equipment replacement costs are illustrated in Table 9.1. Typical equipment configurations for a small, intermediate size, and large hospital are shown in Table 9.2, along with the equipment replacement costs. From the maintenance charges estimated previously, the costs of vendor-supplied service agreements are shown in Table 9.3.

Table 9.1
Average Replacement Costs for Radiological Imaging Equipment[a]

Equipment type	Typical cost
Radiographic/fluoroscopic	$454,000
Radiographic	$175,200
Linear tomographic	$161,500
Dedicated chest	$192,600
Multidirectional tomographic	$330,000
Radiographic mobile	$33,800
Fluoroscopic mobile	$98,000
Special procedures/cardiac catheterization laboratory	$820,000

[a] 1984 dollars.

Table 9.2
Assumed Equipment Configuration for Small, Intermediate, and Large Hospitals

	Small (<150 beds)		Intermediate (<600 beds)		Large (>600 beds)	
	Number	Cost	Number	Cost	Number	Cost
Radiographic/fluoroscopic	1	$454,000	4	$1,816,000	7	$3,178,000
Radiographic	1	$175,200	8	$1,401,600	11	$1,927,200
Radiographic mobile	1	$33,800	5	$169,000	13	$439,400
Linear tomographic			1	$161,500	5	$807,500
Multidirectional tomographic			1	$330,000	1	$330,000
Special procedures/cardiac lab			3	$2,460,000	5	$4,100,000
Fluoroscopic mobile			1	$98,000	5	$590,000
Dedicated chest			1	$192,600	2	$385,200
Total cost:		$663,000		$6,628,700		$11,657,000

Table 9.3
Cost for Vendor Supplied Service Agreements

Type of service agreement	Size of hospital		
	Small	Intermediate	Large
Labor only	$31,500	$314,800	$553,700
Labor plus parts (no glassware)	$41,400	$414,300	$728,500
Labor plus parts (with glassware)	$59,600	$596,500	$1,049,000

Table 9.4
Annual Repair Parts Costs for Typical Radiological Imaging Equipment

	Component costs				Total costs	
	X-ray tubes	TV cameras	XRII	Misc. parts	With glassware	Without glassware
Radiographic/fluoro-scopic	$8,000	$2,000	$6,000	$4,000	$20,000	$4,000
Radiographic	$8,000			$3,000	$11,000	$3,000
Linear tomographic	$8,000			$3,000	$11,000	$3,000
Dedicated chest	$8,000			$3,000	$11,000	$3,000
Multidirectional tom-ographic	$8,000			$3,000	$11,000	$3,000
Radiographic mobile	$2,000			$4,000	$6,000	$4,000
Fluoroscopic mobile	$2,000	$2,000	$4,000	$4,000	$12,000	$4,000
Special procedures/ cardiac cath lab	$16,000	$2,000	$6,000	$6,000	$30,000	$6,000

An estimate of annual costs for repair parts for typical equipment is presented in Table 9.4 and translated into the three example hospitals in Table 9.5.

To maintain an in-house service operation, overhead costs are incurred for service equipment and tools. Test equipment and tools (Table 9.6) reflect an overhead cost of $5,700/yr for the first radiological equipment specialist. Each additional specialist requires approximately $500 of hand tools that represents a $100/yr cost amortized over a 5-yr period.

The total yearly overhead for the first in-house service individual includes expenditures for equipment, training, salary, and fringe benefits, as illustrated in Table 9.7. The salary of $25,000 reflects a salary surveyed by the Society of Radiological Engineering and represents the national average for a skilled radiological equipment specialist. Benefits are computed at 20% of salary. Each additional equipment specialist yields an additional overhead cost of $31,600. A reasonable assumption is that one additional

Table 9.5
Total Annual Repair Costs for Small, Intermediate, and Large Hospitals

Type of service agreement	Size of hospital		
	Small	Intermediate	Large
Labor plus parts (no glass-ware)	$11,000	$91,000	$187,000
Labor plus parts (with glass-ware)	$37,000	$325,000	$617,000

radiological equipment specialist is required for each additional $1.5 million of equipment. This assumption is used by many vendors of radiological equipment.

The costs of vendor and in-house service can be compared for the three different types of maintenance agreements. These comparisons are provided in Table 9.8, 9.9, and 9.10 for small, intermediate, and large hospitals. The costs for the three types of maintenance agreements in the example hospitals are compared in Figures 9.3, 9.4, and 9.5. In these figures, service costs in thousands of dollars are plotted against equipment replacement value in millions of dollars. It is apparent from these curves that in-house service becomes more attractive as the inventory of equipment increases and that the break-even point for the cost effectiveness of in-house service is approximately $1.5 million worth of equipment in all three institutions. However, this analysis does not portray the complete picture for determining the cost effectiveness of in-house service for the following reasons:

1. Because of limited experience and resources, no in-house group can provide 100% of the service required. The smaller the size of the group, the more limited are the experience and resources available within the group. When determining the break-even point, therefore, it is necessary to account for the level of outside consultation and service that must be solicited from vendors for difficult problems.
2. In a small hospital with only one in-house radiological equipment specialist, vendor services are required during

Table 9.6
Test Equipment and Tool Costs for In-House Service Program

Item	Cost
High voltage divider	$13,000
Dosimetry system	$2,500
Storage oscilloscope	$8,000
Hand tools[b]	$1,000
Densitometer	$1,000
Special test objects/phantoms	$3,000
Total cost:	$28,500[a]

[a] Over 5-yr period = $5,700 yearly overhead.
[b] For each additional radiological equipment specialist an additional $500 in hand tools are required = $100 yearly overhead.

Table 9.7
Total Costs for In-House Service Program

	First radiological equipment specialist	Add for each additional radiological equipment specialist
Test equipment overhead	$5,700	$100
Training	$1,500	$1,500
Salary	$25,000	$25,000
Benefits	$5,000	$5,000
Total:	$37,200	$31,600

Table 9.8
Comparison of Costs for In-House Service and Maintenance for Different Types of Service Contracts: Small Hospital[a]

	Labor only		Labor + Parts		Labor + Parts + Glassware	
	Vendor	In-house	Vendor	In-house	Vendor	In-house
Labor	$31,500	$25,000	$41,400	$25,000	$59,600	$25,000
Parts	$11,000	$11,000		$11,000		$11,000
Glassware	$26,000	$26,000	$26,000	$26,000		$26,000
Training		$1,500		$1,500		$1,500
Test equipment overhead		$5,700		$5,700		$5,700
Benefits		$5,000				$5,000
Total:	$68,500	$74,200	$67,400	$74,200	$59,600	$74,200
Vendor-cost less in-house cost	$5,700		$6,800		$14,600	

[a] One radiological equipment specialist.

Table 9.9
Comparison of Costs for In-House Service and Maintenance for Different Types of Service Contracts: Intermediate Hospital[a]

	Labor only		Labor + Parts		Labor + Parts + Glassware	
	Vendor	In-house	Vendor	In-house	Vendor	In-house
Labor	$314,800	$75,000	$414,300	$75,000	$596,000	$75,000
Parts	$91,000	$91,000		$91,000		$91,000
Glassware	$234,000	$234,000	$234,000	$234,000		$234,000
Training		$4,500		$4,500		$4,500
Test equipment overhead		$5,900		$5,900		$5,900
Benefits		$15,000		$15,000		$5,000
Total:	$639,800	$425,400	$648,000	$425,400	$596,500	$425,400
Vendor cost less in-house cost	$214,400		$222,900		$171,100	

[a] Three radiological equipment specialists.

Table 9.10
Comparison of Costs for In-House Service and Maintenance for Different Types of Service Contracts: Large[a]

	Labor only		Labor + Parts		Labor + Parts + Glassware	
	Vendor	In-house	Vendor	In-house	Vendor	In-house
Labor	$ 553,700	$150,000	$728,500	$150,000	$1,049,000	$150,000
Parts	$ 187,000	$187,000		$187,000		$187,000
Glassware	$ 430,000	$430,000	$ 430,000	$430,000		$430,000
Training		$9,000		$9,000		$9,000
Test equipment overhead		$6,200		$6,200		$6,200
Benefits		$30,000		$30,000		$30,000
Total:	$1,170,700	$812,200	$1,158,500	$812,200	$1,049,000	$812,200
Vendor cost less in-house cost	$358,500		$346,300		$236,800	

[a] Six radiological equipment specialists.

vacations and during periods of sick and training leave.

3. Overhead costs associated with the workshop and office space for in-house service should be included in the break-even calculation.

4. Occasionally, service contract discounts can be negotiated with the vendor.

Additional issues to be considered when analyzing the cost effectiveness of the different service alternatives include:

1. Hours of coverage under a vendor contract. Most contracts cover only normal working hours, and an additional fee is charged for work performed outside of this time frame.

2. Distance and response time of the ven-dor. Long distances or slow response times may justify or necessitate in-house service.

3. Vendor reputation for service.

4. Preventive maintenance available under a contract with the vendor. Is a thorough preventive maintenance program provided? Does it ensure patient and operator safety, effective operation of the equipment, and a minimum number of unscheduled breakdowns?

5. Procedures available to monitor the work performed by the vendor.

A final service alternative to consider is use of a vendor on a time and materials basis, rather than a contract basis, for both corrective and preventive maintenance. The merits of this relative method in comparison to the previous approaches depend strongly

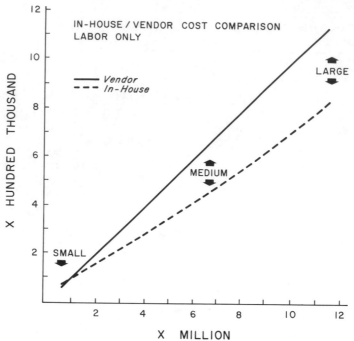

Figure 9.3. Comparison of costs for labor only service contract for small, intermediate, and large hospitals.

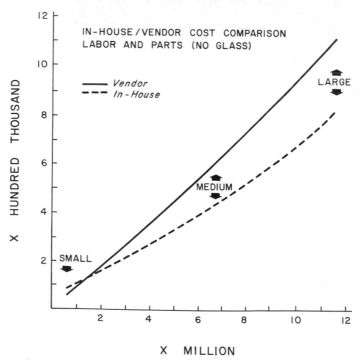

Figure 9.4. Comparison of costs for labor plus parts service contract for small, intermediate, and large hospitals.

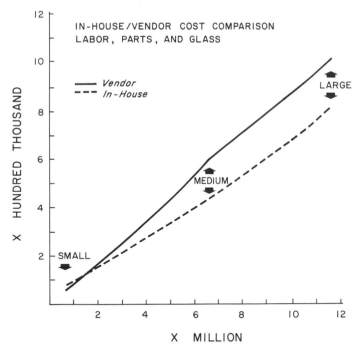

Figure 9.5. Comparison of costs for labor plus parts plus glassware service contract for small, intermediate, and large hospitals.

on the specific institution. For purposes of this discussion, institutional statistics are used from one of the author's institutions.

Commercial vendors were asked to estimate the cost of preventive maintenance procedures on 15 imaging systems. The labor cost for these procedures was $33,000; for biannual preventive maintenance, the cost would be $66,000. To estimate the costs of corrective maintenance, departmental statistics were used that reflect an average of seven requests for corrective maintenance per day, or 1,820 requests per year. The actual repair work per service request averaged 0.8 hr. From these data it is possible to estimate the yearly cost of vendor service on a time and materials basis.

Vendor responses to requests for service required approximately 2 hr of travel, billable at an average rate of $75/hr. The travel cost for 1,820 service calls per year would be $273,000. For an average repair time of 0.8 hr per service call, the actual charge for labor was an additional $109,000/yr. The total cost for vendor service on a time and materials basis for both corrective and twice yearly preventive maintenance is shown in Table 9.11. When these costs are compared

Table 9.11
Total Costs for Vendor Services on a Time and Material Basis for Both Corrective and Preventive Maintenance (PM)

Preventive maintenance	$66,000
+ Travel charges	$273,000
+ Service labor charges	$109,200
+ Projected parts costs	$617,000
Total:	$1,065,200
Corrected total costs for only one PM/system/yr	$1,065,200
	$⟨33,000⟩
Total:	$1,032,000

to those in previous examples, it is apparent that for the large hospital, the cost for vendor service on a time and materials basis is somewhat less than that for vendor contract service. Of course, contract service has one additional advantage; it reduces the vulnerability of the institution to high service costs associated with the catastrophic breakdown of radiological equipment.

In summary, it appears that in-house service becomes cost-effective when the replacement value of the equipment exceeds about $2 million and that one additional individual can be added to the in-house service force for each $1.5 million above this baseline amount.

Several other factors are worthy of consideration when evaluating service alternatives. First, the average response time for in-house service is generally less because the individual is present on site, and no travel is involved. This is frequently an advantage because minor problems can be corrected rapidly with little equipment downtime. Second, when in-house radiological equipment specialists are based administratively in the department, accountability problems may be substantially reduced because these individuals are part of the radiology "team" and are motivated to maintain equipment in top order.

Considerations in Preventive and Corrective Maintenance

Some additional considerations are worthwhile concerning corrective and preventive maintenance. While these comments are directly primarily to in-house service programs, the concepts are applicable to other forms of service.

EMERGENCY SERVICE

A maintenance group must be managed effectively to ensure: (1) sufficient staff; (2) satisfactory shift scheduling; (3) adequate spare parts inventory; (4) complete and accurate system documentation; and (5) a method of self-evaluation.

Staffing Needs

To determine an institution's need for maintenance staffing, past service records should be analyzed to determine the average daily breakdown frequency, daily peak breakdown frequency, and the probability of failure of multiple systems within the same time period. These rates should be examined critically to determine if they can be decreased. For example, a more extensive or frequent preventive maintenance program might eliminate some unexpected failures of a system or subsystem. This elimination might be accomplished by refurbishing, upgrading, or, perhaps, replacing the system or subsystem. Once unexpected breakdowns are reviewed and minimized, sufficient staffing for a shift can be determined by assessing:

1. The desirability of staffing for peak or for average failure frequencies, depending on financial considerations and departmental work load.
2. The responsiveness of local vendor service for backup.
3. The numbers, sophistication, and age of the various imaging systems.
4. From the standpoint of patient care, the desirability of rapid in-house responsiveness under the worst conditions.

There are no general rules for the number of staff per shift for a particular institutional setting. Factors influencing the number of staff desired per shift include:

1. Past emergency service history.
2. Emergency service program objectives based on considerations of the institutional environment and finances.
3. Periodic review of the program to ensure that objectives are being met.

Shift Scheduling

Two considerations are important in the evaluation of adequate scheduling. The first is that systems with a partial failure often cannot be surrendered for repair until the patient load declines, usually late in the afternoon. The second is the "evening callback syndrome." This syndrome occurs when large numbers of inpatients are scheduled in the early evening hours, as is often the case for CT procedures. These tendencies create a scheduling dilemma, since maintenance may be needed at both 8:00 A.M. and 7:00 P.M. If left unchecked, this situation has one of three outcomes:

1. A high level of vendor-provided service occurs during periods of premium billing rates.
2. Small problems are not repaired and cascade into larger problems.
3. Disillusionment and fatigue of the in-house equipment specialist occurs because of extensive overtime.

To address these staffing considerations, the manager should identify a satisfactory staff schedule as well as the number of staff required per shift. This identification should reflect the past service history, present condition of the equipment, and subjective and objective institutional considerations as they pertain to patient care.

Spare Parts Inventory

In a radiological facility of moderate to large size with different brands and types of imaging equipment, it is financially impractical to carry a spare parts inventory to meet all potential failures of equipment. In addition, the space allocated for in-house maintenance usually is inadequate for a massive inventory. Nevertheless, there are procedures available to an in-house equipment manager to reduce equipment downtime caused by the unavailability of parts. A few of these procedures are:

1. Before purchasing an equipment system, the spare parts inventory and the locations of parts depots should be determined for each potential vendor.
2. Institutions in the vicinity with similar equipment should be identified, and the service record of the vendors should be evaluated.
3. The equipment manufacturer should be asked for recommendations on an in-house spare parts inventory.
4. An adequate supply of basic electronic components that are compatible with the equipment should be maintained.
5. X-ray tubes should be standardized as much as possible throughout the department, so that a spare tube or two can be kept on site and quickly installed.
6. The purchase of radiological imaging systems comprised of components similar to those already in use in the institution should be considered. Among these components are controls, tables, microprocessors, and computers. If past performance of these systems has been acceptable and if they are still state-of-the-art and compatible with current clinical needs, then not only are larger quantities of different parts justifiable, but also spare parts can be cannibalized from systems replaced on a cyclical schedule.
7. Finally, and perhaps most importantly, the repair parts frequently used should be identified, and the stock of those

with high failure rates should be replenished.

Equipment System Documentation

Nothing is more frustrating than inaccurate or incomplete documentation of a radiological system. A mechanism to circumvent this problem is the possession of two complete sets of system documentation, including all available training and service manuals. At least one set should be on site at the time of installation, and the other should be delivered before final payment is approved. One set of systems documentation can be filed permanently in the shop for ready access, and the other can be kept in a locked filing cabinet with limited access.

Evaluation of Corrective Maintenance

A method should be devised to evaluate the corrective maintenance aspects of the service program. There should be three main objectives in this evaluation: (1) to detect repetitive or excessive subsystem failures for each system so that appropriate corrective procedures can be implemented; (2) to determine that the spare parts inventory is adequate; (3) to assure that personnel scheduling optimizes responsiveness to system failure.

The format utilized for evaluation of corrective maintenance should permit:

1. Rapid identification of systems with excessive downtime.
2. Evaluation of the effectiveness of the preventive maintenance program.
3. Evaluation of the responsiveness to failure.
4. Formulation of capital equipment replacement budgets based on failure trends.
5. Projection of more accurate fiscal operating budgets.
6. Evaluation of the radiological equipment specialist program for expertise and efficiency.

This information acquired can be invaluable in the certificate of need process required for system replacement.

Evaluation of Preventive Maintenance

All components of the preventive maintenance program should be based on internally defined objectives. The objectives should be based on characteristics of the institution, such as the types of equipment used, patient services provided, availability of revenue, and qualified maintenance personnel. The frequency of performance of preventive maintenance checks should include consideration of the clinical applications of the equipment, patient volume, and the level of care exercised by the users. The manager of a preventive maintenance program should match preventive maintenance frequencies and procedures to fit the working environment so that unscheduled breakdowns can be minimized and patient and operator safety can be maximized. These goals must reflect, of course, constraints of the resources available to the program and the availability of time on the equipment.

Because of the high daytime work load of most clinical units, it often is desirable to establish a preventive maintenance shift over the period from later afternoon to late evening. This shift can be covered by one or two individuals who rotate quarterly with daytime personnel. By utilizing this scheduling approach, it is possible to reduce conflicts in room utilization and to extend corrective maintenance coverage to roughly 18 hr/day at no significant increase in cost.

References

1. Establishment and administration of a maintenance and service program for radiological imaging equipment. In: *Proceedings of the American Association of Physicists in Medicine Symposium*, Midwest Chapter, Chicago, Oct 26–27, 1979.
2. Barnes GT, McDonal L: When is in-house service cost effective? In: *Proceedings of the Society for Photooptical Instrumentation Engineers*. Bellingham, WA, 1980, vol 233, pp 286–290.
3. Brown WJ, Randall MG: An alternate to vendor supplied service. In *Proceedings of the Society for Photooptical Instrumentation Engineers*. Bellingham, WA, 1977, vol 127, pp 142–144.

CHAPTER TEN

Prospects for the Future

WILLIAM R. HENDEE, Ph.D.

Over the past decade, radiology has been one of the fastest growing areas of health care. In the 3 years between 1978 and 1981, for example, annual domestic purchases of imaging equipment alone more than doubled from $665 million to more than $1.4 billion. By 1986 annual expenditures are expected to rise another 80% to a level of perhaps $2.5 billion in 1982 dollars (1). Most of this growth rate is attributable to the infusion of new technology into radiology over the past decade. Most of this technology is based upon computers and the processing of digital imaging data, and its refinement and extension to other imaging problems (as well as the development of additional new technologies) is expected to continue over the next decade.

The development of technological innovations and their introduction into clinical radiology require large investments of capital by both developers and clinical institutions. For a number of reasons, investments probably will continue in spite of current and projected economic constraints. First, improved diagnostic methods usually permit earlier detection and treatment of disease with the likelihood of increased effectiveness and reduced cost and morbidity. Many of the newer imaging methods are replacing more invasive radiological and surgical procedures, thereby reducing the extent of hospitalization and the consequent cost to the patient. Finally, diagnostic imaging usually is a profitable venture for a hospital; therefore, the incentive is present to maintain a state-of-the-art imaging facility in an effort to attract patients and revenue into the institution. This incentive must be balanced against the increased economic constraints existing in society in general and in the health care field in particular. An appropriate balance will require that sound decisions be made regarding equipment purchase and that technical verification be conducted to ensure that the purchased equipment satisfies clinical needs both upon installation and over extended use. The development of approaches to satisfy these objectives is the theme of this book.

The precarious nature of estimating the course of radiology over the next few years is evident from consideration of the innovations introduced into radiology over the past 10 yr. A decade or so ago, transmission computed tomography was just being introduced into radiology, and gray scale and real-time ultrasound were virtually unheard of in the clinical arena. Digital subtraction angiography had not been introduced clinically, and interventional angiographic procedures were under development in only a few centers. Computers were just beginning to satisfy a need in clinical nuclear medicine, and nuclear magnetic resonance was unheard of outside of the laboratories of chemists and physicists. In radiation therapy, ^{60}Co units were the mainstay for most treatments of cancer, whereas today linear accelerators occupy the locations of most of the ^{60}Co units formerly in use. Radiology has come a long way in 10 yr, and predictions of the future of radiology are uncertain for even a period as short as a decade. Still, such predictions are necessary if a reasonable course is to be charted between innovations and economics, subject to whatever changes may be dictated by future unforeseen events.

ROENTGENOGRAPHY

The introduction of digital data processing techniques into conventional roentgenography ultimately may have a greater impact than any other innovation introduced into radiology over the past decade (2). To date, this introduction has yielded a variety of microprocessor-based management systems for patient information, as well as an improved approach to visualization of contrast-filled vessels (digital subtraction angiography or DSA). It appears fairly certain that DSA is just the beginning of digital data collection and display in roentgenography and that with solution of certain "front end" (i.e., x-ray detector) and "back end" (i.e., data storage and retrieval) problems, none of which are intractable at the physics and engineering levels, digital techniques will expand to most fluoroscopic and many roentgenographic procedures. With this expansion, the networking of various imaging modalities in different areas of a hospital, and even among institutions, should be possible. With this networking approach to the transmission and display of diagnostic images, an essential ingredient in the establishment of a successful radiology program will be the compatibility among various radiologic imaging and viewing devices. This compatibility, together with the need for continuous supervision of the imaging systems and their interactions with various display devices, will require a rather sophisticated level of physics and engineering involvement.

Display of digitized roentgenographic images on video terminals will provide the viewer with the opportunity to alter the brightness and contrast of images in a manner now possible with other imaging modalities, such as computed tomography, nuclear medicine, ultrasound, and nuclear magnetic resonance. This capability should reduce the need for repeated exposures in roentgenography while offering an increased capability to extract useful information from the image. It will also present the opportunity to mask information in the image and to introduce artifacts that may be mistaken for patient pathology. Considerable scrutiny will be required of these potential problems and their possible effect on the viewer's impression of the image.

COMPUTED TOMOGRAPHY (CT)

After a decade of phenomenal success in which over 2600 CT units were installed in the United States alone, computed tomography is expected to encounter its first major challenge with the introduction of imaging systems employing the principle of nuclear magnetic resonance (NMR). For a variety of reasons, however, computed tomography is expected to survive this challenge, even though some slowing in new and replacement installations might be anticipated.

Among the reasons contributing to the survival of computed tomography are the somewhat higher cost of NMR units, the constraining posture of regulatory and reimbursement agencies towards NMR, and conceivably the high demand for access to NMR units that will encourage the retention of CT units for those examinations where NMR does not yield a decided advantage.

One advantage of CT over NMR is a more rapid scan time. The superior low contrast resolution of static NMR images compared to CT may produce an increased emphasis on CT as a dynamic imaging modality. This emphasis could increase the use of CT to follow the progression of contrast media through various structures and possibly in an enhanced interest in "real-time" CT scanners such as the cardiac CT scanners under construction at Mayo Clinic and the University of California at San Francisco. Another possible development in CT is its use as a quantitative index of tissue composition and pathology (3). Because of variations in CT numbers between scanners for the same test material, and even in the same scanner from one moment to the next, quantitative transmission computed tomography has not been used to date to any significant degree. Nevertheless, the potential of quantitative CT as a clinically useful tool is recognized by many investigators, and this approach could become an important part of CT in the future clinical environment. The use of quantitative CT data as a diagnostic index will require the frequent normalization of CT data to objects of known composition and will depend strongly on the involvement of physicists and chemists in the data accumulation and interpretive processes.

NUCLEAR MAGNETIC RESONANCE

The most exciting radiologic imaging modality to emerge over the past few years is nuclear magnetic resonance (4). This technique, which employs static and time-varying magnetic fields combined with radiofrequency alternating magnetic fields to obtain data from a region of tissue in vivo, yields electronic signals that are related not only to the atomic composition of the tissue region but also to molecular bonding configurations within the region which affect the way the signals decay with time. Because the signals are relatively weak, imaging times are rather long (a few minutes); during one imaging period, however, data can be collected for an entire volume of tissue, rather than for a cross-sectional slice of tissue, such as in computed tomography or ultrasound. Magnets with rather high field strength are used to overcome the relatively poor signal to noise ratios of NMR units; in many NMR units, these magnets are superconductive in an effort to overcome the high consumption of electricity associated with resistive magnets.

There is little question but that superconductive NMR units represent the most sophisticated technology of all imaging systems developed to date. NMR imaging units pose some interesting siting considerations within the hospital, as they must be located so that magnetic materials such as steel beams, elevators, etc. do not perturb the uniform magnetic field required for satisfactory images. In addition, they require a level of physics and engineering involvement that surpasses that needed with virtually any other imaging modality.

NUCLEAR MEDICINE

Nuclear medicine was the first imaging modality to utilize computers and to apply computer technology to the study of physiology and function rather than anatomy and form. Because of its sophisticated technology, nuclear medicine has captured the imagination and involvement of physicists and engineers for many years. In all likelihood, the utilization of nuclear medicine for the study of physiologic processes will continue to grow, especially if two evolving technologies develop as expected.

The first of these evolving technologies is the detection of primary and metastatic cancer cells by the use of radiolabeled monoclonal antibodies (5). This technology promises to provide a method for targeting radioactive "missiles" that will seek out cancer cells and reveal their presence by the emission of radiation once the antibodies are attached to the cells. Although radiolabeled antibodies are very promising, considerable work remains to be done before they become useful in routine clinical work. First, the specificity of the antigen-antibody reaction must be improved for artifically created antibodies

so that they yield a satisfying target to non-target ratio for imaging. Second, improved methods must be developed to tag the antibodies with radioactivity without interfering with the affinity of the labeled antibodies for the antigen. Third, nuclear medicine instrumentation must be improved to yield a greater affinity for the "hot spot" imaging methodology that labeled antibodies offer.

The second technology, positron emission tomography, has been available for a number of years but has not been adopted into widespread clinical use because it is inordinately expensive and because few clinical applications have been developed that provide clinical information that is not obtainable by other means (6). Still, positron-emitting radionuclides such as ^{11}C, ^{13}N, and ^{15}O may present few labeling or affinity problems for monoclonal antibodies, and the use of positron imaging with its inherently increased sensitivity could overcome some of the limitations of present imaging techniques applied to radiolabeled antibodies. Radiolabeled antibodies and positron emission tomography will require an extensive commitment to routine monitoring of the technology and to frequent verification of the integrity of the results.

ULTRASOUND

In the late 1970s and early 1980s, ultrasound was the fastest growing segment of the diagnostic imaging market, with a doubling of sales between 1978 to 1982. Between 1975 and 1982, the number of ultrasound examinations performed in the United States increased ten-fold. Today, ultrasound is second only to roentgenography in its frequency of clinical use. To a large measure these rapid growths in sales and utilization are a reflection of the introduction of gray scale and real-time ultrasound systems over the mid-to-late 1970s. Among other factors influencing the growth of ultrasound are the relatively low cost of ultrasound equipment, the apparent lack of risk accompanying the levels of ultrasound intensity used clinically, and the diffusion of ultrasound equipment throughout a number of medical specialties rather than its confinement to radiology. Although the latter influence continues to grow, the overall rates of growth in ultrasound sales and utilization appear to be plateauing to some degree, and a diminished growth rate probably can be anticipated over the next few years.

Two emerging clinical applications of ultrasound are dedicated neonatal units and ultrasound systems designed for use during operative procedures (7). Neonatal units utilize the ultrasonic transmission properties of the soft neonatal skull to permit ultrasonic visualization of the newborn brain. Intraoperative ultrasound units are beginning to be used for direct visualization of the internal structures of organs during surgery. Another application of ultrasound that is receiving considerable attention at present is intrauterine surgery under ultrasonic guidance. For example, shunts for cerebrospinal fluid in hydrocephalic fetuses have been positioned under ultrasonic guidance.

Because of its relatively low cost, its real-time characteristics, and its diffusion among many medical specialties, ultrasound instrumentation has not been challenged severely by the advent of newer, relatively expensive modalities, such as computed tomography and nuclear magnetic resonance. There is little reason to believe that the relative independence of ultrasound from challenge by other modalities will change significantly over the next few years; consequently, ultrasound should remain a viable part of the imaging arena for a number of years.

Every prognostic indicator available sug-gests that the technology of radiology will exhibit unparalleled development and growth over the next decade. This development and growth reflects the progression of radiology into the computer-electronic era and will require an increased involvement of physicists and engineers in the radiologic process. They also will require careful attention to the wise selection and performance evaluation of radiologic equipment to ensure that limited funds are spent wisely and that purchased equipment performs reliably and well.

References

1. Brown PW, Campbell-White A: *The U.S. Diagnostic Imaging Industry, Industry Study.* San Francisco, Hambrecht and Quist, 1982.
2. Fullerton GD (ed): *Electronic Imaging in Medicine.* New York, American Institute of Physics, 1983.
3. Hendee WR: Advances in transmission computed tomography. In Hamilton B (ed): *Medical Diagnostic Imaging Systems.* New York, Frost and Sullivan, 1982.
4. Morgan CJ, Hendee WR: Magnetic resonance imaging. I. Physical principles. II. Clinical applications. *West J Med* 141:638–648, 1984.
5. Hendee WR: The impact of future technology on oncologic diagnosis: oncologic imaging and diagnosis. *Int J Radiat Oncol Biol Phys* 9:1851–1865, 1983.
6. Hendee WR: *The Physical Principles of Computed Tomography.* Boston, Little, Brown, 1983.
7. Rubin JM, Dohmann GJ: Intraoperative neurosonography: the surgeon's eye into the brain. *Diagn Imaging* Sept:26–30, 1982.

Brief Description of Radiologic Modalities

WILLIAM R. HENDEE, Ph.D., RAYMOND P. ROSSI, M.S.,
VICTOR M. SPITZER, Ph.D., ANN L. SCHERZINGER, Ph.D.,
ROBERT K. CACAK, Ph.D., and GEOFFREY S. IBBOTT, M.S.

ROENTGENOGRAPHY

Roentgenographic Imaging

Since the discovery of the x-ray by Roentgen in 1895, roentgenographic imaging has provided medicine with one of its most valuable tools to assist in the diagnosis and treatment of disease. Stated simply, the objective of roentgenographic imaging is the production of images of internal body structures that contribute to a diagnosis which is useful in the clinical management of the patient.

The fundamental aspects of the roentgenographic imaging process are depicted in Figure A.1. A source of x rays is used to irradiate the portion of the patient to be examined. The x rays are differentially attenuated (some are absorbed, some are scattered, and some are transmitted) within the patient, depending on the physical properties (i.e., physical density and atomic number) of each region of the patient. This differential attenuation produces a two-dimensional array of x-ray intensities that reflects the internal structure of the irradiated region of the patient. Since x rays cannot be detected by the human senses; they must be converted to some form of image for viewing and interpretation by the physician. This conversion is accomplished in an image receptor that provides either a direct visible image or a latent image that can be processed in some manner to yield a visible image. In roentgenography, the two most common forms of image receptors are a combination of intensifying screens and film and the electrooptical image intensifier.

In an intensifying screen-film combination, the x-ray image is converted to light in the intensifying screens, and the light image is recorded as a latent image on the film. By photographic processing, the latent image is rendered visible as a distribution of opaque silver granules on an otherwise transparent plastic film base. This distribution of opaque granules yields an image of the internal anatomy of the patient. In an electrooptical image intensifier, the x-ray image is converted to a light image that may be viewed directly through lenses and mirrors or indirectly by use of closed circuit television. With either approach, the image also may be recorded on film.

The next step in the roentgenographic process involves interpretation of the visible image by the physician to arrive at a clinical diagnosis. Many factors are involved in this interpretation, including comparisons of the image mentally to the appearance of normal and abnormal images in the physician's memory, weighted by knowledge of the patient's symptoms and clinical history.

Production of Roentgenographic Images

There are several techniques for producing roentgenographic images. Among the more common methods are radiography, fluoroscopy, computed tomography and, most recently, digital radiography. In conventional radiography, static, life-size or magnified images are obtained of the anatomical region of interest. Usually, screen-film combinations are used to produce single images or sequential images separated by short intervals of time. Radiographic images have high spatial and temporal resolution, but only moderate contrast resolution. To produce conventional radiographs, the x-ray source frequently is positioned above the patient, and the image receptor is located below the patient.

Fluoroscopy is a dynamic imaging tech-

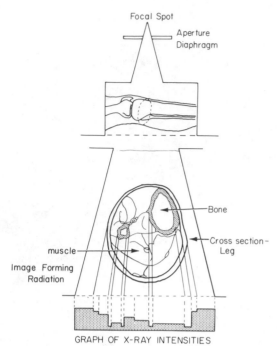

Figure A.1. Fundamental aspects of the radiological imaging process.

nique that requires instantaneous (i.e., real-time) detection, conversion, visualization, and, sometimes, interpretation of the x-ray image. Electrooptical image intensifiers usually are used in conjunction with closed circuit TV chains and small format film recording cameras. The x-ray source usually is located below the patient and the image intensifier above, although exceptions to this geometry are not infrequent. Fluoroscopy is used primarily to provide impressions of the structures under study and to localize regions of interest. For final interpretation and diagnosis, selected portions of the fluoroscopic image usually are recorded on film. Fluoroscopic images yield moderate spatial resolution, high temporal resolution, and moderate contrast resolution.

Computed tomography, introduced into clinical medicine in 1972, represents one of the major breakthroughs in roentgenographic imaging. In this imaging technique, an x-ray source rotates around the patient in a plane perpendicular to the patient's long axis. To intercept the x-ray beam transmitted through the patient, a bank of stationary detectors may surround the patient; alternately, an array of detectors may rotate with the x-ray source but on the opposite side of the patient. In comparison to conventional radiography and fluoroscopy, a narrow pencil or fan beam of x-rays is used. As the x-ray source rotates around the patient, many measurements are obtained of the differential attenuation of x rays in the patient. These measurements are stored in computer memory. After the measurements have been completed they are submitted to a mathematical routine (i.e., an algorithm) in the computer to produce an image representing the transverse anatomy of the patient. This image is displayed on a TV monitor and recorded on film. The attenuation data are stored in the computer and can be manipulated in many ways to yield a variety of reconstructed images. Computed tomographic images provide moderate spatial resolution, poor temporal resolution, and excellent contrast resolution.

Digital imaging systems are relatively new to roentgenographic imaging. These systems share certain characteristics with CT scanners in that the radiological image is stored in digital form in a computer and can be manipulated in many ways prior to being displayed and recorded.

Two approaches to digital radiography currently are under development. The first approach, referred to as digital fluoroscopy, uses a conventional image intensifier to produce a light image of the two-dimensional array of x-ray intensities emerging from the patient. This light image is viewed by a high resolution, low noise television camera, and the resultant analog signal from the camera is transmitted to an analog to digital converter. Here the signal is digitized and stored for further processing in a computer. The processed image is displayed on a television monitor and may be recorded on film as a permanent record.

The second approach to digital radiography, termed scan projection radiography, employs a narrow fan- or pencil-shaped x-ray beam and a one-dimensional array of radiation detectors, usually scintillation or semiconductor detectors. In this approach, the image is accumulated one line at a time by pulsing the x-ray beam, with the patient moved in increments between pulses. X rays transmitted through the patient are detected and converted into digital data for processing by a computer. From the computer-processed data, images are reconstructed, manipulated, and recorded in a fashion similar to CT, except that they represent coronal and sagittal, rather than transverse projections of the patient.

Digital radiography currently is in its infancy, and its ultimate role in radiology remains to be determined. Already, however, digital radiography appears to offer significant advantages in angiography, including the performance of subtraction studies with less invasiveness and far greater ease compared to analog (i.e., film) subtraction methods. It also appears to provide contrast resolution enhanced over that available with conventional film techniques.

Examples of Common Roentgenographic Imaging Techniques

Common examinations likely to be encountered in roentgenography include the following.

CHEST

Roentgenographic examination of the chest is by far the most common procedure in radiology, accounting for 35 to 50% of the examinations in a typical radiology de-

partment. The most frequently used projections are the P-A (posterior-anterior) and lateral, as illustrated in Figure A.2. Chest roentgenography is used to identify and characterize lesions produced by tuberculosis and cancer prior to the identification of these diseases by clinical examination. Preoperative and postoperative chest roentgenograms are used to assess respiratory function and the possible consequences of anesthesia following surgery. Chest roentgenography also is used to evaluate the functional capability of the diaphragm and to identify cardiac problems. To minimize magnification of the heart, radiographic examination of the chest normally is performed at long distances (e.g., 1.85 m) between the x-ray source and the image receptor.

SKULL

Among other applications, skull radiography is used to assess trauma of the skull and facial bones and to evaluate the sinuses. Examples of A—P (anterior-posterior) and lateral skull roentgenograms are shown in Figure A.3. Many skull examinations previously conducted with conventional roent-

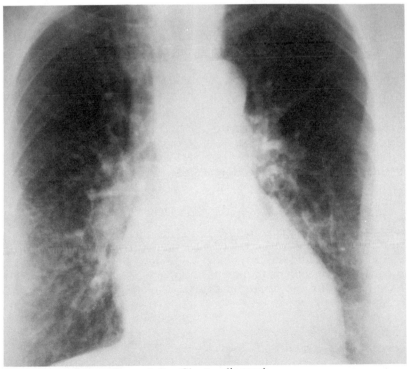

Figure A.2. Chest radiograph.

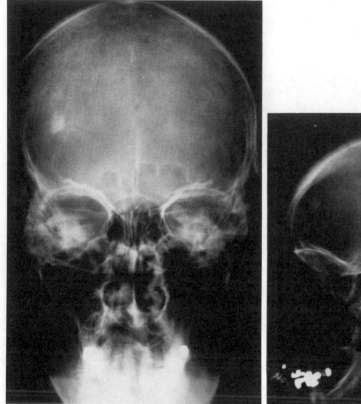
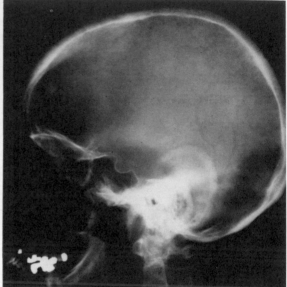

Figure A.3. (*Left*) Frontal skull radiograph. (*Right*) Lateral skull radiograph.

genographic techniques now are performed with computed tomography.

GASTROINTESTINAL (GI) TRACT

X-ray examination of the gastrointestinal tract may be performed to determine the presence of a gastric or duodenal ulcer, to verify the existence of cancer in the GI tract, and to study the function of the esophagus, colon, or rectum. Many other applications of roentgenography in the GI tract exist. Examples of upper and lower GI radiographs are shown in Figure A.4. GI examinations usually involve both fluoroscopic examination to study the flow of barium contrast agent through the GI tract, and radiographic imaging with intensifying screens and film for detailed evaluation of the anatomical areas of interest.

UROGRAPHY

This x-ray technique is used extensively for evaluation of the kidneys, ureter, blad-

der, and urethra. In urography an iodine contrast agent is employed to enhance the contrast between the structures of interest and the surrounding tissues. The agent is injected intravenously and excreted by the kidneys, with a series of radiographs taken at time intervals after injection. An example is shown in Figure A.5 of a urographic image taken 10 min following the injection of a contrast agent.

EXTREMITIES

The most common reason for x-ray examination of the upper and lower extremities is to determine the presence of fracture following trauma. A fracture in the forearm is revealed in Figure A.6. Extremity imaging may be employed also to evaluate invasive bone disease. Because of the very fine structure in the distal skeleton, an image receptor capable of providing high resolution usually is employed for extremity imaging.

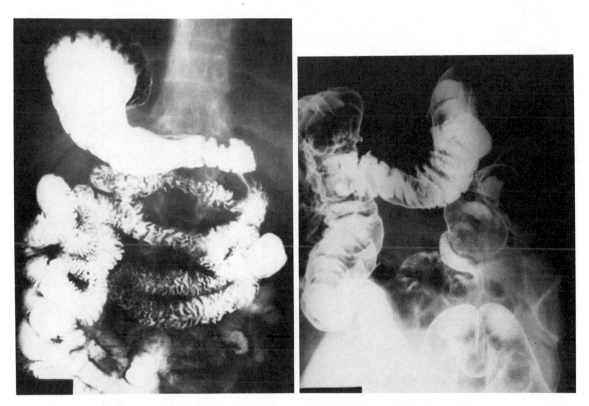

Figure A.4. (*Left*) Upper GI radiograph. (*Right*) Lower GI radiograph.

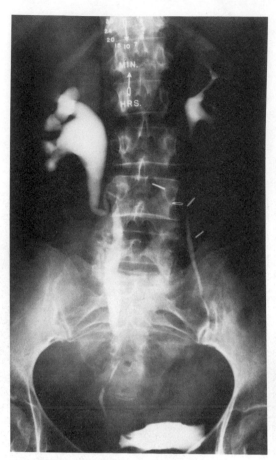

Figure A.5.   An excretory urogram radiograph.

ANGIOGRAPHY

Angiography is an x-ray technique used to image the vascular structure of any part of the body. Angiographic procedures usually are conducted in a sterile environment and are considered invasive in nature. A special device known as a catheter is introduced into an artery or vein near the vascular area to be evaluated. Then an iodine contrast agent is injected (usually under pressure), and a rapid sequence of radiographs is obtained. Roentgenographic images demonstrate the flow of the contrast agent (and therefore, blood) in both the arterial and venous phases of flow and facilitate the identification of arterial obstructions and the determination of the integrity of the vessels involved in the blood supply to an organ or tumor. Often this information is critical to surgical intervention. An example of a single image from a cerebral angiographic sequence is shown in Figure A.7.

COMPUTED TOMOGRAPHY

Computed tomography (CT) is utilized widely in the evaluation of the skull and brain. This technique has the advantage of distinguishing subtle differences in tissues and is particularly useful in skull trauma. An example of a CT image is shown in Figure A.8. Computed tomography also is

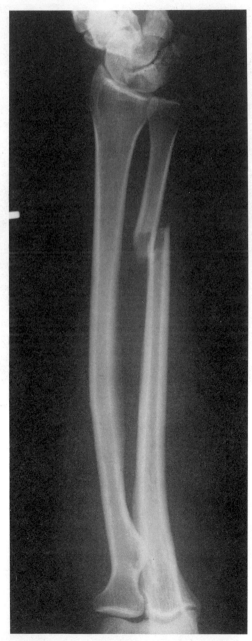

Figure A.6.   A radiograph of the forearm revealing a fracture.

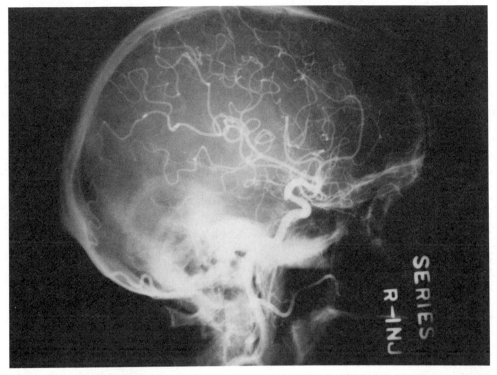

Figure A.7.   Example of a cerebral angiographic image.

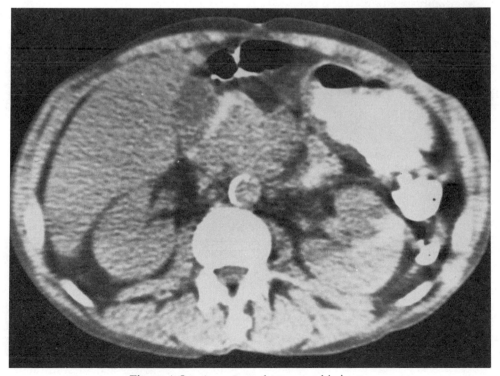

Figure A.8.   A computed tomographic image.

useful for imaging other areas of the body and has the distinct advantage of being less discomforting for the patient compared to many alternate roentgenographic procedures.

NUCLEAR MEDICINE

Nuclear medicine includes methods for diagnostic imaging, nonimaging radioassay techniques, and some therapeutic procedures. The common link between these applications is the utilization of radioactive nuclides or radioisotopes. The therapeutic use of radionuclides (e.g., the use of iodine-131 for treatment of thyroid conditions, including cancer) requires no major equipment beyond a survey meter and a radioisotope calibrator. Nonimaging diagnostic procedures may require automatic sample counting equipment for radioimmunoassay measurements or a single crystal scintillation probe and associated electronics for measurement of thyroid uptakes. The instrumentation required for nuclear medicine imaging is considerably more complicated.

Diagnostic nuclear medicine imaging utilizes the injection, ingestion, or inhalation of a radioisotope into the body and detection of the subsequent locations of the radioisotope to measure physiologic and morphologic characteristics of the body. This detection process yields an image of the distribution of the radioisotope throughout the body. The radioisotope is attached (tagged) to a pharmaceutical or chemical structure designed to concentrate in a specific organ or region of the body. The pharmaceutical is tagged in tracer quantities with the radioisotope, and consequently there is little or no harmful effect on the system under study.

A theoretical advantage of nuclear medicine is its potential to produce 100% contrast between a labeled area and the surrounding environment. A contrast of 100% is seldom achieved in practice because of the less than optimum specificity of currently available pharmaceuticals for complete extraction by a single organ or tissue. The goal of 100% contrast is also hampered by the inability of most radiopharmaceuticals to accept a perfect tag, i.e., a tag that adheres and remains bound exclusively and totally to the desired pharmaceutical.

In addition to its high contrast advantages, nuclear medicine also provides the capability to quantify the functional integrity of an organ and the changes in organ function with time. Some major applications of nuclear medicine imaging are included in Table A.1; representative images are shown in Figures A.9A through D.

The most common item of imaging equipment in nuclear medicine is the scintillation camera (sometimes referred to as a gamma

Table A.1
Applications of Nuclear Medicine Imaging

Target	Isotopes/pharmaceuticals used	Measurement
Blood	^{99m}Tc-pertechnetate	Volume, flow
Brain	^{99m}Tc-DTPA,[a] ^{123}I or ^{133}Xe	Blood flow and distribution
Bones	^{99m}Tc-methylene diphosphonate	Tumor uptake
Heart	^{99m}Tc-pertechnetate or labeled blood cells, ^{201}Tl	Blood flow, volume, infarction
Kidneys	^{99m}Tc-DTPA, DMSA,[b] or ^{131}I-hippuran	Tubular and cortical function
Liver/spleen	^{99m}Tc-sulfur colloid or red blood cells	Size, shape, tumor involvement, focal concentrations
Lungs	^{133}Xe-gas, ^{99m}Tc-aerosols, ^{99m}Tc-microspheres	Emboli caused defects, ventilation, perfusion
Thyroid	^{123}I, or ^{131}I, or ^{99m}Tc-pertechnetate	Tumor uptake, function
Abcess	^{67}Ga-citrate	Focal concentrations
Tumors	^{123}I-monoclonal antibodies, ^{67}Ga-citrate	Tumor uptake

[a] DTPA, diethylenetriamine pentaacetic acid.
[b] DMSA, dimercaptosuccinic acid.

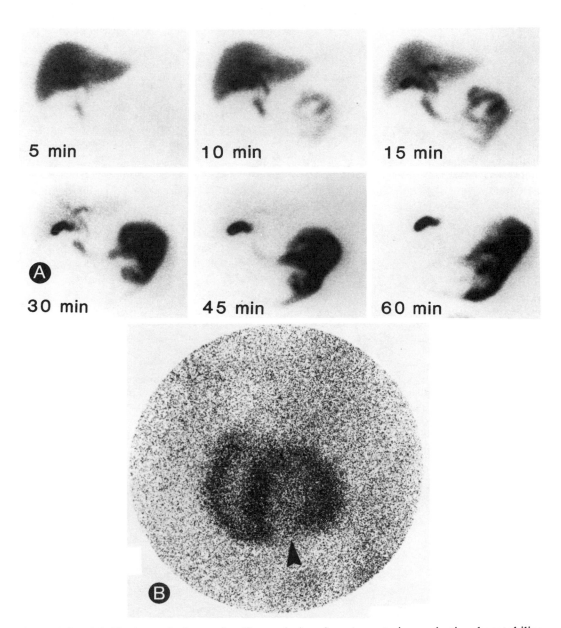

Figure A.9. (*A*) Nuclear scintigram for diagnostic imaging. An anterior projection hepatobiliary study using ^{99m}Tc-diethyl-IDA demonstrates normal physiology with no cardiac blood pool and a very low background at 5 min. By 10 min the biliary tract, duodenum, and gallbladder are visible. At 45 min all activity cleared by the hepatocytes has been excreted into the biliary tract, indicating a normal hepatobiliary transit time. (From Kuni CC, Klingensmith WC III: *Atlas of Radionuclide Hepatobiliary Imaging*. Copyright © 1983 by Year Book Medical Publishers, Inc., Chicago.) (*B*) Thallium-201 is taken up by muscle tissue. This left anterior oblique myocardial thallium-201 image collected just after treadmill stress demonstrates a large defect involving the inferolateral left ventricular wall (*arrow*). The defect did not fill in before the patient was reimaged 3 hr later, indicating that the area of decreased activity is due to irreversible ischemia (infarction). The image contains 200,000 counts and required 7 min to accumulate.

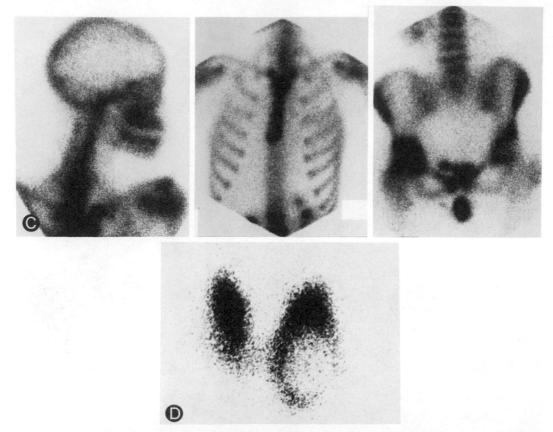

Figure A.9. (*C*) The two views on the left of this bone scan demonstrate normal bone uptake of the ^{99m}Tc-MDP in the head and chest area (*left* and *middle*). The bottom of the center image also shows normal hot spots or high uptake in the kidneys. However, abnormal increased uptake of the radiopharmaceutical is shown in the right hip (anterior pelvis image at the right). Diagnosis was septic arthritis of the right hip. Images required from 1 to 3 min to accumulate and contain 700,000 counts. (*D*) This thyroid image was taken with iodine-123 using a pinhole collimator at 3 inches from the patient's neck in an anterior projection. In 4 min 50,000 counts were obtained. The image demonstrates a normal right lobe and a large cold nodule on the lower left lobe of the thyroid. The nodule was mobile and smooth but not tender on palpation. Cold nodules are most commonly attributable to colloid cysts, adenoma, carcinoma, or nontoxic nodular goiter. A diagnosis of colloid cyst was surgically proven.

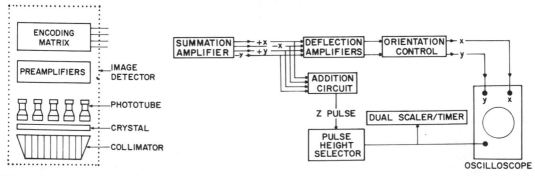

Figure A.10. Functional diagram of the scintillation camera. Ionizing radiation from the patient which passes through the collimator channels may be converted to light in the crystal. This light is converted to electric current and amplified in the phototubes. An encoding matrix determines position of the original ionizing radiation. The electric pulses are then passed to amplification, shaping and energy selection circuits (*right*) for control of the electron beam in the oscilloscope. Here, the electronic signals are converted back into light for viewing or photography. The oscilloscope might be replaced by or multiplexed with a computer.

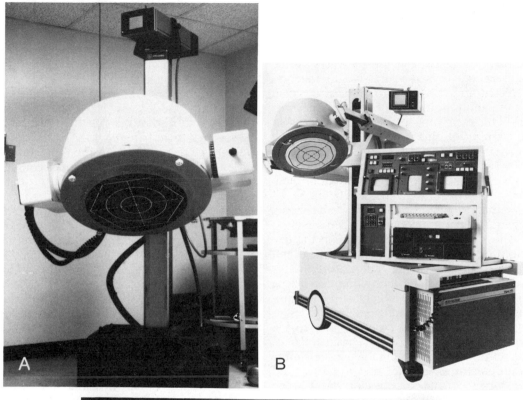

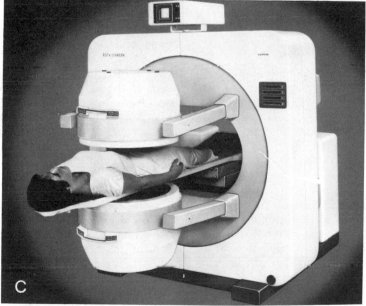

Figure A.11. (*A*) Standard large field of view (15-inch diameter) general purpose camera. The electronics console is out of view. (*B*) Mobile small field of view (10-inch diameter) high resolution camera. This unit also has an onboard computer. (Courtesy of Technicare.) (*C*) Tomographic (rotating) camera system with dual large field of view detector. (Courtesy of Siemens Medical Systems.)

or Anger camera). Major camera components are outlined in Figure A.10. Radiation (gamma- or x-rays) emitted from the body is absorbed by the sodium iodide crystal. Absorption of the radiation releases visible light in the crystal which is subsequently detected and converted to an electric signal by the photomultiplier tubes above the crystal. This electronic pulse is then processed to form a dot on the output display device, normally a cathode-ray tube. An image of the radioisotope distribution is formed from an accumulation of a large number of these distinct events. The image may be displayed on either an analog cathode-ray tube or as a digital image on a computer video screen.

The spatial relationship between the distribution of optical density in the image and the distribution of the radioisotope in the patient is defined by the collimator placed in front of the scintillation crystal. The simplest and most common collimtor design utilizes lead channels perpendicular to the crystal face. Variations in the basic design of the scintillation camera include mobile units and detector assemblies that rotate around the patient for the collection of tomographic data. These variations in scintillation camera design are shown in Figures A.11*A* through *C*.

ULTRASOUND

Diagnostic ultrasonic techniques are commonly used in many areas of medicine, including radiology, obstetrics, gynecology, opthalmology, neurology, gastroenterology, and cardiology. The widespread acceptance of ultrasound reflects in part its ability to obtain images noninvasively with no known bioeffects.

Ultrasonic images display information that is related to the acoustic properties of tissues, rather than to the attenuation of x rays as displayed by conventional roentgenography. In ultrasound, images are formed by the transmission of mechanical vibrations through tissue at frequencies (1 to 15 MHz) above the audible range of sound. These ultrasonic pulses are generated by a piezoelectric crystal housed within an ultrasound transducer, with the frequency of the sound and the shape of the sound beam determined by the characteristics of the transducer. The ultrasonic pulses propagate through different tissues at characteristic speeds and are

partially reflected at interfaces between different tissues in the body. Although reflection is slight ($\sim$1%) at soft tissue interfaces, it can approach 100% at interfaces between soft tissues and air or bone. Because of the highly reflective characteristics of air and bone, the use of ultrasound is limited to regions not "hidden" by these materials. The reflected ultrasound (i.e., the "echoes") travel back to and are recorded by the transducer. The pulse-echo transition time on the order of fractions of a millisecond, coupled with the assumed speed of sound in tissue, is used to identify the location of the interface in the tissue sample. In ultrasonic imaging, limited use is also made of through-transmission techniques by which a continuous or pulsed ultrasonic wave is generated by one transducer while a second transducer, located on the opposite side of the patient, is used to record the sound transmitted through the tissue. A third technique, Doppler imaging, yields information on blood flow by utilizing the frequency shift resulting from the reflection of an ultrasonic wave off moving targets.

Four basic types of instrumentation are commonly employed for diagnostic applications of ultrasound. These types are A-mode, static and real-time B-mode, M-mode, and Doppler scanners.

The simplest technique, A-mode, provides a one-dimensional cathode-ray tube (CRT) trace of the echoes arising from interfaces seen from one position of the transducer (Fig. A.12). The A-scan trace is a plot of echo-strength vs. echo depth along the ultrasonic beam and requires only a CRT for display. For permanent records, the trace is recorded on Polaroid film. The A-mode methodology is most useful when the anatomy studied is relatively simple, so that it is possible to identify the echoes associated with anatomic structures of interest. Present applications of the A-mode technique include the detection of midline shifts of the brain and the identification of structures and masses in the eye. In addition, A-mode traces are provided on other types of ultrasonic instrumentation to assist in setting sensitivity controls and to provide more detailed echo information.

A B-mode imaging system (Fig. A.13*A*) provides a two-dimensional image of a section of patient anatomy. This image is ob-

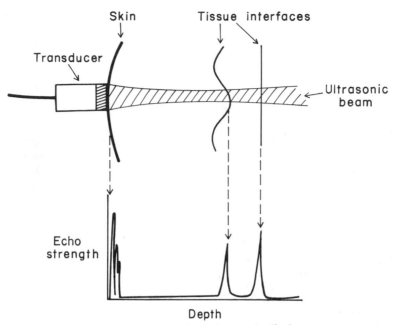

Figure A.12.   Generation of A-mode display.

tained by sweeping the transducer over the skin and recording the depth and intensity of echoes corresponding to a given position of the transducer (Fig. A.13*B*). The position measurement necessitates rigid attachment of the transducer to the ultrasound unit, making standard B-scanners too bulky for mobile use. The accuracy of the position measurement is called the scan arm registration and directly affects the resolution of the image. At each position of the transducer, depth and echo intensity are recorded, resulting ultimately in a static image of the anatomical plane of interest. In this image, the brightness of each spot represents the intensity of the echo received from that location. Figure A.13*C* presents a longitudinal image through the abdomen of a normal subject. This image reveals strong reflections from the diaphragm and kidney border and collecting systems and weaker echoes from the tissue parenchyma. With B-mode systems currently available, the most current image is stored in computer-type memory and is accessible for sophisticated image processing. Images are recorded permanently on x-ray film in a multiformat camera. B-mode units have traditionally been the primary diagnostic unit in the ultrasound department for abdominal, obstetrical, gynecological, and fetal brain studies.

Real-time ultrasound images are produced by obtaining B-mode images rapidly in succession (10 to 40 images/sec). Real-time units differ from B-mode scanners primarily in the configuration of the transducer. The real-time transducer head is designed to perform sequential scans automatically when held stationary over the area of interest. With some units this automation is accomplished by rapid mechanical oscillation or rotation of one or more transducer crystals within the transducer head (Fig. A.14*A*). This technique is referred to as sector scanning because the region imaged resembles a pie-shaped segment of tissue. Other units produce real-time images by electronic sequencing across a linear array of crystals in the transducer head (Fig. A.14*B*). With either approach, images can be produced rapidly enough that the motion of heart valves, organs, and contrast agents can be visualized. These rapid displays are also useful for searching for organs of interest. In real-time units, a rigid scan arm is not required to record the position of the transducer, and real-time systems can be constructed to be portable. Also, the selection of scan planes is easier. The need to produce images rapidly, however, limits the lateral field of view, the number of lines per image, and/or the depth of the image.

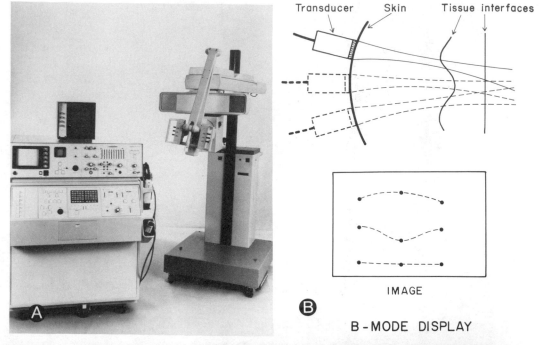

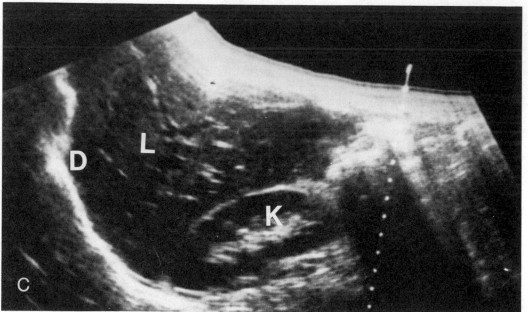

Figure A.13. (*A*) Static B-mode ultrasound imaging scanner. (*B*) Generation of a B-mode image. *Solid dots* on the image represent echoes received from the three positions of the transducer illustrated. A continuous image (*dashed lines*) is generated by a continuous sweep of the transducer over the skin. (*C*) B-mode image of a longitudinal section through the right side of the abdomen. Patient head is to the *left*, feet to the *right*. *L*, liver; *K*, kidney; *D*, diaphragm.

Hence, somewhat poorer spatial image quality results when temporal resolution is improved. Real-time units are available in a wide variety of configurations from a simple hand-held model with a 2- × 2-inch display screen and no permanent record or sensitivity control, to more sophisticated units with all of the image processing options of B-

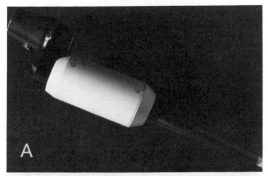

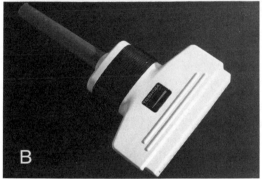

Figure A.14. Real-time sector head transducer. (*B*) Real-time linear array transducer.

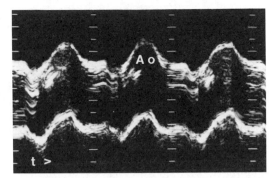

Figure A.15. M-mode trace obtained through adult heart. LA = left atrium, *Ao*, Aortic root. Vertical axis is depth in the patient; horizontal axis is time.

mode scanners. In real-time units, single images can be recorded with a standard camera, or the entire examination can be recorded on videotape. Because of their ability to image moving structures, their mobility, low cost (at least for some simpler units), and recent advances in image quality, real-time units are capturing a major share of the market formerly held by static B-mode units.

Another approach to B-mode units is the water path, rapid scan units exemplified by the Octoson and by dedicated ultrasound breast scanners. The water path provides coupling between the patient and the transducer(s). These units perform static B-mode scans automatically and rapidly, but not at real-time rates.

A measurement principle similar to B-mode is used to obtain M-mode (motion mode) information. However, the displayed information is the echo pattern from tissue interfaces at one position of the transducer as a function of time. In this approach, stationary objects present a straight line on the display, while moving objects yield a fluctuating path. M-mode systems are widely used in cardiology to study valvular

or heart wall motion; a typical trace obtained from such a study is shown in Figure A.15.

Although stand-alone M-mode instruments are still available, it is becoming more common to see M-mode as an optional module for real-time B-mode units. In such a combined system, one can obtain a real-time image of the heart along with an M-mode trace to facilitate more accurate placement of the transducer. Problems with these units arise in coupling the real-time frame rates of 10 to 40 images/sec with the 1000 pulse/sec pulse repetition frequency required for high resolution M-mode studies. Manufacturers have developed various ways to accomodate these problems.

Doppler units are used mainly to detect abnormalities in blood flow through peripheral blood vessels. Blood flow causes shifts in the Doppler frequency in the audible range, and the simpler Doppler units present this information through a loudspeaker. More sophisticated units present a visual display of the average frequency, or even the entire spectrum of frequencies, obtained as a function of time. In addition, Doppler units can be combined with B-mode units to produce images of vessels superimposed on the surrounding stationary tissues. These systems, termed duplex units, suffer from problems similar to those of combined M- and B-mode systems.

COMPUTED TOMOGRAPHY
CT Scanner Test Phantoms

A number of tests have been designed to measure various aspects of CT scanner performance. Many of the tests described and referred to in Chapters 7 and 8 utilize phantoms or test objects to qualify a variety of performance parameters. Advantages of using phantoms include their ease of use, their applicability to most CT scanners, and their use without disrupting the electronic and mechanical integrity of the CT scanner. Most phantoms are designed to simulate human tissue composition and to provide quick interpretation of measurements; however, some test objects require more extensive mathematical analysis of the data.

There are a number of CT phantoms available commercially. A compilation of phantom manufacturers is maintained by the American Association of Physicists in Medicine (AAPM).* Before purchasing a phantom, the buyer should study the features of each and determine which phantom provides the test objects relevant to his or her application. A description of test objects and phantoms found to be useful for the tests described in Chapters 7 and 8 follows. This list is intended only to be representative of some types of test objects and is not intended to be all-inclusive.

LOW CONTRAST RESOLUTION

The low contrast resolution test object measures the ability of a CT scanner to discriminate small objects surrounded by media of similar x-ray attenuation. One type of test phantom is shown in Figure A.16 and consists of a 2.54-cm (1-inch) thick plate of polystyrene, approximately 20 cm (8 inches) in diameter, encased in a cylindrical acrylic shell. The polystyrene has ten sets of holes, with each set containing four holes aligned on a radial projection. The size of the holes is constant within a set, but each set ranges from 3 to 8 mm. The acrylic shell is filled with a solution of methanol and water, allowing the solution to fill the holes in the polystryene. The test pattern consists of these solution-filled holes and a polystyrene "background."

The difference in x-ray attenuation characteristics between the polystyrene and the solution is determined by the concentration

of the methanol. For low methanol concentrations (~100% water), the attenuation of the solution is greater than the polystyrene, and the holes appear lighter than the background in the CT image. For high methanol concentrations (e.g., 50%-50% mixture), the attenuation of the solution is less than the polystyrene, and the holes appear darker than the background. At intermediate concentrations, the holes and the background have very similar attenuations and, if desired, all holes may be rendered invisible in the image by carefully selecting the concentration of methanol. For most low contrast tests, a desirable concentration is one that shows about half of the sets of holes in the image. A test consists of scanning the test object and determining the smallest set of holes in which all four holes can be clearly discriminated. Increased noise often obscures holes near the center of the phantom, so that all of the holes in one set cannot be seen, while smaller holes in adjacent sets near the phantom periphery can be visualized. The decreased visibility of the holes in the center of the phantom is caused by statistical imprecision of the smaller number of x-ray photons there. Increasing the radiation dose generally increases the visibility of these holes; hence this low contrast test must be specified in relation to a specific radiation dose.

HIGH CONTRAST RESOLUTION

A high contrast spatial resolution test pattern is used to determine the ability of a CT scanner to image small objects with substantial differences in x-ray attenuation from the surroundings. Often, the high contrast resolving power of a CT system is expressed in terms of its spatial frequency response or modulation transfer function (MTF). The MTF may be calculated from: (a) a square-wave response function obtained with a star pattern similar to those used in conventional diagnostic radiology; (b) an edge-response function obtained with a test pattern consisting of two dissimilar materials with a well-defined edge separating them; or (c) a point-response function obtained with a small high density wire to serve as a point object (or "impulse"). Unfortunately, most of these techniques involve somewhat

---

* AAPM Report prepared by the Task Group on CT Image Descriptors (in preparation). This report includes a section describing CT scanner phantoms available commercially.

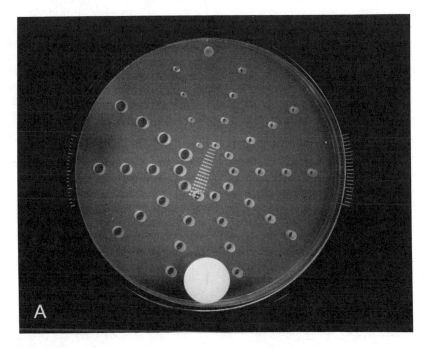

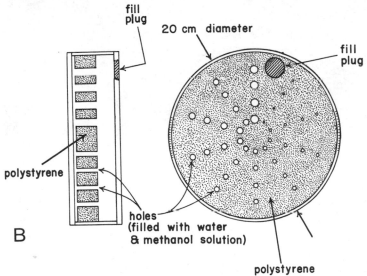

Figure A.16. Photo of low contrast CT phantom. (B) Schematic of low contrast hole phantom. Hole sizes are: 3, 4, 4.5, 5, 5.5, 6, 6.5, 7, 7.5, and 8 mm. (A and B, Courtesy of Ultra-Cal, Inc., 3014 Laurashawn Lane, Escondido, CA 92026.)

lengthy analyses of the data to determine a MTF.

A simpler technique for determining resolution of a CT scanner is to determine its resolving power in terms of its ability to visualize small objects in the image. This technique is much less elegant than determining a complete MTF, but it is easier and suffices for most applications. The procedure is simply to scan a test pattern with sets of holes of various sizes, each set containing holes of a particular diameter, and visually to determine the smallest set in which all holes can be discriminated. The size of this set is a measure of the resolving power of the CT scanner. Figure A.17 shows one type of test pattern in which there are 17 sets of holes, with each set containing five round holes. The sizes of the holes range from 1.1 to 0.41 mm. For convenience, this test pattern is incorporated in the same phantom section as the low contrast test pattern.

PATIENT DOSIMETRY

Many techniques have been proposed for measuring the radiation dose received by patients undergoing CT scanner examinations. Some researchers have used film (1) and thermoluminescent dosimeters (TLDs) (2, 3) to determine dose profiles, while others have developed special types of ionization chambers to measure the same quantity (4). More recently, a different type of variable, the CT Dose Index (CTDI), has been proposed (5–7). This index has the advantage of being measured accurately, quickly, and simply, with a long, pencil-type ionization chamber. The CTDI also has the advantage of being easily converted to the clinically relevant quantity, Multiple Scan Average Dose (MSAD). The latter quantity is an accurate measure of the average dose to a specified location within a patient receiving a series of closely spaced scans. The size of

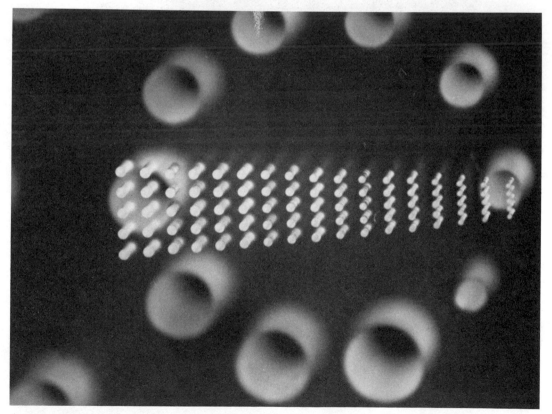

Figure A.17. Close up photo of high contrast test object. Hole sizes range from 0.41 to 1.09 mm. (Courtesy of Ultra-Cal, Inc.)

the phantoms shown in Figures A.18 and A.19 are suggested by investigators at the Center for Devices and Radiological Health (2).

The head phantom is 16 cm in diameter, 14.4 cm long, and has six holes to accommodate a pencil ionization chamber. The four peripheral holes are equidistantly

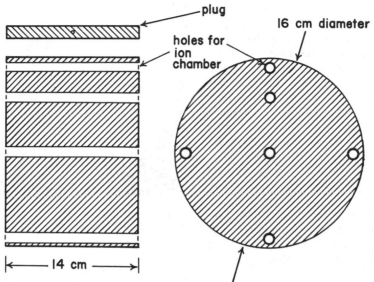

Figure A.18. Schematic drawing of "head" dosimetry phantom. Pencil type ionization chamber is inserted in holes for measurements. (Courtesy of Ultra-Cal, Inc.)

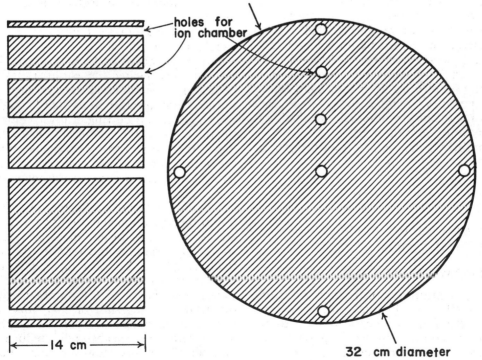

Figure A.19. Schematic drawing of "body" dosimetry phantom. Pencil type ionization chamber is inserted in holes for measurements. (Courtesy of Ultra-cal, Inc.)

placed on a 14-cm diameter. The fifth hole is at the center, and the sixth hole is on a diameter of 9.9 cm. By moving the ionization chamber from one hole to the next, initiating a single scan, and recording the integrated current (charge) at each location, a reasonably comprehensive map of patient dose throughout the head may be determined. Somewhat more definitive dose distributions may be obtained by rotating the phantom about its axis as necessary. Several plugs are provided for those holes not occupied by the ionization chamber. Each plug has a small hole (centered end-to-end) that is visible in the CT image if the x-ray beam is intersecting the center of the phantom.

The body phantom is constructed in a fashion similar to the head phantom, except that the diameter is 32 cm. There is a total of seven holes in this phantom, with the four peripheral holes on a 30-cm diameter. The CTDI from either size dosimetry phantom is determined from the equation:

$$CTDI = \frac{f \, C_f \, C_{TP} Q}{t}$$

where f = f-factor (rad to roentgen conversion) $\cong$ 0.94 rad/R for CT scanner x-ray energies; C_f = ionization chamber calibration factor (in r-mm/coulomb); C_{TP} = temperature pressure factor = $(273.15 + T)760/295.15 \, P$; T = temperature (in °C); P = pressure (in mm Hg); Q = total charge from the ionization chamber for a single scan (coulombs); and t = nominal slice thickness of the x-ray beam (in mm).
The MSAD is determined from the expression:

$$MSAD = CTDI \frac{(t)}{BI}$$

where BI = bed increment or distance between scans (in mm).

UNIFORMITY SECTION

This phantom section is simply a cylindrical shell of acrylic filled only with water (Fig. A.20). For most applications, a 20-cm diameter section can be employed. The phantom is scanned, and the average and standard deviation of the CT numbers are determined within a specified area (usually

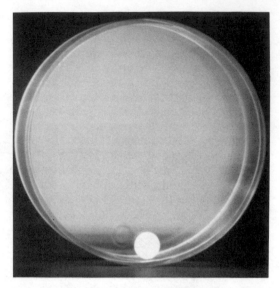

Figure A.20.   Uniformity CT phantom section. (Courtesy of Ultra-Cal, Inc.)

called the "region of interest" or ROI) selected on the video monitor, using software provided by the scanner manufacturer. The capability of calculating averages and standard deviations within ROIs is usually provided.

Ideally, the average CT number of water should be zero at all locations within the phantom. However, as the ROI is moved off the axis and nearer the periphery of the phantom, deviations in the average CT number may occur, due to "hardening" of the x-ray beam occurring near the center of the phantom. If the CT number is lower or higher in the center than near the periphery, the terms "cupping" and "capping," respectively, are used to describe this phenomenon.

For most techniques, fluctuations of the CT numbers, producing pixel to pixel variations, or "noise" in the image, are due to statistical variations inherent in the relatively small number of x rays penetrating the phantom and striking the detectors. The standard deviation of CT numbers within the ROI is a measure of this noise and usually increases near the center of the phantom, where increased absorption reduces the number of photons. However, some manufacturers will "shape" the x-ray fan beam by inserting a filter that is thicker at the edges of the beam. These filters are designed to harden and partially attenuate the edges of the fan beam relative to the beam at the center of the fan. The latter effect produces a more uniform dose distribution throughout the patient. Inclusion of such a filter, however, may modify the behavior of the average CT number and standard deviation from that described above.

One technique for assessing the image noise characteristics of a CT scanner is to measure the standard deviation as a function of x-ray fluence (8). If the standard deviation σ is graphed against the x-ray fluence, measured in milliampere seconds × slice thickness, the curve decreases approximately as the latter product to the $-\frac{1}{2}$ power. At extremely large milliampere seconds × slice thickness, it has been shown that the fluctuations due to photon statistics become less important relative to the electronic noise inherent in the scanner, and the curve decreases at a much slower rate (9).

Other tests that may be performed with the uniformity section include the "calibration" of CT numbers. Inside a phantom filled with water, the CT number should be zero, and outside the phantom (in air) the CT number should be −1000. These two calibration points arise because of the definition of CT number:

$$CT \text{ number } (x) = 1000 \left(\frac{\mu_x - \mu_w}{\mu_w} \right)$$

where CT number (x) is the CT number of a scanned material; μ_x is the linear attenuation coefficient of material x; and μ_w is the linear attenuation coefficient of water. Note that if $\mu_x = \mu_w$ (i.e., the material is water), the CT number is zero. If the material measured is air, $\mu_x \cong 0$, and the CT number is −1000. If $\mu_x = 2 \mu_w$, then the CT number equals +1000. Coincidentally, the density and composition of dense bone produces a linear attenuation coefficient approximately twice that of water. The CT number, in this case, is approximately +1000; however, dense bone is not a true calibration point.

The CT number of water may be measured as a function of many other variables present in a CT scanner. Some of these variables include: (a) algorithm type; (b) slice width; (c) milliamperage; (d) kilovoltage

peak; (e) phantom size; (f) scan speed; and (g) phantom position. In all cases, the average CT number of water should remain constant at zero for the ideal scanner; however, in practice, some deviations are usually tolerated.

CT NUMBER LINEARITY/ EFFECTIVE ENERGY

The phantom section used to determine effective energy consists of 24 large (1-inch diameter) plastic pins immersed in water as is shown in Figure A.21. There are four pins each of six types of plastic. The four pins of each type of plastic are positioned on a series of diameters spaced at 30°. Each plastic type consists of pins at various depths from the surface of the phantom. The CT number at each depth for each plastic may be easily measured from a single image of this phantom using the "region of interest" feature available on most scanners. Measured CT numbers plotted on a graph against the linear attenuation coefficients are x-ray energy-dependent, and therefore the coefficients at one energy presumably will yield a more linear graph than at other energies. By adjusting the energy and refitting the CT numbers, the best linear fit, exemplified by a maximum in the correlation coefficient, may be observed. The corresponding value of energy represents the effective energy of the x-ray beam (10, 11). Because of the variability in density of plastics, a sample of the plastic used in the phantom is helpful in determining the density of the material. The mass attenuation coefficients may be determined from the elemental composition of the plastic in conjunction with the published tables (12).

ALIGNMENT AND ARTIFACTS

This section of the phantom, shown in Figure A.22, consists of an acrylic shell containing five aluminum pins, each 6 mm in diameter, spaced several centimeters apart in a "+" pattern. This phantom section is also filled with water. Geometrical misalignment of the CT scanner will produce dark streak artifacts emanating from one or more of the pins. The streaks may resemble a dark "comet," with the head of the comet located at one or more of the pins and all of the tails pointing in one particular direction.

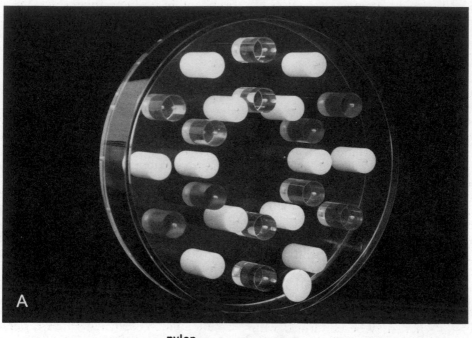

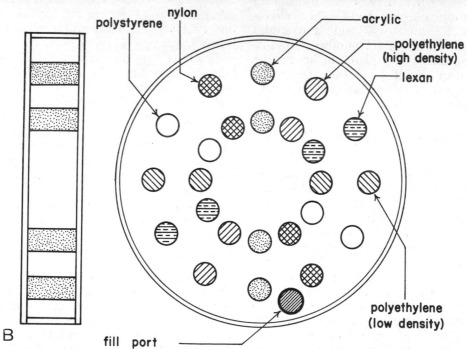

Figure A.21. (*A*) Photo of linearity CT phantom section, used for determing effective energy and CT number dependences. (Courtesy of Ultra-Cal, Inc.) (*B*) Schematic figure of linearity phantom.

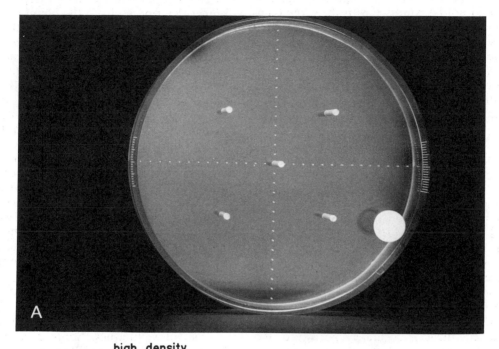

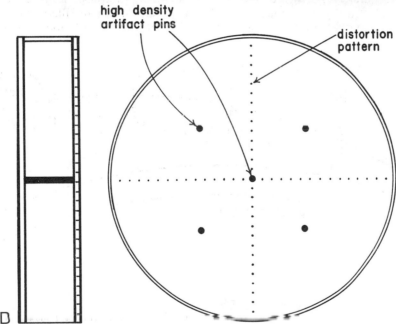

Figure A.22. (*A*) Photo of artifact/distortion CT phantom. (Courtesy of Ultra-Cal, Inc.) (*B*) Schematic drawing of artifact/distortion CT phantom, showing high density aluminum pins and +-shaped pattern of holes for determining distortion.

The geometrical misalignment artifacts should not be confused with the more common high density artifact exhibited to a lesser or greater extent by most scanners. The high density artifacts appear as dark streaks occurring on lines defined by two or more of the pins. A qualitative assessment of the high density artifacts may be made from a visual examination of the image.

SPATIAL DISTORTION

On one surface of the alignment and artifacts phantom section is a large "+," consisting of 1-mm holes spaced 1 cm apart (shown in Fig. A.22). This pattern may be used to test for reconstruction distortions and distortions occurring in the video monitor and hard copy camera system. To test the spatial accuracy of the reconstruction algorithm, the distance-measuring devices present on the video monitor viewing system are used to measure the distance between two holes in the "+" pattern. If the reconstructed image is accurately portrayed, the distance between selected pairs of holes in the "+" pattern as measured from the image

will closely approximate the corresponding distance determined from the phantom.

Even if the reconstruction algorithm is accurate, the image on the video monitor may contain distortion. Overall vertical and horizontal distortion may be determined by measuring the vertical and horizontal diameters of a circular phantom on the video monitor with a ruler or caliper. All diameters should measure the same, although they may be somewhat smaller than the true phantom size. The holes in the "+" pattern may prove helpful in determining other distortions in the video image. Similar distortion measurements should be performed on the hard copy film. Distortion measurements are particularly important if the CT scanner images are used for tumor and organ localization in radiation treatment planning.

BEAM WIDTH MEASUREMENTS

The determination of x-ray beam width or "sensitivity profile" may be performed by a variety of techniques. Some procedures consist of scanning an air-filled hole, a metal plate (13), or wire (8, 14) inclined through

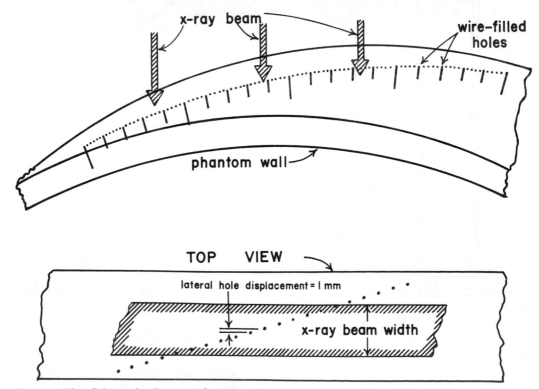

Figure A.23. Schematic diagram of arrangements of holes in the wall of the phantom section.

the x-ray beam at a well-known angle (for example, at 45° to the beam). From a measurement of the apparent width of the plate or wire on the image, the true width of the beam that is utilized to reconstruct the image may be determined. This width should reflect any changes in collimator setting selectable by the CT scanner operator. Note that the beam width may vary slightly from the center to the outer edge of the image (15, 16). Other techniques for determining beam width include scanning the x-ray beam through a series of wire-filled holes (as shown in a schematic of a phantom wall in Fig. A.23) or small beads inclined across the beam (17).

RADIATION THERAPY

The goal of radiation therapy is to deliver radiation accurately to a target volume identified by a radiation therapist. Accuracy is required in both the amount of radiation delivered and in the location to which it is delivered. As a result, the equipment used to deliver the radiation, as well as the equipment used to plan the radiation treatment, must be properly calibrated so that the radiation dose is known accurately. It is also essential that devices used to locate the patient with respect to the radiation beam are properly aligned. The achievable accuracy is in some part determined by the equipment itself, but maintenance of the equipment to the manufacturer's specifications requires an appropriate quality assurance program.

Treatment Unit

Radiation therapy treatment equipment is frequently divided into three categories. These are: superficial x-ray generators, orthovoltage x-ray generators, and megavoltage treatment units. The first two categories will not be addressed in any detail here. These units are generally quite simple, and selection is fairly straightforward. Megavoltage treatment units are frequently broken up into two groups: isotope units and linear accelerators (Fig. A.24). By far, the most common isotope unit is the cobalt unit, and other isotope units will not be discussed here. The cobalt unit consists of a source of radioactive cobalt, mounted in a protective shield in such a way that the source can be

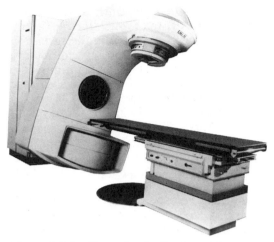

Figure A.24. Example of a linear accelerator.

moved from the shielded position to an exposed position. The shielded housing is mounted on an arm or gantry so that the location of the source may be adjusted with respect to the patient. A port or collimator is provided to direct the beam of radiation toward the patient when the source is in the exposed position. The useful radiation produced by such a source is gamma radiation; however, these gamma rays behave in a manner very similar to the x rays produced by some of the other treatment machines. One major distinction between cobalt units and linear accelerators is that the radiation from the cobalt unit is essentially monoenergetic and of a fixed energy. In comparison, the x rays produced by linear accelerators describe a spectrum of energies, and different linear accelerators may produce radiation of different maximum energies. The x rays are produced by accelerating electrons to high energy (for example, 4 million electron volts [4 MeV]) and allowing the electrons to strike a target. The x rays thus produced have a maximum energy equal to the electron beam energy and are described by this energy (e.g., 4 MV). The beam of x rays from a 4-MV linear accelerator is quite comparable to the beam of gamma rays from a cobalt unit.

The choice of beam energy is frequently a compromise between cost, penetrating power of the radiation, the availability of other modalities such as electrons, and the degree of skin sparing. In general, the higher the beam energy, the more penetrating the radiation. At the same time, as the energy increases, the depth at which the maximum dose is deposited moves from the surface to a depth of as much as several centimeters. For example, the depth of maximum dose of a cobalt unit is 0.5 cm. However, the depth of maximum dose of a 10-MV x-ray beam is approximately 2.5 cm. As a result, while a higher energy beam is frequently desirable to treat deeply seated tumors, the choice of such a beam may result in underdosing of very superficial structures (Figs. A.25 and A.26).

As might be expected, accelerators which produce beams of higher energy frequently are more expensive and more complex than are accelerators which produce beams of lower energy.

Another type of electron accelerator, called a betatron, is frequently found in radiation therapy departments. The betatron differs in that electrons are accelerated in a circular orbit, rather than in a straight line as in linear accelerators. Other differences

are that higher energies frequently are achieved in betatrons than with linear accelerators, at dose rates which are frequently lower.

The dose delivery from cobalt units is regulated by a timer. Since the radiation is produced by the decay of a long-lived radioactive source, the dose rate from a cobalt unit is essentially constant, decreasing only slowly over time. Therefore, delivery of a required dose is conducted by calculating the time required to deliver that dose and adjusting the timer appropriately. The beam is switched on by the operator and is turned off automatically when the treatment time has elapsed.

In contrast, the dose rate from a linear accelerator is not fixed and may vary during a treatment. In fact, the dose rate may be adjusted by the operator. It is, therefore, not practical to regulate treatments with a timer. Instead, linear accelerators incorporate dose monitoring devices which provide a continual indication at the console of the dose that

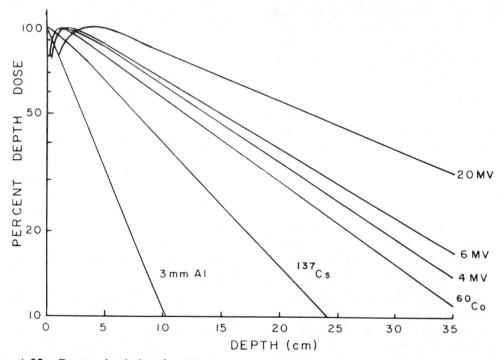

Figure A.25. Percent depth dose for 100-sq cm area x- and γ-ray beams of different energies, plotted as a function of depth in water. The SSD is 100 cm for all beams except for the 3.0-mm Al HVL (SSD = 15 cm) x-ray beam and for the ^{137}Cs beam (SSD = 35 cm). (Reproduced with permission from Hendee WR: *Radiation Therapy Physics.* Copyright © 1981 by Year Book Medical Publishers, Inc., Chicago.)

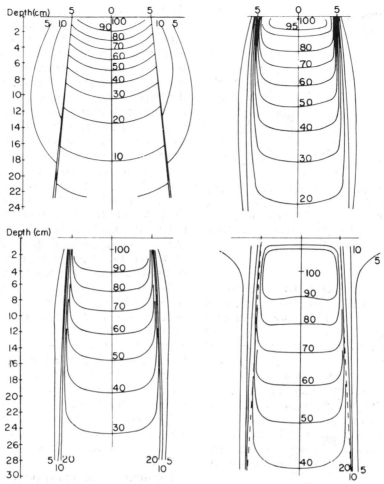

Figure A.26. Four isodose distributions. (*Upper Left*) Orthovoltage x-rays (200 kVp, 10 × 10 cm, 50 cm source-skin distance (SSD), 2.0 mm Cu half value layer (HVL). (*Upper Right*) ^{60}Co γ-rays (10 × 10 cm, 80 cm SSD). (*Lower Left*) X rays from a 6-MV linear accelerator (10 × 10 cm, 100 cm SSD). (*Lower Right*) 20-MV x rays from a betatron (10 × 10 cm, 100 cm SSD). (Reproduced with permission from Hendee WR: *Radiation Therapy Physics.* Copyright © 1981 by Year Book Medical Publishers, Inc., Chicago.)

has been delivered. When the monitor agrees with a dose selector switch which has been adjusted by the operator for this treatment, the beam is turned off. Maintaining the accuracy of these dose-monitoring devices is one of the roles of a quality assurance program.

As was mentioned earlier, delivering a dose accurately is only one of the goals of radiation therapy. The other goal is to deliver this dose of radiation to precisely the correct location. Achieving this accuracy is accomplished by the use of a simulator and a treatment planning computer but is also dependent upon aspects of performance of

the treatment unit. Most treatment units are equipped with a light localizer, which consists of a light bulb mounted inside the collimator in such a way that a beam of light is projected through the collimator in exactly the same location as will the radiation beam when the unit is turned on. When a patient is positioned for treatment, the patient, the treatment couch, and the gantry are adjusted so that the light localizer is aligned with anatomic landmarks or with indelible markings inked on the patient's skin. This ensures that the radiation beam is passing through the patient's skin at the correct location. However, it does not ensure that the beam

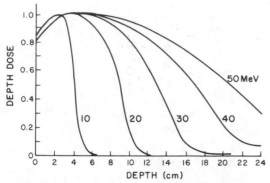

Figure A.27. Central axis depth dose curves for electron beams of selected energies. (Reproduced with permission from Hendee WR: *Radiation Therapy Physics.* Copyright © 1981 by Year Book Medical Publishers, Inc., Chicago.)

is passing through deeper structures as intended. To make sure that the patient is indeed positioned correctly, most treatment rooms are equipped with optical or laser projection systems which project beams of light from the walls or the ceiling of the treatment unit, to intersect at a common point known as the isocenter. The isocenter is the intersection of the central axis of the radiation beam with the axis of rotation of the treatment unit gantry. Therefore, the beam is always aimed directly at the isocenter, regardless of gantry angle or collimator angle.

Some linear accelerators are designed to deliver beams of electrons as an alternative to x-ray beam therapy. Electron beams differ from x-ray beams in that in general they are far less penetrating. In addition, the dose from electron beams is fairly uniform over a plateau of several centimeters and then decreases very rapidly. The width of the plateau region is determined by the beam energy. The dose to the skin surface is quite high, almost equaling the maximum dose. Electron beams provide very little skin sparing (Fig. A.27).

Simulators

To determine the target volume to be treated, a physician makes use of a variety of diagnostic modalities, such as diagnostic radiology, CT, ultrasound, etc. He must then translate this information into a three-dimensional representation of the patient and the target volume. The target volume, which is frequently located deep within the patient, must next be related to external anatomic landmarks. These landmarks are used to position the patient for treatment. However, it is highly desirable to be able to verify that the target volume is indeed encompassed by the treatment beam. This is frequently done by exposing radiographs of the patient in the treatment beam. These may be port films (films made before or after the treatment, requiring a small additional dose) or verification films (films actually exposed during the treatment). Due to the high energy of the treatment beams, these films are of poor diagnostic quality and exhibit very little contrast. As a result, it is often difficult to determine that the target volume is actually encompassed in the treatment beam.

The radiation therapy simulator (Fig. A.28) is a device which is designed to provide high quality port films and enhance the treatment planning process. A simulator is essentially a radiographic (and sometimes fluoroscopic) x-ray machine, mounted on a mechanical frame which is geometrically identical to a treatment unit. A simulator must have a treatment couch which is essentially identical to that of a treatment unit, and a light localizer and laser or optical side lights comparable to those in the treatment room.

Simulation is generally performed prior to the patient's first treatment or before major changes in the treatment. The patient is positioned on the simulator couch in the position that will be used for treatment. From a remote control room, the radiation therapist views the patient under fluoroscopy and localizes the target volume. From this remote control room adjustments may be made in the location of the treatment couch, the angle of the treatment beam, and the size and shape of the radiation field. Once the radiation therapist is satisfied that the radiation fields are encompassing the intended target volume, the position of all adjustable parameters is noted, and indelible ink marks are placed on the patient's skin to indicate the location of the various localizer lights. Radiographs are then taken which show, with diagnostic radiographic quality, the location of the radiation fields in comparison with the patient's anatomy. The patient is now ready for treatment.

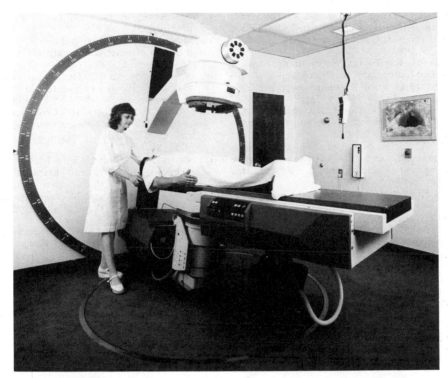

Figure A.28. Example of a radiation therapy simulator. (Courtesy of Varian Associates, Palo Alto, CA.)

Treatment Planning Computer

The treatment planning computer also is an important piece of equipment in the treatment planning process. The purpose of the treatment planning computer is to calculate and display the dose distribution resulting from a proposed treatment configuration so that the ideal treatment plan may be chosen.

Most modern treatment planning computers are general purpose minicomputers which are incorporated into a package with appropriate peripheral devices and supplied with software for performing dose calculations. A computer must be provided with data or programmed with appropriate algorithms which accurately characterize the radiation beams from the treatment units for which dose calculations are to be done. Supplying the data or verifying the accuracy of the algorithms is the responsibility of a physicist. When a treatment plan is to be performed, information specific to the individual patient is obtained such as the external contour and the internal anatomy in a transverse plane containing the tumor. Such information would easily be obtained from a CT scan. These data are entered into the computer via a digitizing device or sometimes through direct digital interfaces with the CT scanner or other modality. The transverse information is displayed on the treatment planning computer screen, and representations of radiation treatment beams may be superimposed on the contour. The computer than calculates the resulting dose distribution from the selected treatment field arrangement. The radiation therapist or a treatment planning technologist determines whether or not the displayed distribution is acceptable. If not, changes in the locations of the treatment beams, their relative weights, or other alterations are introduced, and the dose distribution again is calculated. This process is repeated until an optimal plan is achieved. The treatment plan arrived at in this fashion is frequently transferred to some sort of hard copy. This information is then used in positioning the patient for treatment.

References

1. Dixon RL, Ekstrand KE: A film dosimetry system for use in computed tomography. *Radiology* 127:255–258, 1978.

2. Shope TB, Morgan TJ, Showalter CK, et al: Radiation dosimetry survey of computed tomography systems from ten manufacturers. *Br J Radiol* 55:60–69, 1982.
3. Jucious RA, Kambic GX: Radiation dosimetry in computed tomography. In: *Proceedings of the Society for Photooptical Instrumentation Engineers.* Bellingham, WA, 1977, vol 127, pp 286–295.
4. Moore MM, Cacak RK, Hendee WR: Multisegmented ion chamber for CT scanner dosimetry. *Med Phys* 8:640–645, 1981.
5. Suzuki A, Suzuki MN: Use of a pencil-shaped ionization chamber for measurement of exposure resulting from a computed tomography scan. *Med Phys* 5:536–539, 1978.
6. Spokas JJ: Dose descriptors for computed tomography. *Med Phys* 9:288–292, 1982.
7. Shope TB, Gagne RM, Johnson GC: A method for describing the doses delivered by transmission x-ray computed tomography. *Med Phys* 8:488–495, 1981.
8. Cacak RK, Hendee WR: Performance evaluation of a fourth generation computed tomography (CT) scanner. *Proceedings of the Society for Photooptical Instrumentation Engineers.* Bellingham, WA, 1979, vol 173, pp 194–207.
9. Cohen G, DiBianca FA: Information content and dose efficiency of computed tomography scanners. In Haus AG (ed): *The Physics of Medical Imaging,* New York, American Institute of Physics, 1979, pp 356–365.
10. Miller MR, Payne WH, Waggner RG, et al: Determination of effective energies in CT calibration. *Med Phys* 5:543–545, 1978.
11. White DR, Speller RD: The measurement of effective photon energy and 'linearity' in computerized tomography. *Br J Radiol* 53:5–11, 1980.
12. Hubbell JH: Photon mass attenuation and mass energy-absorption coefficients for H, C, N, O, Ar and seven mixtures from 0.1 keV. *Radiat Res* 70:58–81, 1977.
13. Schneiders NJ, Bushong SC: CT quality assurance: computer assisted slice thickness determination. *Med Phys* 7:61–63, 1980.
14. Schneiders NJ, Bushong SC: An improved method for determining CT image slice thickness. *Med Phys* 8:516–519, 1981.
15. Brooks RA, Di Chiro G: Slice geometry in computer assisted tomography. *J Comput Assist Tomogr* 1:191–199, 1977.
16. Bracewell RN: Correction for collimator width (restoration) in reconstructive x-ray tomography. *J Comput Assist Tomogr* 1:6–15, 1977.
17. Weaver KE, Goodenough DJ: Imaging factors and evaluation: computed tomography scanning. In Haus AG (ed): *The Physics of Medical Imaging,* New York, American Institute of Physics, 1979, pp 309–35.

Types of CT Scanner Geometries

ROBERT K. CACAK, Ph.D.

INTRODUCTION

CT scanners were introduced to routine clinical practice in the early 1970s, and improvements have come rapidly since then. Several geometrical arrangements of the x-ray tube and detectors relative to the patient have evolved in the space of just a few years. Most of the impetus for this evolution arose because of the demand for faster scan times and increased spatial resolution. Parallel to the evolution in geometry was a corresponding increase in computer memory size, speed, and sophistication to satisfy the demand for faster image reconstruction. In addition, an increase in computer size and speed was required to handle correspondingly larger amounts of data generated within the shorter scan times by a greater number of detectors.

It is sometimes convenient to categorize CT scanners according to their geometry. The term "generation" is also applied occasionally to distinguish the various geometries, although most manufacturers appear reluctant to apply these terms to their equipment, presumably because of the connotation of a relative ranking that may be attached to this terminology. In truth, a "fourth generation" scanner does not have an innate advantage over "third" and "second" generation CT scanners or vice versa, and each geometry should be evaluated on its own merits. Table A.2 lists some advantages and disadvantages of some of the currently available geometries, and a short description of each of the geometries follows.

Pencil-Beam, Translate-Rotate (First Generation)

Historically, this was the first type of scanner to be used on patients. The x-ray beam is a narrow pencil beam that is "scanned" along a line A through the cross section of a patient, as shown in Figure A.29. On the opposite side of the patient is a single detector that moves in synchrony with the x-ray source along a line A'. At the completion of a scan, both the source and detector are rotated slightly around the patient. Then, another scan of source and detector along lines B and B', respectively, is performed. The scanning procedure is repeated at many small angular increments until the x-ray source and detector are approximately 180° from their initial positions. This scanning procedure is slow and usually requires a few minutes to complete. To reduce the time for a series of closely spaced slices, two detectors are often employed, one slightly above and one slightly below the plane of Figure A.29. To immobilize the head during the relatively lengthy procedure and to maintain the x-ray intensity at a moderate level at locations where no part of the head is in the beam, a water-filled cap that completely encloses the patient's head is often employed. It is not practical to scan bodies with this geometry because of the unavoidable motion of the body (e.g., breathing, peristalsis) during the scan procedure.

Fan-Beam, Translate-Rotate (Second Generation)

Not long after the pencil-beam geometry was introduced, the need for a faster CT scanner and a scanner that could accommodate bodies was recognized. To achieve faster scan times, the pencil beam of the earlier geometry is broadened into a fan beam with a divergence of about 30°, as shown in Figure A.30. A series of several (20 to 60) detectors is used to intercept the x-ray beam. The detectors and the x-ray source are scanned linearly across the patient, as shown in Figure A.30. At the end of the scan, the detectors and source are rotated to a new position, and another scan is performed. In contrast to the small angular increment of the pencil-beam, translate-rotate system, the fan-beam rotation is a few

Table A.2
Comparison of CT Scanner Geometries

Geometry	Advantages	Disadvantages
1. Pencil beam, translate-rotate (first generation)	Simple one-detector data acquisition system. Inexpensive.	Slow; not practical for bodies. Mechanically complex.
2. Fan beam, translate-rotate (second generation)	High resolution. Moderately priced.	Mechanically complex. Scan speeds less that 5 sec are difficult
3. Rotate-rotate (third generation)	High resolution.	Detector drift can cause artifacts. Somewhat lower detector efficiency.
4. Stationary detector (fourth generation)	Continuous calibration of detectors. Fewer moving parts.	More detectors needed to achieve high resolution. More expensive.
5. Completely stationary (fifth generation)	No moving parts. Very fast scan times.	Still somewhat unsettled technology.

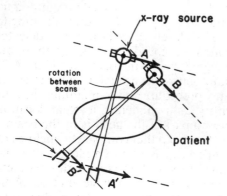

Figure A.29. Pencil beam, translate rotate geometry (first generation).

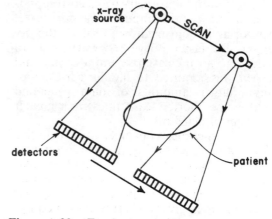

Figure A.30. Fan beam, translate rotate geometry (second generation). After each scan, the x-ray tube and detector array are rotated a few tens of degrees before the successive scan.

tens of degrees between each scan. Therefore, the source and detectors require only a few translations to complete the data acquisition necessary for one image, and the total scan time is correspondingly reduced. Scan times for this geometry may be as short as 5 sec, although times of 20 sec are more typical.

Rotate-Rotate (Third-Generation)

This type of geometry completely eliminates the translate or "scan" part of the motion described in the first two sections. The x-ray beam is a wide, fan-shaped beam, and a series of many (often, a few hundred) detectors arranged in a curved array intercepts and measures the x-ray beam after passing through the patient. The geometry for this system is shown in Figure A.31. The

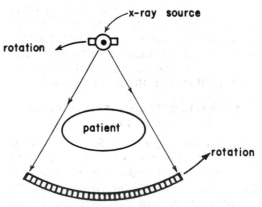

Figure A.31. Rotate-rotate geometry (third generation).

x-ray source and detector array are smoothly rotated 360° about the patient without any translational motion. Because of the simpler rotate-only motion, somewhat faster scan times (2 to 10 sec) are typical.

Stationary Detector Array (SDA) (Fourth Generation)

Historically, this geometry was introduced about the same time as the rotate-rotate geometry. This geometry also has a wide fan beam; however, the array of moving detectors is replaced by a large ring of stationary detectors, as shown in Figure A.32. This system has the advantage of fewer moving parts, and the data cables from the detectors to the computer do not move or flex.

A disadvantage of this system is that only a fraction of the detectors are used at any one time. Therefore, to achieve spatial resolution comparable to other geometries, more total detectors are required.

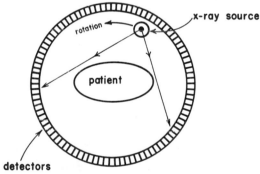

Figure A.32. Stationary detector array geometry (fourth generation).

Stationary Geometries (Fifth Generation)

The desire to image the heart in various phases of its beating cycle and to monitor the rapid flow of contrast media through various organs has stimulated the development of CT scanners with scan times in the few milliseconds range. Conventional scanner geometries are not satisfactory for these very fast data accumulation times for two reasons. First, the number of x rays that can be obtained from a single, conventional x-ray tube in a few milliseconds is too low to provide an image with reasonable noise characteristics. Second, rotating a relatively heavy x-ray tube and perhaps a detector system around a patient on a diameter of a few feet in a few milliseconds is a reasonably difficult engineering problem.

Various schemes have been proposed to bypass the above problems. One of these consists of installing several conventional x-ray tubes and a detector system around the patient and firing the x-ray tubes in rapid sequence (1).

Another scheme has been proposed that encloses a large tungsten ring (i.e., an x-ray tube anode) in a bell-shaped vacuum tube (2) and includes a ring of detectors around the patient. The patient is positioned in the center of the anode ring, and the high energy electron beam is focused to a small point on the anode where x rays are produced. The position and focusing of the electron beam are controlled magnetically, resulting in a CT scanner design with no moving parts. The focal spot from which the x-rays emanate may be scanned around the ring in a

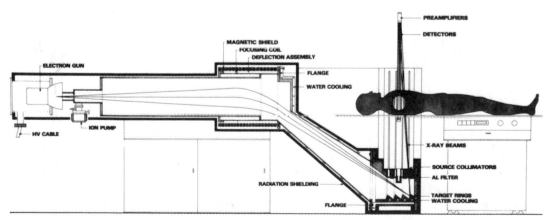

Figure A.33. Schematic diagram of a completely stationary (fifth generation) CT scanner. (Courtesy of Imatron, Inc.)

few milliseconds. A modification of this design has been built and is being offered by one manufacturer.* A schematic diagram of this system is shown in Figure A.33.

---

* Imatron, Inc., 454 Carlton Court, South San Francisco, CA 94080.

References

1. Ritman EL, Kinsey JH, Robb RA, Harris LD, Gilbert BK: Physics and technical considerations in the design of the DSR. *Am J Roentgenol* 134:369–374, 1950.
2. Iinuma TA, Tateno Y, Omegaki Y, Watanabe E: Proposed systems for ultrafast computed tomography. *J Comp Assist Tomogr* 1:494–499, 1977.

Index